Biomedical Membranes and (Bio)Artificial Organs

World Scientific Series in Membrane Science and Technology: Biological and Biomimetic Applications, Energy and the Environment

Series Editor: Joel R Fried *(University of Louisville, USA)*

Membranes can be biological, such as lipid bilayer membranes that encapsulate a human cell, or synthetic membrane that may be polymeric, biomimetic, or inorganic. Common to both is the ability to regulate transport of an ion or a molecule such as water, a fixed gas, or polynucleotides as examples. Membranes find important applications when they can be selective on the basis of size, charge, or polarity. These applications are found in nearly all aspects of our economy and have great importance in medical areas as described in the first volume of our book series, Biomedical Membranes and (Bio)artificial Organs, edited by Professor Dimitrios Stamatialis of the University of Twente in the Netherlands. Another very important application for synthetic membranes is the separation of mixtures of gases that is the focus of Volume 2, Membranes for Gas Separations, edited by Professor Moises Carreon of the Colorado School of Mines. Forthcoming book coverage includes the use of membranes in water treatment, applications of biomimetic membranes that mimic the structure of biological membranes, the use of molecular simulations to study transport properties, applications for ceramic and metallic membranes, the use of membranes in energy and environment applications including fuel cells, and the design and application of membrane systems in the chemical, petrochemical, and pharmaceutical industries. These areas have great technological, economic, and medical importance. It is our expectation that this new book series on Membrane Science and Technology that will provide an authoritative and contemporary coverage of these important topics.

Published

Vol. 2 *Biomedical Membranes and (Bio)Artificial Organs*
edited by Dimitrios Stamatialis

Vol. 1 *Membranes for Gas Separations*
by Moises A Carreon

World Scientific Series in Membrane Science and Technology:
Biological and Biomimetic Applications, Energy and the Environment Vol. 2

Biomedical Membranes and (Bio)Artificial Organs

Editor

Dimitrios Stamatialis

University of Twente, The Netherlands

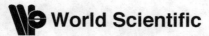

NEW JERSEY • LONDON • SINGAPORE • BEIJING • SHANGHAI • HONG KONG • TAIPEI • CHENNAI • TOKYO

Published by

World Scientific Publishing Co. Pte. Ltd.

5 Toh Tuck Link, Singapore 596224

USA office: 27 Warren Street, Suite 401-402, Hackensack, NJ 07601

UK office: 57 Shelton Street, Covent Garden, London WC2H 9HE

Library of Congress Cataloging-in-Publication Data
Names: Stamatialis, Dimitrios, editor.
Title: Biomedical membranes and (bio) artificial organs / [edited by] Dimitrios Stamatialis.
Other titles: World scientific series in membrane science and technology ; v. 2.
Description: New Jersey : World Scientific, 2017. | Series: World scientific series in membrane science and technology, volume 2 | Includes bibliographical references.
Identifiers: LCCN 2017015007 | ISBN 9789813221758 (hc : alk. paper)
Subjects: | MESH: Membranes, Artificial | Bioartificial Organs
Classification: LCC QH601 | NLM QT 37 | DDC 571.6/4--dc23
LC record available at https://lccn.loc.gov/2017015007

British Library Cataloguing-in-Publication Data
A catalogue record for this book is available from the British Library.

About the book cover image:
Confocal microscopy image of proximal tubule epithelial cells cultured on polymeric hollow fiber membranes. In blue the DAPI staining of cell nuclei and in green the zonula occludens-1 immunostaining for cell tight junctions. Taken by Dr. Natalia Chevtchik (co-author of chapter 5 of this book).

For any available supplementary material, please visit
http://www.worldscientific.com/worldscibooks/10.1142/10549#t=suppl

Desk Editor: Kalpana Bharanikumar

Typeset by Stallion Press
Email: enquiries@stallionpress.com

Printed in Singapore

I would like to thank from the bottom of my heart, my family, my wife Ellie and my boys Daniel and Thomas, for their continuous support (and patience) during the book preparation and far beyond!
I would also like to thank, Mrs Steffi Olbrich for her assistance in the book editing.

Dedicated to my parents, Fotios and Maria, and to my grandmother Kaliope, who I am sure is watching from up there smiling, as always...

Preface

In the coming years, due to the aging of the population and the low availability of donor organs, there will be urgent need for bioengineered organs to assist, mimic or replace failing patient organs. The developed organs could be:

— artificial: based on new biomaterials and novel designs;
— bioartificial: combining biomaterials and biological cells.

Membranes play, and will continue to play, an important role in the development of these organs. The examples are endless. For the treatment of chronic kidney disease, patients are treated at the hospital 3 times a week with an artificial kidney, a hollow fiber membrane device which removes the toxins from their blood. Membranes are used for blood oxygenation regularly during heart surgeries, and most of the drug-delivery systems are based on thin membranes for the controlled delivery of the active substances to the patients.

For the last 15 years, I have been giving lectures on these topics to undergraduate and graduate students of our University, students of biomedical engineering, chemical engineering or technical medicine. The learning material was mostly based on scientific literature, research papers and reviews. All these years, however, I have been missing a book which would comprehensively address the development of biomedical membranes and their applications for (bio)artificial organs. When was I approached by Prof. Fried to edit such a book, I accepted really quickly.

And here it is! It covers the state-of-the-art and main challenges for applying synthetic membranes in these organs. It consists of 11 chapters, written by world renowned experts in the fields of membrane technology, biomaterials science and technology, cell biology, medicine and engineering.

Every chapter describes the clinical needs and the materials, membranes and concepts required for the successful development of the bioartificial organs. It also highlights the importance of accomplishing an integration of engineering with biology and medicine to understand and manage the scientific, industrial, clinical and ethical aspects of these organs.

The book is suitable for undergraduate and graduate students in biomedical engineering, materials science and membrane science and technology, as well as, for professionals and researchers working in these fields.

I hope you will enjoy reading it as much as we enjoyed preparing it.

Dimitrios Stamatialis
Bioartificial Organs Group,
Department of Biomaterials Science and Technology,
MIRA Institute, University of Twente, The Netherlands
March 2017

About the Editor

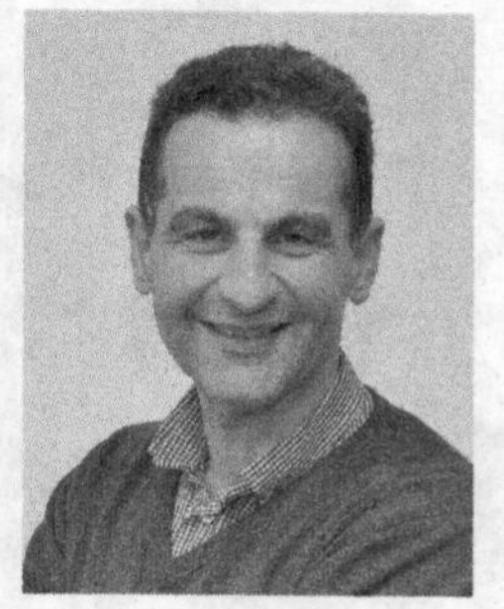

Prof. Dimitrios Stamatialis is a full Professor, chair of (bio) artificial organs at the University of Twente, NB Enschede, the Netherlands.

He is the author of more than 130 scientific publications and holds 7 patents. He is involved in numerous national and international research projects leading to products and applications, some of which have been licensed to companies.

He is extensively involved in international activities including being a member of the EU Tox group, a working group dealing with coordination of European research on uremic toxins; an editor of the *International journal of artificial organs*, the official journal of the European Society of artificial organs; and a coordinator of the EU Marie Curie ITN project "BIOART" focussing on the development of prototype devices for the treatment of kidney and liver disease.

He teaches various BSc and MSc courses at the MIRA Institute for Biomedical Engineering and Technical Medicine at the University of Twente.

Contents

Chapter 1
Controlled Drug Release Systems: Mechanisms and Kinetics

M. Sanopoulou* and K. G. Papadokostaki

Institute of Nanoscience and Nanotechnology,
National Center for Scientific Research "Demokritos",
15310 Ag. Paraskevi, Athens, Greece
**m.sanopoulou@inn.demokritos.gr*

1.1 Introduction

The terms "controlled drug delivery" and "controlled drug release" encompass a variety of medication dosage forms that aim at regulating the temporal and spatial delivery of therapeutics. Since its first appearance in the 1960s, the scientific and technological field is continuously expanding to cover not only macroscopic-scale membrane-based devices intended to regulate the release rate over extended periods of time, but also more sophisticated systems, such as nanocarriers and drug–polymer conjugates for targeted and site-controlled delivery [Hoffman, 2008]. However, currently the majority of approved controlled release (CR) products are devices in which a polymeric layer (usually in the form of a membrane surrounding the drug or a matrix containing it) regulates the drug release rate. Thus, polymeric membranes have found one of their major applications in the CR medical area. Different classes of polymers (elastomers, hydrogels, erodible, sensitive to external stimuli such as temperature and pH) and numerous formulation designs have been exploited in CR products. In all cases, a main requirement for a CR device is delivery of a sustained dose rate, between an upper and a lower limit, for a sufficiently prolonged time. The approach to the ideal case of zero-order kinetics, providing a constant rate of release, is mainly determined by the physicochemical mechanism of release and the design of the device. The basic mechanisms that control the release of the drug molecules through the polymeric layer are osmosis, diffusion, chemical degradation, swelling and dissolution, with diffusion playing a dominant role in many CR systems. Diffusion-controlled systems are mainly of the reservoir and the matrix designs. Reservoir systems typically provide uniform release rates, but simple matrix systems, operating by a purely diffusive transport, yield release rates that decline with time. However, in many practical cases, drug diffusion is often coupled with other rate-controlling processes, and the resulting release kinetics often favors the stabilization of the release rate. Thus, fundamental understanding of the mechanisms underlying the drug release process is important in the design and development of a CR formulation, especially in respect to the achievement of the desired release profile.

This chapter starts with an overview of the basic mechanisms of release in polymer-based CR systems. It then focuses on systems where diffusion plays a dominant role in determining the kinetics of release and provides examples of relevant medical formulations. Matrix systems are described in more detail, with an emphasis on mechanisms and conditions that tend to stabilize the rate of release.

1.2 Release Mechanisms

1.2.1 *Osmosis*

Osmotic delivery systems are based on the principle of osmosis that occurs when a membrane permeable to water but not to particular solutes separates two solutions of different solute concentrations. In the simple design of an elementary osmotic pump, a core of concentrated drug solution is contained in a semi-permeable membrane. Osmotically driven water influx into the core, through the semi-permeable membrane, displaces drug molecules through an orifice of the device (Fig. 1.1).

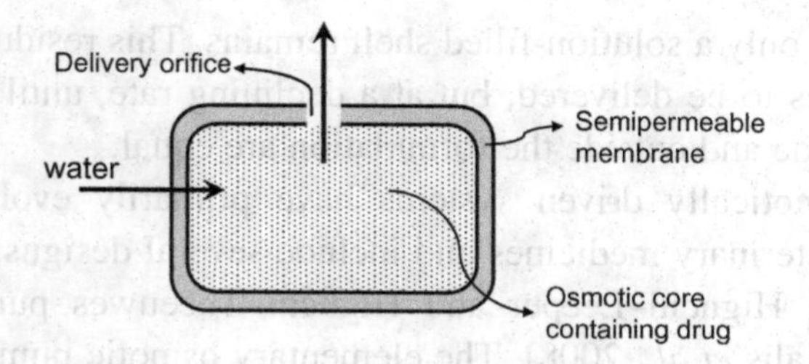

Figure 1.1. Schematic representation of an elementary osmotic pump.

In general, the osmotic volume flow rate of water, dV/dt, across a semi-permeable membrane of thickness L and area A can be described by

$$\frac{dV}{dt} = \frac{AL_P(\sigma\Delta\pi - \Delta P)}{L}, \tag{1.1}$$

where L_p is the (hydraulic) water permeability of the semi-permeable membrane and σ its osmotic reflection coefficient (which is equal to 1 for completely selective membranes, i.e. membranes permeable to water but completely impermeable to the osmotic agent or drug). $\Delta\pi$ is the osmotic pressure difference across the semi-permeable membrane and ΔP is the hydrostatic pressure difference between the two sites of the semi-permeable membrane.

The effective drug release rate through the orifice of osmotic pumps, dQ_t/dt, can be derived from the volume flow rate of liquid drug solution, dV/dt, as

$$\frac{dQ_t}{dt} = \frac{dV}{dt}C, \tag{1.2}$$

where C is the drug concentration of the core solution. Combining Eqs. (1.1) and (1.2) and for $\Delta\pi \gg \Delta P$, we obtain

$$\frac{dQ_t}{dt} = \frac{Ak\Delta\pi}{L}C, \tag{1.3}$$

where $k = L_p\sigma$. According to Eq. (1.3), the release process continues at a constant rate until the entire solid drug inside the formulation has been dissolved and only a solution-filled shell remains. This residual dissolved drug continues to be delivered, but at a declining rate, until the osmotic pressures inside and outside the formulation are equal.

Oral, osmotically driven systems have primarily evolved for the delivery of veterinary medicines and include several designs, namely the Rose–Nelson, Higuchi–Leeper and Higuchi–Theeuwes pumps [Baker, 2004; Stamatialis *et al.*, 2008]. The elementary osmotic pump developed by Alza Corp. under the name OROS® is commercially available for a number of drugs such as nifedipine and verapamil for the treatment of hypertension, and more recently paliperidone for schizophrenia [Conley *et al.*, 2006].

1.2.2 *Diffusion*

Diffusion refers to the transport of molecules under a concentration (or activity) gradient. In order to diffuse through a polymeric medium, drug molecules have to be in the dissolved (mobile) state. For unidirectional transport in the x-direction, the diffusion flux J due to the concentration gradient $\partial C/\partial x$ is given by Fick's first law:

$$J = -D\frac{\partial C}{\partial x}, \tag{1.4}$$

where D is Fick's diffusion coefficient.

By combining Eq. (1.4) with the mass balance equation, we obtain

$$\frac{\partial C}{\partial t} = \frac{\partial J}{\partial x}. \tag{1.5}$$

Fick's second law, known as the diffusion equation, is derived as

$$\frac{\partial C}{\partial t} = \frac{\partial}{\partial x}\left(D\frac{\partial C}{\partial x}\right). \tag{1.6}$$

Operation of diffusion-controlled CR systems involves partitioning of the dissolved drug molecules between the polymer phase and the external aqueous environment. The partition coefficient, K, is an equilibrium property and is defined as the ratio of the dissolved solute concentration in the polymer phase, C, to solute concentration in the aqueous external phase, c:

$$K = \frac{C}{c}. \tag{1.7}$$

The permeability coefficient of the polymer, P, is the product of the thermodynamic parameter K and the kinetic parameter D.

According to the irreversible thermodynamics approach, diffusion occurs under an activity gradient $\partial\alpha/\partial x$ (instead of a concentration gradient), due to a chemical potential driving force. The expression for the flux J is given by [Flynn *et al.*, 1974; Petropoulos *et al.*, 1992, 2012]:

$$J = -D_{\mathrm{T}} S \frac{\partial a}{\partial x}, \tag{1.8}$$

where D_{T} is the thermodynamic diffusion coefficient and S is the solubility coefficient that defines partitioning of the diffusing molecules between the polymer and the external phase, in terms of the activity of the latter phase. On the basis of Eq. (1.8), the diffusion equation is given by

$$\frac{\partial C}{\partial t} = \frac{\partial}{\partial x}\left(D_{\mathrm{T}} S \frac{\partial a}{\partial x}\right). \tag{1.9}$$

For an ideal system (D, S const.), $D = D_{\mathrm{T}}$ and Eq. (1.9) reduces to Eq. (1.6).

1.2.3 *Polymer Swelling*

Swelling refers to the volume increase of a polymeric medium due to the absorption of water from the surrounding aqueous phase. Synthetic and natural hydrogels can absorb many times their weight in water. In glassy hydrogels, the slow structural relaxations of the swelling polymer affect the kinetics of water uptake, which in turn influences the release of the drug. Swelling-controlled systems strictly refer to the cases where water not only activates the release of the drug, but is also the rate-controlling mechanism of drug release. This is usually a limiting case, and in a broader sense the term is used to denote systems where polymer swelling is one of the controlling mechanisms operating at times comparable with those of the release process. This subject is further discussed in Section 1.4.2.

1.2.4 *Polymer Erosion and Degradation*

Polymers susceptible to hydrolytic or enzymatic degradation when in contact with the physiological environment are also used to control the rate of drug release. Biodegradable polymers include both synthetic and natural products. The most common synthetic biodegradable polymers are poly(lactic acid) and copolymers of lactic and glycolic acids that degrade by hydrolysis of ester linkages. In biodegradable proteins (e.g. collagen and gelatin) and polysaccharides (as chitosan and alginates), degradation is usually effected by enzymes. Erosion may proceed from the surface or the bulk of the polymer, or a combination of the two [Peppas & Narasimhan, 2014; Siegel & Rathbone, 2012]. Erodible devices may be controlled by more than one mechanism (such as water and drug diffusion, swelling, chemical degradation or dissolution of the polymer), and the interplay between these processes may lead to zero-order release kinetics.

To identify conditions of a constant rate of release, Hopfenberg [1976] assumed that a zero-order process, characterized by a single rate constant, is the rate-determining process taking place at the boundary between the unaffected polymer phase and the degraded or swollen material. The rate constant, k_0, may correspond to a single physical or chemical phenomenon or to the superposition of several processes, and the rate of drug release is assumed to be proportional to the surface of the eroding polymer that is allowed to change with time t. The fractional amount of drug released, Q_t/Q_∞, is then given by the expression

$$\frac{Q_t}{Q_\infty} = 1 - \left(1 - \frac{k_0 t}{C_0 L}\right)^n, \tag{1.10}$$

where C_0 is the uniform initial drug concentration and L the radius of a sphere or a cylinder or the half-thickness of a plane sheet. The factor n is equal to 3, 2 or 1 for spheres, cylinders or plane sheets, respectively. It is thus evident that a zero-order release profile will only be attained from a planar erodible device.

1.2.5 *Release Activated by External Stimuli*

In these systems, the drug release is controlled by external stimuli such as temperature, pH, ionic strength, an electric field, electromagnetic radiation or UV light. Hydrogels that respond to such external stimuli undergo drastic conformational changes upon narrow variation of the variable around a given critical point. Depending upon the polymer, the system can either shrink or swell upon a change in any of these environmental factors. For most of these polymers, which are also called responsive or "smart", the structural changes are reversible and repeatable upon additional changes in the external environment [Siegel, 2014]. One of the most famous and studied responsive polymers that finds applications in drug delivery has been poly(*N*-isopropyl acrylamide) due to its low critical solution temperature in water at 32°C, close to body temperature.

In most cases, during operation of a CR device, more than one of the mechanisms described above are involved, and the rate of drug release results from coupling of the corresponding transport processes. In what follows, we first describe predominantly diffusion-controlled systems and then matrix systems where the interplay between diffusion and other processes may favor the approach to a constant rate of release (zero-order kinetics).

1.3 Diffusion-Controlled Systems: Design and Formulations

1.3.1 *Matrix and Reservoir Systems*

The basic designs for diffusion-controlled drug release devices are the reservoir and the matrix systems. Figure 1.2 presents the two designs incorporated in the multi-layer structures of transdermal patches.

In the reservoir system, the rate-controlling polymeric membrane encapsulates the drug reservoir, the latter in a liquid or solid suspension. The release process involves (i) partitioning of the drug between the reservoir phase and the membrane, (ii) diffusion through the membrane

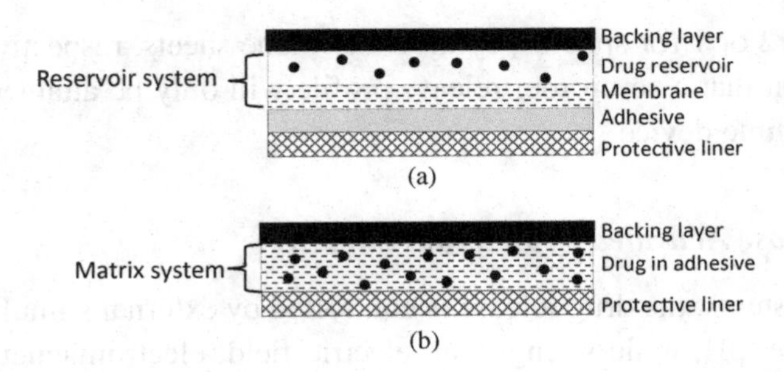

Figure 1.2. Schematic representation of (a) reservoir and (b) matrix designs incorporated in transdermal formulations. Not to scale.

and (iii) partitioning between the membrane phase and the external releasing medium. For a saturated reservoir containing an excess of non-dissolved drug, the flux through the polymer membrane remains constant until the drug concentration falls below the saturation limit. Thus, after an initial transient period, for the major part of the release process and on the basis of Eqs. (1.4) and (1.7), the constant release rate per unit area (in the case of planar geometry), for a concentration-independent system, is given by

$$\frac{dQ_t}{dt} = \frac{D(C_S - C_L)}{L} = \frac{DK(c_S - c_L)}{L} = \frac{P(c_S - c_L)}{L}, \tag{1.11}$$

where C_S and C_L represent the drug concentrations within the membrane surface at the high concentration side (C_S = drug saturation) and at the low concentration side (usually zero), respectively; c_S and c_L are the corresponding equilibrium concentrations in the adjacent solution and the product DK is the permeability coefficient, P, of the membrane.

The uniformity of the release rate is the biggest advantage of reservoir systems. On the other hand, the membrane has to be free of defects to avoid dose dumping and is thus costly to fabricate.

In the simpler design of matrix-controlled release (MCR) systems, the polymer matrix is initially homogeneously loaded with the drug and serves both as the depot of the drug as well as the rate-controlling layer. Matrix systems can be in different geometrical structures such as slabs, cylinders and rods, or more elaborate designs. Simple matrix systems are easy to fabricate, but as will be discussed below, they usually suffer from a declining dose rate.

1.3.2 *Pharmaceutical Formulations*

Matrix and reservoir designs are used in various formulations intended to deliver the therapeutic agent by different administration routes. The limited examples of Table 1.1 are meant to show the broad spectra of pathological conditions and duration of treatment by various formulations relatively recently developed. Types of formulations include the following.

- *Subcutaneous implants*. Subcutaneous implants, usually in the form of small, thin, flexible rods or "matchsticks", are mainly designed for long-term treatments as they require a minor procedure for both insertion and removal. The most known product, Norplant and Norplant II (Jadelle), was developed by the Population Council in the 1970s for contraception purposes. These poly(dimethylsiloxane)-based devices, in the form of capsules, rods or covered rods, were tested in large groups of women and found capable of continuously releasing levonogestrel for up to 6 years with varying degrees of rate uniformity, depending mainly on the architecture of the device [Robertson *et al.*, 1983]. Examples of recent therapeutic implant applications are shown in Table 1.1.
- *Ophthalmic systems*. Ocular inserts and implants are used for the treatment of eye disorders. Ocusert® (Alza Corp.), introduced in the 1970s, is a reservoir system of ethylene–vinyl acetate membrane inserted in the *cul de sac* of the eye and releasing pilocarpine to the tear fluid for a week, at a constant rate. Long-term drug delivery implants are an alternative to repeated injections or systemic administration in order to treat disorders of the posterior segment of the eye (Table 1.1) [Wang *et al.*, 2013].
- *Drug eluting stents*. Apart from implantable devices that deliver therapeutic agents as a primary function, drug-eluting stents, classified as combination products, are a relatively new technology in the treatment of coronary artery disease. Stents are small-wire metal meshes in the form of a tube, used to keep the artery open after angioplasty. In order

Table 1.1: Examples of diffusion-controlled drug-delivery products.

Active ingredient	Product name/company	Formulation	Design/material	Use	Treatment duration
Histerlin acetate	Supprellin®LA/Indevus Pharm.	Subcutaneous implant	Reservoir/PHEMA, PHPMA	Children with central precocious puberty	12 months
Fluocinolone-acetonide	ILUVIEN®/Alimera Sciences, Inc.	Intravitreal implant	Reservoir/polyimide tube, PVA	Diabetic macular edema	36 months
Dinoprostone (prostaglandin E2)	PROPESS®/Ferring Pharm.	Vaginal insert	Matrix/PEG	Initiation of cervical ripening	24 h
Everolimus	XIENCE™ V/Abbot	Drug-eluting coronary stent	Matrix/P(VDF-HFP)	Prevention of artery restenosis after angioplasty	28 days
Rotigotine	NEUPRO®/UCB, Inc.	Transdermal patch	Self-adhesive matrix/ silicone adhesive	Parkinson's disease-primary restless legs syndrome	24 h
Granisetron	Sancuso®/ProStrakan Inc.	Transdermal patch	Self-adhesive matrix	Chemotherapy-induced nausea and vomiting	7 days
Rivastigmine	EXELON®/Novartis Pharm. Corp.	Transdermal patch	Matrix/P(BMA-co-MMA)	Dementia associated with Alzheimer's or Parkinson's disease	24 h
Buprenorphine, under development (PHASE III)	Probuphine®/TITAN Pharmaceutics	Subcutaneous implant	Matrix/P(EVA)	For treatment of opioid dependence	6–12 months

PHEMA: poly(hydroxyethyl methacrylate); PHPMA: poly(hydroxypropyl methacrylate); PVA: poly(vinyl alcohol); PEG: polyethyleneglycol; P(VDF-HFP): poly(vinylidene fluoride-co-hexafluoropropylene); P(BMA-co-MMA): poly(butyl methacrylate-co-methyl methacrylate); P(EVA): poly(ethylene vinyl acetate).

to reduce restenosis of the artery due to hyperplasia reaction at the stented site, stents coated with polymeric layers containing anti-restenotic drugs have been developed (Table 1.1). Research and development in this area is currently very active, aiming at the improved efficacy and safety through stent design and choice of polymer and drug [Khan *et al.*, 2012; Puranik *et al.*, 2013].

- *Vaginal inserts*. In addition to steroid-releasing subcutaneous implants, intravaginal rings offer another option for contraception and hormone replacement therapies in women [Brache & Faundes, 2010], while under research is the development of rings delivering anti-HIV microbiocides [Malcolm *et al.*, 2010]. Flexible silicone elastomers are mainly used in the form of matrix or reservoir systems, due to their well-established biocompatibility, inertness and ability to release in a predictable manner small lipophilic steroid molecules.
- *Transdermal patches*. Percutaneous absorption of drugs, originally through topical application of ointments and gels, is particularly advantageous in comparison to oral delivery for those drugs that are prone to pre-systemic, first-pass hepatic metabolism. Extended-release transdermal drug-delivery systems (TDDS), commonly known as patches, are multi-layer devices consisting of a reservoir or a matrix system sandwiched between an impermeable backing layer and an adhesive one (Fig. 1.2). In addition, a protective layer (overlapping or peripheral to the adhesive one) is added, to be removed before application of the patch. In a structurally simpler type of matrix patch, the adhesive layer serves also as the drug matrix (matrix-in-adhesive patch). Approximately three-fourths of commercially available TDDS products are matrix type [Banerjee *et al.*, 2014], many of them in the matrix-in-adhesive design. About 20 drugs are currently approved in the United States and Europe in TDDS formulations for use, among others, in hormonal replacement therapy, chronic pain relief, smoking cessation and certain types of dementia [Paudel *et al.*, 2010; Wiedersberg & Guy, 2014].

The majority of these drugs are small, moderately lipophilic molecules in order to overcome the skin's resistance to permeation (see Section 1.6). In addition, most formulations contain chemical enhancers (e.g. amphiphilic molecules or alcohols) which aim at disrupting the ordered structure of the stratum corneum and at increasing the drug partitioning into the skin [Barry, 1991]. Physical methods increasing skin permeability include ionophoresis or sonophoresis [Stamatialis *et al.*, 2008]. However, for the efficient delivery of hydrophilic molecules, macromolecules or vaccines, more invading methods are under research/development, such as thermal ablation skin pre-treatment or the use of microneedles [Paudel *et al.*, 2010].

- *Oral tablets*. Among CR solid oral dosage forms, hydrophilic matrix systems are among the most widely used, due to their ease of manufacture by direct compression or granulation of the polymer with the active ingredient. Matrix materials broadly used in the pharmaceutical industry are mainly the cellulose ethers hydroxypropylmethyl cellulose and hydroxypropyl cellulose, polyacrylic acids crosslinked with a polyfunctional compound (known as carbomers) as well as alginates. The drug-release profile can be modulated by modifying the swelling properties of the crosslinked polymers or by the concurrent dissolution of the linear polymers [Nokhodchi *et al.*, 2012].

1.4 Mechanisms and Kinetics in Matrix Systems

1.4.1 *Purely Diffusion-controlled Systems*

The simplest case of solute release from a matrix device applies to purely diffusive transport through the matrix to the external aqueous phase. In order to diffuse through a polymeric medium, drug molecules have to be in the dissolved (mobile) state. Since, in many MCR systems, the initial drug load exceeds the solubility limit in the polymer phase, they are classified according to the state of the drug in the polymer as (i) unsaturated or saturated systems and (ii) supersaturated ones. In the first case, the initial solute concentration, C_0, is lower or equal to the limit of solubility of the solute in the matrix, C_S, and all of solute load is in the "dissolved state" and hence fully mobile. In supersaturated systems, $C_0 > C_S$, and part of the solute load is dispersed in the matrix.

For matrices homogeneously loaded to $C_0 \le C_S$, the release kinetics is described by the diffusion equation. Fick's second law (Eq. (1.6)) is solved analytically for different geometries (slabs, spheres, cylinders) with different initial and boundary conditions. Here, we consider the simplest case of a thin film of thickness $2L$ with negligible edge effects, where the release process in the surrounding aqueous phase takes place under perfect sink conditions and in the absence of mass-transfer limitations due to boundary layers adjacent to the surface of the film. Under these initial and boundary conditions, the time evolution of the solute concentration profile is shown in Fig. 1.3(a). Fickian kinetics of solute release can be approximated by the following expressions for the fractional amount of solute released, Q_t/Q_∞, applicable to early-, and late-, time kinetic regime, respectively

$$\frac{Q_t}{Q_\infty} = 2\left(\frac{Dt}{\pi L^2}\right)^{1/2} \quad \text{for} \quad 0 \le \frac{Q_t}{Q_\infty} \le 0.6 \tag{1.12}$$

and

$$\ln\left(1 - \frac{Q_t}{Q_\infty}\right) = \ln\frac{8}{\pi^2} - \frac{D\pi^2 t}{4L^2} \quad \text{for} \quad 0.4 \le \frac{Q_t}{Q_\infty} \le 1.0. \tag{1.13}$$

The release kinetics from supersaturated matrices is addressed by the Higuchi model. Higuchi [1961], in a two-page communication, introduced a simple equation that became the basis for kinetic analysis of most pharmaceutical CR systems. The equation was originally derived for ointments and later extended to solid matrices [Higuchi, 1963]. According to Higuchi, for a matrix of thickness $2L$, loaded to $C_0 \gg C_S$, where a large part of the solute load is immobilized in a state of fine dispersion, the amount of drug released per unit area is

$$Q_t = \left(2DC_S\left(C_0 - \frac{C_S}{2}\right)t\right)^{1/2} \tag{1.14}$$

and the fractional amount, Q_t/Q_∞, is given by

$$\frac{Q_t}{Q_\infty} = \left(\frac{2DC_S\left(1 - \frac{C_S}{2C_0}\right)t}{L^2 C_0}\right)^{1/2} \approx \left(\frac{2DC_S t}{L^2 C_0}\right)^{1/2}. \tag{1.15}$$

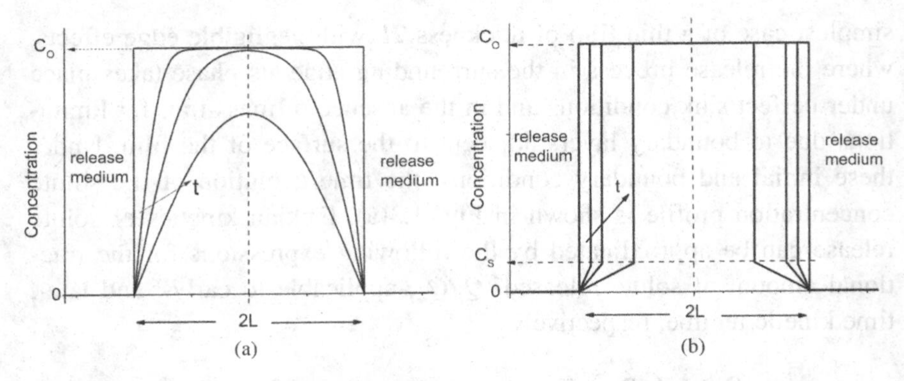

Figure 1.3. Time evolution of (a) Fickian and (b) Higuchi concentration profiles in thin films of thickness $2L$, initially containing solute concentration (a) $C_0 \leq C_S$ or (b) $C_0 > C_S$, respectively. Release occurs from both faces of the film and the concentration at the film boundaries is maintained at zero.

According to the Higuchi model, a moving boundary divides the matrix in an inner core loaded with concentration C_0 and an outer layer of dissolved drug. The dissolved drug molecules are released to the external phase by Fickian diffusion through the outer layer, under a concentration gradient. The boundary moves inward as the undissolved drug is converted to the dissolved form as shown in Fig. 1.3(b). Equation (1.14) was derived assuming that (a) the presence of dispersed solute has no material effect on the transport properties of the matrix and (b) instantaneous equilibrium exists between dissolved (mobile) and dispersed (immobile) solute.

The main characteristics of Fickian and Higuchi kinetics are the following:

(1) Both Eqs. (1.12) and (1.15) predict $t^{1/2}$ kinetics. As a result, the rates of release are continuously declining in both cases. However, the validity of Eq. (1.12) applies up to $Q_t/Q_\infty \sim 0.6$, but that of Eq. (1.15) extends well beyond this value, and the decline at later stages of the process is less marked in the supersaturated case.
(2) In the Fickian case, the release kinetics is governed by the diffusion coefficient D. Higuchi kinetics (Eq. (1.15)) is equivalent to Fickian

kinetics for the short-time regime (Eq. (1.12)), governed by an effective diffusivity $D_{eff} \approx (\pi/2)DC_S/C_0$.

(3) For a particular solute–polymer system characterized by constants D and C_S, the rate of release is independent of the initial load C_0 as long as $C_0 < C_S$ [Eq. (1.12)]. On the other hand, if $C_0 \gg C_S$, the rate of release will tend to decrease with increasing solute load [Eq. (1.15)].

Analogous expressions for Fickian and Higuchi kinetics for other geometries can be found in Crank [1975] and various review articles [see, e.g. Siepmann & Siepmann, 2012].

The plots of Fig. 1.4 compare Fickian and Higuchi release kinetics from thin films. The initial high dose rate characterizing both cases (Figs. 1.4(b) and (c)) is usually called "burst" effect and is inherent in purely diffusion-controlled kinetics. [In real CR devices, an initial "burst" is also produced by drug particles that have migrated from the bulk of the matrix to the surface during storage and are rapidly released when the device comes in contact with the releasing environment.] The overall declining rate of purely diffusion-controlled simple matrix systems is the main disadvantage of these CR devices, as the "holy grail of CR technology has long been the achievement of a constant, or zero order, release rate" [Paul, 2011]. A constant rate of release is required for safe and efficient medication. On the other hand, a device characterized by a declining dose rate, as well as by other kinds of inefficient design, can be wasteful and raise hazardous issues to health and/or environment. For example, according to an FDA document, currently marketed transdermal patches may retain 10–95% of the initial drug load after the intended period of application to the skin [FDA Guidance for Industry, 2011]. This raises potential safety issues, such as adverse pharmacological effects, if the patient failed to remove the patch at the end of the prescribed period. A discarded patch containing residual drug is potentially dangerous not only for the patient, but also for other persons, as well as pets. To reduce the potential risks, the FDA document advises the developers and producers to adopt a "quality of design" approach in order to minimize the amount of residual drug remaining in the patch after use. Thus, for several reasons, it is important to maximize the efficiency of a matrix device, i.e. the fractional amount of embedded drug that can be delivered

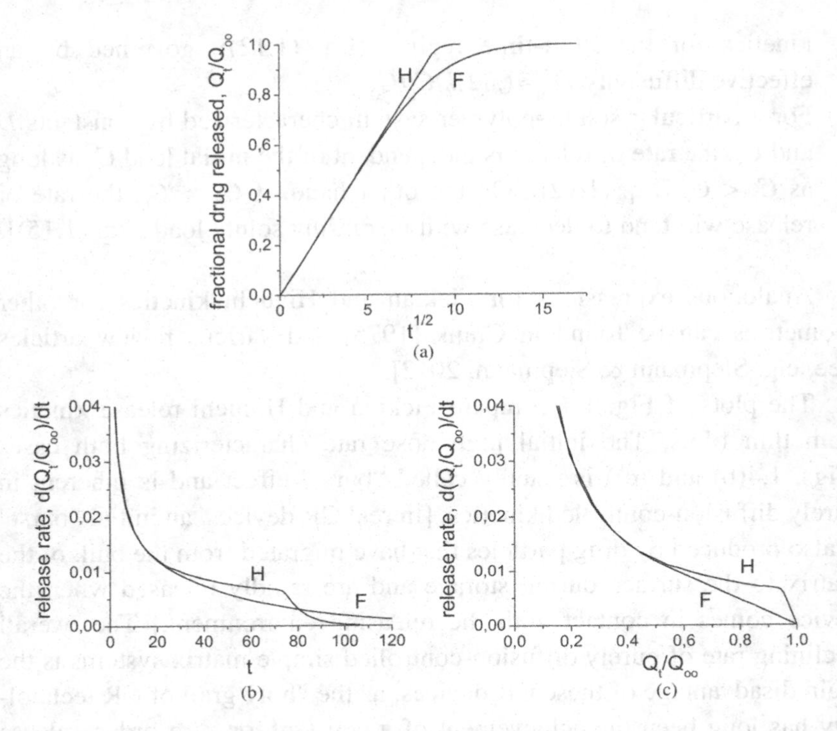

Figure 1.4. Fickian (F) and Higuchi (H) release kinetics from a thin-film device of thickness 2*L*. The kinetic curves are plotted on a Q_t/Q_∞ vs $t^{1/2}$ plot (a) and the corresponding rates of release, expressed here as $d(Q_t/Q_\infty)/dt$, are plotted on a *t* scale (b) and on a Q_t/Q_∞ scale (c). Curve F refers to an unsaturated polymer–solute system characterized by diffusivity *D*. Curve H refers to a supersaturated system with an effective diffusivity D_{eff} equal to *D* and thus, on the basis of Eqs. (1.12) and (1.15), characterized by the same initial rate as curve F. Data represent numerical calculations taken and adapted from Papadokostaki *et al.* [2008].

within the required therapeutic dose rate. The efficiency of a device, thus defined, can be easily evaluated by plotting the rate of release vs the fractional amount of drug released (as done in Fig. 1.4(c)), instead of vs *t* (Fig. 1.4(b)). In addition, such plots facilitate the comparison, in terms of efficiency, between different devices.

Matrix systems exclusively functioning by a diffusion mechanism are a limiting case. Examples include the transport of lipophilic small molecular weight (MW) steroids or even weakly polar drugs through poly(dimethylsiloxane) (PDMS) [Malcolm *et al.*, 2004; Panou *et al.*, 2014; Robertson *et al.*, 1983]. In most practical systems, diffusion is accompanied by other rate-controlling mechanisms during the release process, mainly associated with the ingress of solvent (water) in the matrix, either due to the hydrophilic nature of glassy hydrogels or due to the osmotic action of hydrophilic additives in a hydrophobic elastomeric matrix. The concurrent operation of mechanisms other than diffusion can lead to deviations from $t^{1/2}$ kinetics of release, resulting in a more uniform release rate even in simple matrix devices.

Two such mechanisms, usually found in MCR systems, are discussed below.

1.4.2 *Swelling-induced Polymer Relaxation Effects*

In contrast to non-polar hydrophobic elastomers, hydrophilic polymers, as those used in matrix tablets, absorb substantial amounts of water upon immersion in an aqueous environment. The kinetics of the drug release from a hydrogel matrix is usually affected by the swelling kinetics of the initially dry polymer, offering possibilities of attaining a uniform rate of release.

Penetration of water in glassy hydrogels usually deviates from Fickian kinetics. Non-Fickian kinetics observed in glassy polymer–swelling agent systems is commonly attributed to the slow viscous structural relaxations of the swelling polymer in response to penetrant-induced osmotic stresses, which occur on time scales comparable to those of the diffusion process. Another physical cause for anomalous kinetic behavior is the development of mechanical constraints imposed on local swelling. During the sorption process, differential swelling stresses, acting transverse to the direction of diffusion, are generated by the constraints imposed by the dry and rigid inner core of the polymer sample on the outer swollen and plasticized regions [Crank, 1975; Sanopoulou & Petropoulos, 2001]. Both phenomena described above may co-exist during transport of a swelling agent in a glassy polymer.

Polymer relaxation effects during water penetration in hydrogels arise from the fact that glassy polymers ($T_g > T$) are characterized by slow macromolecular mobility. Thus, the long-range re-arrangements of the polymer structure in order to accommodate the water molecules may be sufficiently slow to exercise a substantial, or even a controlling, influence on the course of the sorption process. The swelling process may be regarded as viscoelastic volume dilation of the polymer under an osmotic stress induced by the penetrating water. The rate of polymer relaxation is governed by a relaxation frequency, β (reciprocal relaxation time $\tau = 1/\beta$) and may be comparable to the rate of diffusion, governed by D_w/L^2, where D_w is the diffusion coefficient of water. The kinetics of water uptake is determined by the relative rates of these two processes, expressed by the dimensionless parameter $\beta L^2/D_w$. More often in CR literature, the reciprocal of $\beta L^2/D_w$ is used [defining the corresponding ratio of diffusion and relaxation times], which is called the diffusion Deborah number *De* [Vrentas *et al.*, 1975; Wu & Peppas, 1993]:

$$De = \frac{D_w}{\beta L^2}. \tag{1.16}$$

For $De \ll 1$ or $De \gg 1$, the kinetics of water sorption are Fickian. For intermediate values of *De*, the relaxation process occurs at times comparable to the diffusion process and deviations from Fickian kinetics occur. A semi-empirical power law is used to describe these deviations [Crank, 1975]:

$$\frac{Q_t}{Q_\infty} = kt^n, \tag{1.17}$$

where k is a constant and n is indicative of the sorption kinetics. For a thin film under semi-infinite conditions (i.e. for $Q_t/Q_\infty < 0.6$), Fickian diffusion is characterized by $n = 0.5$. Increasing values of $n > 0.5$ denote increasing deviations from Fickian kinetics with $n = 1$ for Case II (or zero-order) kinetics and $n > 1$ for Supercase II kinetics.

Case II diffusion is considered a limiting form of deviation from Fickian kinetics found in glassy polymer–penetrant systems. It is characterized by a sharp penetrant front that propagates in the polymer with a constant velocity and by small concentration gradients (flat *C* profile) in the swollen polymer behind the front, as a consequence of rapid diffusion of the incoming penetrant to the relaxing front. The possibility of attaining zero-order release kinetics from a purely relaxation-controlled CR matrix is illustrated by a model system studied by Hopfenberg and Hsu [1978].

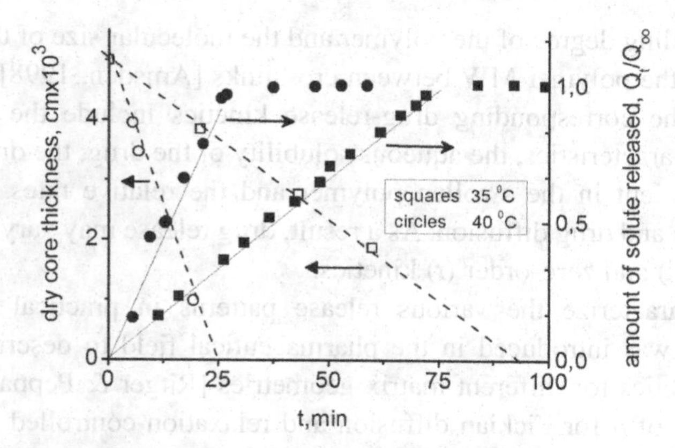

Figure 1.5. Relaxation-controlled, zero-order release kinetics of Sudan red (full points), loaded to polystyrene films, in *n*-hexane solvent. Open points represent the corresponding diminishing thickness of the dye-containing dry polymer core. Data taken and adapted from Hopfenberg and Hsu [1978].

The release kinetics of a dye (Sudan red) from polystyrene thin-film matrices to *n*-hexane (a swelling agent of polystyrene) was studied at different temperatures and solute loads (Fig. 1.5). Photomicrographs of the cross-sections of loaded matrices at different time intervals of the release process revealed a sharp penetrant front, propagating at a constant velocity in the film and separating the dry film core, uniformly loaded with the dye, and the swollen and dye-depleted outer layer. Due to the fast diffusion of both solvent and solute in the swollen layer, both *n*-hexane penetration and drug release were controlled by the constant rate of relaxations at the moving boundary. As a result, the release of the dye exhibits zero-order kinetics, with a constant delivery rate over the entire release process.

In hydrogel-based MCR systems, both water penetration and drug release usually exhibit some degree of deviation from Fickian kinetics, resulting in a more uniform rate of release as compared to purely diffusion-controlled systems. The equilibrium swelling and the kinetics of water uptake in hydrophilic polymers, such as poly(2-hydroxyethyl methacrylate-co-methyl methacrylate) (P(HEMA-co-MMA)) and poly(vinyl alcohol) (PVA) varies with the crosslinking density of the polymer network [Brazel & Peppas, 1999; Hasimi *et al.*, 2008]. In turn, the diffusion coefficient of solutes in amorphous crosslinked hydrogels depends mainly on the swelling degree of the polymer and the molecular size of the solute relative to the polymer MW between crosslinks [Amsden, 1998]. Factors affecting the corresponding drug-release kinetics include the polymer network characteristics, the aqueous solubility of the drug, the drug diffusion coefficient in the swollen polymer and the relative rates of water penetration and drug diffusion. As a result, drug release may vary between Fickian ($t^{1/2}$) and zero-order (t) kinetics.

To characterize the various release patterns in practical systems, Eq. (1.17) was introduced in the pharmaceutical field to describe drug-release kinetics for different matrix geometries [Ritger & Peppas, 1987]. The values of n for Fickian diffusion and relaxation-controlled transport vary with the matrix geometry. Values of n for thin-film geometry are stated above. For a sphere and a cylinder, Fickian kinetics is characterized by $n = 0.43$ and $n = 0.45$, respectively. Intermediate cases between purely diffusion-controlled and purely relaxation-controlled processes are characterized by $0.43 < n < 0.85$ for spheres and $0.45 < n < 0.89$ for cylinders.

An example of the variety of release kinetics that can be obtained under the concurrent operation of diffusion and polymer relaxation processes is given by Brazel and Peppas [1999] who studied the water uptake, and drug release, kinetics from P(HEMA-co-MMA) and PVA hydrogels of different initial crosslinking densities of the polymer networks. Depending on the polymer characteristics [composition of P(HEMA-co-MMA), degree of hydrolysis of PVA and crosslinking density of polymer network], the equilibrium swelling of the matrices varied widely and the kinetics of water uptake were characterized by n values ranging from 0.5 to 1.2. Drug release from these matrices also varied between Fickian and zero-order kinetics depending on the MW of the diffusing drug and the network characteristics of the polymer matrices.

Finally, if the polymer is soluble in water, the rate of polymer dissolution accompanying swelling may also play a role in the release process. An example is given by the work of Colombo *et al.* [1999] who used a water-soluble, colored drug to visualize the concurrent swelling, erosion and drug diffusion fronts in hydroxypropyl methyl cellulose matrix tablets. The release kinetics were discussed in relation to the relative rates of these processes and, for various drug loads, the rate of release was reasonably uniform over extended periods of the release process.

To summarize, hydrophilic polymers, due to coupling of diffusion with the polymer swelling process, offer many possibilities of stabilizing an otherwise diffusion-controlled drug-release rate.

1.4.3 *Osmotic Effects*

Except from osmotic pumps, the principle of osmosis is also exploited in matrix systems to promote drug release. For instance, the suitability of siloxanes, and particularly of PDMS, as a carrier material for long-term release of small MW steroids has been well established several decades ago. This, in conjunction with the biocompatibility characteristics of the polymer, has prompted much research efforts on methods to expand the application of PDMS-based CR devices in a broader range of pharmaceuticals such as hydrophilic drugs and proteins. Methods to promote the release process of water-soluble drugs include chemically induced hydrophilicity in PDMS, by covalent grafting or copolymerization, and the addition of osmotic excipients.

Additives of mild osmotic action, such as low MW sugars and polyethylene glycols, have a moderate effect on release rate if present at low contents since the water-filled areas in the matrix are isolated. Water-soluble drugs may exert an osmotic action themselves, as in the case of clonidine hydrochloride or proxyphylline loaded to PDMS disks and slabs [Carelli *et al.*, 1987; Soulas & Papadokostaki, 2011a]. The osmotically driven release mechanism from hydrophobic matrices has been studied in detail in the case of inorganic salts of high osmotic action (NaI, NaCl) embedded in the form of particles in PDMS elastomers [Schirrer *et al.*, 1992; Soulas *et al.*, 2009]. The mechanism proposed by Carelli *et al.* [1987, 1989] and successfully applied for low salt loads by Schirrer *et al.* [1992] is shown schematically in Fig. 1.6. PDMS surrounding the salt particles acts as a semi-permeable membrane. Although the water uptake by PDMS is very low, diffusion of water molecules is rapid. When water reaches a salt particle, the latter starts to dissolve and an osmotic pressure, π, starts to build up inside the swollen cavity. Swelling of the cavity is resisted by a retractive force exerted by the surrounding polymer. The osmotic pressure may be high enough to result in mechanical failure of the surrounding polymer, creating microcracks. The cracks spread

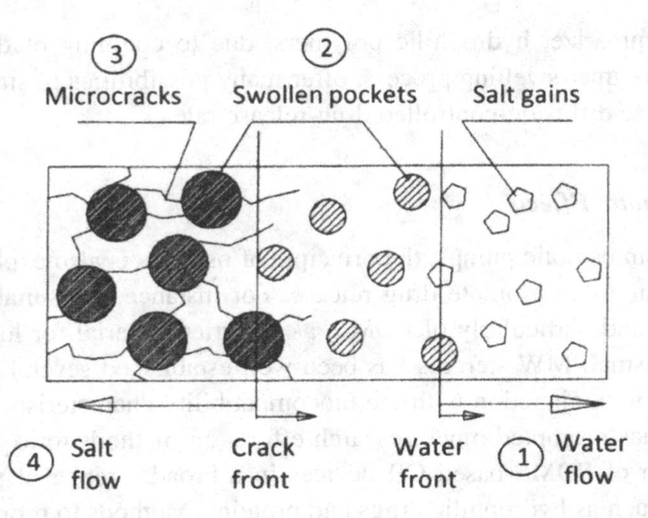

Figure 1.6. Schematic representation of the release mechanism of a highly osmotic solute dispersed in a hydrophobic matrix involving water diffusion, swelling of the solute cavities, creation of microcracks and solute flow toward the surrounding water. Taken from Schirrer *et al.* [1992], with permission of Springer.

through the matrix to neighboring cavities and eventually form an interconnecting network filled with water, through which the dissolved salt is released.

Amsden *et al.* [1994] proposed a mechanism based on rupture of the swollen cavity wall at its thinnest point, thus forming a system of interconnected cavities providing fast access of dissolved salt to the exposed surface. This process is expected to become increasingly less plausible as the salt load decreases and the cavity walls become thicker and hence less susceptible to rupture. Finally, for polymers other than highly hydrophobic elastomers, the osmotically driven release may not necessarily involve mechanical failure of the polymer encapsulating the cavity wall. In moderately hydrophilic matrices (as cellulose acetate), the osmotic action of the solute may create superhydrated polymer zones surrounding the solute cavities, wherein the water concentration is higher than that expected in the absence of the solute. These zones of enhanced hydration will eventually expand and merge to create a network of water-rich pathways extending to the surface of the matrix, as schematically shown in Fig. 1.7 [Babasola *et al.*, 2013; Petropoulos *et al.*, 2012].

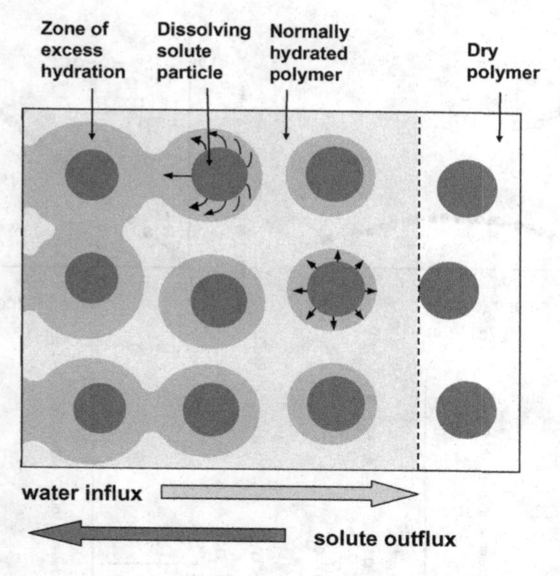

Figure 1.7. Schematic representation of the mechanism of osmotically induced swelling, involving zones of excess polymer hydration, wherein solute transport is facilitated. Thin arrows show preferred microscopic transport direction of solute. Taken and adapted from Petropoulos *et al.* [2012].

The osmotically driven release from hydrophobic elastomers is affected by the size and shape of osmotic particles, the osmotic activity, solute solubility and solute load, mechanical properties of the polymer and device geometry (slab, cylinder or disk) [Amsden, 2007; Carelli *et al.*, 1987; Soulas *et al.*, 2009]. However, by proper control of these factors, strong deviations from diffusional ($t^{1/2}$) release kinetics occur, leading to a stabilization of the release rate. An illustrative example is given in Fig. 1.8, concerning the release of proxyphylline from PDMS matrices. Proxyphylline, a water-soluble drug, results in osmotically driven water uptake upon immersion of the PDMS matrix in water. The osmotic effect of proxyphylline is mild and does not materially affect the diffusion-controlled release of the drug, exhibiting $t^{1/2}$ kinetics. The addition of NaCl particles, as a highly osmotic excipient, in the drug-loaded matrices has a dramatic effect on the amount of imbibed water. The microcrack mechanism outlined above eventually forms an interconnecting network filled with water, through which both the dissolved salt, as well as

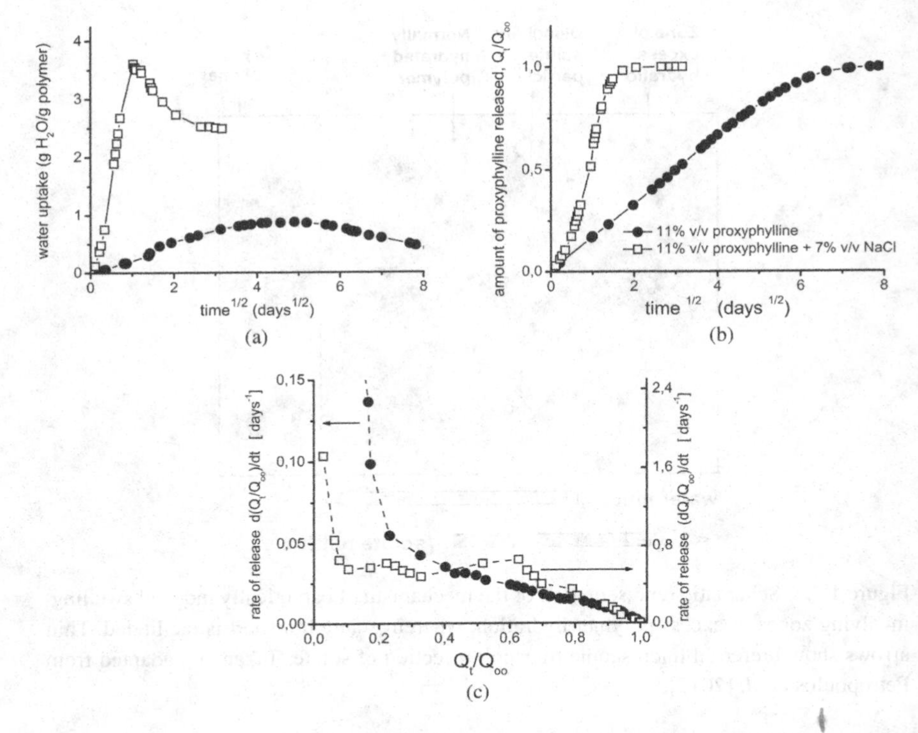

Figure 1.8. Effect of NaCl on (a) water uptake, (b) proxyphylline release kinetics and (c) proxyphylline rate of release, from PDMS matrices. In all plots, circles refer to matrix loaded to 11% (v/v) proxyphylline and squares to matrix with the same drug load plus 7% (v/v) NaCl particles. Data taken and adapted from Soulas and Papadokostaki [2011b].

proxyphylline, is released [Soulas & Papadokostaki, 2011b]. The drug's release profile is characterized by a strong rise in release rate, after an initial gestation time needed for the microcrack network to form, leading to S-shaped release curves on a $t^{1/2}$ scale. This form of marked deviations from diffusion kinetics leads to a more uniform rate of proxyphylline release.

The concept of osmotically driven release has been exploited in order to facilitate the release of bioactive macromolecules, such as proteins, from elastomeric matrices. Proteins often do not possess substantial osmotic pressure themselves, to initiate crack formation. For example, the osmotic pressure of saturated bovine serum albumin (BSA) solution is lower than 10 atm [Gu *et al.*, 2005], to be compared with the corresponding values of 402 atm for NaCl and 263 atm for KCl [Amsden *et al.*, 1994]. To enhance the osmotic effects, Carelli *et al.* [1989] prepared PDMS matrices in the form of disks and cylinders, with various loads of granules composed of BSA and NaCl in two w/w ratios. With the higher NaCl:BSA ratio granules, BSA release occurred at a uniform rate for extended portions of the release curve. The same was observed for the release of NaCl, although at a faster rate. The results indicated that the release of both solutes involved both diffusion and convection. Other examples of uniform-rate macromolecular release with the aid of osmotic excipients is the release of interferon-γ, co-lyophilized with BSA and trehalose (osmotic pressure = 98 atm), from a photo-crosslinked biodegradable elastomer [Gu *et al.*, 2005], and of BSA, co-lyophilized with trehalose, from viscous liquid hydrophobic polymers based on 5-ethylene ketal ε-caprolactone [Babasola *et al.*, 2013].

1.5 Modified Matrix Designs

In addition to the transport mechanisms described above, the uniformity of dose rate of diffusion-controlled matrix devices can be improved by modifying the design of the matrix. In most cases, the modification aims at either a spatial distribution of the permeation properties of the matrix and/or the initial solute load properties or at modifying the matrix surface area available for release. Lee [1986] has examined theoretically the effect of different initial drug concentration profiles from planar, cylindrical and spherical geometries, on the release kinetics and identified cases that provide approach to zero-order kinetics. The applicability of this concept was demonstrated experimentally by partial solute extraction from loaded PHEMA hydrogel beads, in order to generate a sigmoidal initial drug concentration profile. Since glassy matrices are generally characterized by more uniform release profiles than purely diffusion-controlled systems, particular attention has been given to minimize the initial burst effect from the former without altering the long-term release rate. For example, surface crosslinking and surface solute extraction from initially uniformly loaded cylindrical PVA disks has been applied for this purpose [Huang *et al.*, 2002].

The spatial distribution of permeability properties or solute initial load can also be achieved by multi-layer matrices. Such composite MCR devices afford the possibility of distributing solute load and permeability properties independently of each other. As shown by both theoretical calculations and experimental work, a uniform rate of release can be achieved by judicious choice of the design parameters of the multi-layer device (drug load, polymer permeability, relative thickness of the layers) [Charalambopoulou *et al.*, 2001; Kim & Lee, 1992; Lu & Anseth, 1999; Papadokostaki *et al.*, 2008, 2009].

Finally, coating of loaded matrices of various geometries with a polymeric layer is also a broadly used method of modulating release rate. In most of these cases, the geometry of the uncoated device results in multi-dimensional diffusion and the partial coating aims at modulating the release rate by altering the releasing surface of the device. The Geomatrix™ system is a flexible technology to achieve a zero-order release rate from hydrophilic matrix tablets by coating the drug-loaded core matrix with one or two barrier layers [Conte & Maggi, 1996]. The coating can be applied by a multi-layer compression process during tablet manufacture. The layers serve to modulate the hydration rate of the system and/or to reduce the tablet-releasing surface. In addition, more than one coated tablet unit can be placed in a gelatin capsule to obtain different dosages.

The above techniques are also suitable for achieving other than uniform release rate CR profiles. For example, the realization that the 24-h circadian rhythms of various biological processes influence the occurrence or the intensity of symptoms of several diseases has led to increasing interest in CR systems capable of a pulsatile drug release to synchronize with the circadian rhythms in order to improve the efficacy treatment [Mandal *et al.*, 2010]. In addition, delivering two drugs simultaneously or sequentially is also pursued.

1.6 Transport Phenomena Affecting *In Vitro–In Vivo* Correlations

The previous sections refer to the kinetics of release resulting from mechanisms operating during transport of the drug through the polymer matrix. The *in vivo* levels of drug concentration in the organism may also be determined by other factors related to the physiological environment where drug release will actually take place. For example, the surrounding tissue in implants, or stagnant aqueous boundary layers next to the CR device surface, may offer resistance to mass transfer and alter the release kinetics, resulting in poor *in vitro*/*in vivo* correlations. The resistance of skin to transport of solutes is another example. The synthetic polymeric layer of a TDDS controls only partly the delivery rate of the drug, as upon application of the patch the drug molecules, toward their route to systemic circulation, are first confronted with the natural barrier imposed by the skin. Stratum corneum, the uppermost layer of epidermis, is mainly responsible for the barrier properties of the skin. Human stratum corneum is a (10–20 μm in the dry state) multi-layer structure consisting of keratin-rich corneocytes embedded in an intercellular lipid phase. The tortuous diffusion path through this structure is mainly held responsible for the low diffusivities of small molecules in stratum corneum. For example, D values of small MW steroids, calculated from permeation experiments across human epidermis, assuming a thickness of hydrated, rate-controlling stratum corneum of 40 μm, are in the order of 10^{-11}–10^{-13} cm^2/s [Scheuplein *et al.*, 1969] to be compared with corresponding values of 10^{-7} cm^2/s for PDMS and 10^{-9} cm^2/s for EVA copolymers [Roseman, 1980]. Thus, it is not surprising that most drugs administered by passive diffusion by TDDS have MW between 162 (for nicotine) to 357 (for oxybutyn) and moderate lipophilicity, expressed by $\log K_{o/w}$ values between 1 and 4, respectively.

1.7 Conclusions

The development of CR devices constitutes a significant progress toward the efficient and safe drug therapy and is continuously evolving to new therapeutic approaches. Here, we focused on systems where diffusive transport through a polymeric medium plays an important role in the release process, and we provided examples of the vast medical applications of predominantly diffusion-controlled systems, with emphasis to matrix products. Matrix systems are relatively simple to manufacture and safe against dose dumping. They are also challenging in respect to the main requirement of a CR device to deliver the drug load at a uniform rate within the therapeutic window of the drug. Despite their wide spread in the form of various therapeutic formulations, there is still room for substantial improvement in their design and operation. Optimum design, in turn, can greatly benefit from the knowledge of the complex transport mechanisms operating during the release process. Here, we discussed two common mechanisms operating in parallel with the diffusion process in many practical systems that can, under proper conditions, favor the stabilization of the release rate: relaxation-controlled swelling of glassy hydrophilic polymers and osmotic effects activated by hydrophilic excipients in elastomeric matrices. The full exploitation of this kind of fundamental knowledge in industrial design of CR products is not an easy task due to the complexity of the transport phenomena and the great number of physicochemical, as well as geometrical, variables that determine the kinetics of release. It can be expected that advanced realistic computer modeling will be extensively applied in the future as a tool both at the stage of materials selection of the matrix and at the stage of adjusting device parameters to ensure optimum operational conditions.

List of Abbreviations

BSA	bovine serum albumin
CR	controlled release
MCR systems	matrix-controlled release systems
P(BMA-co-MMA)	poly(butyl methacrylate-co-methyl methacrylate)
PDMS	poly(dimethylsiloxane)
PEG	polyethyleneglycol
P(EVA)	poly(ethylene vinyl acetate)
PHEMA	poly(hydroxyethyl methacrylate)
P(HEMA-co-MMA)	poly(2-hydroxyethyl methacrylate-co-methyl methacrylate)
PHPMA	poly(hydroxypropyl methacrylate)
PVA	poly(vinyl alcohol)
P(VDF-HFP)	poly(vinylidenefluoride-co-hexafluoropropylene)
TDDS	transdermal drug-delivery systems

References

Amsden B (1998). Solute diffusion within hydrogels. Mechanisms and models, *Macromolecules*, 31, pp. 8382–8395.

Amsden B (2007). Review of osmotic pressure driven release of protein from monolithic devices. *J Pharm Pharm Sci*, 10, pp. 129–143.

Amsden BG, Cheng Y-L and Goosen MFA (1994). A mechanistic study of the release of osmotic agents from polymeric monoliths. *J Control Release*, 30, pp. 45–56.

Babasola IY, Zhang W and Amsden BG (2013). Osmotic pressure driven protein release from viscous liquid, hydrophobic polymers based on 5-ethylene ketal ε-caprolactone: potential and mechanism. *Eur J Pharm Biopharm*, 85, pp. 765–772.

Baker RW (2004). *Membrane Technology and Applications*, 2nd Edn. (John Wiley and Sons).

Banerjee S, Chattopadhyay P, Ghosh A, Datta P and Veer V (2014). Aspect of adhesives in transdermal drug delivery systems. *Int J Adhes Adhes*, 50, pp. 70–84.

Barry BW (1991). Lipid–protein-partitioning theory of skin penetration enhancement. *J Control Release*, 15, pp. 237–248.

Brache V and Faundes A (2010). Contraceptive vaginal rings: a review. *Contraception*, 82, pp. 418–427.

Brazel CS and Peppas NA (1999). Mechanisms of solute and drug transport in relaxing, swellable, hydrophilic glassy polymers. *Polymer*, 40, pp. 3383–3398.

Carelli V, Di Colo G, Guerrini C and Nannipieri E (1989). Drug release from silicone elastomer through controlled polymer cracking: an extension to macromolecular drugs. *Int J Pharm*, 50, pp. 181–188.

Carelli V, Di Colo G and Nanipieri E (1987). Factors in zero-order release of clonidine hydrochloride from monolithic polydimethylsiloxane matrices. *Int J Pharm*, 35, pp. 21–28.

Charalambopoulou GCh, Kikkinides ES, Papadokostaki KG, Stubos AK and Papaioannou ATh (2001). Numerical and experimental investigation of the diffusional release of a dispersed solute from polymeric multilaminate matrices. *J Control Release*, 70, pp. 309–319.

Colombo P, Bettini R and Peppas NA (1999). Observation of swelling process and diffusion position during swelling in hydroxylpropyl methyl cellulose (HPMC) matrices containing a soluble drug. *J Control Release*, 61, pp. 83–91.

Conley R, Gupta SK and Sathyan G (2006). Clinical spectrum of the osmotic-controlled release oral delivery system (OROS), an advanced oral delivery form. *Curr Med Res Opin*, 22, pp. 1879–1892.

Conte U and Maggi L (1996). Modulation of the dissolution profiles from Geomatrix® multi-layer matrix tablets containing drugs of different solubility. *Biomaterials*, 17, pp. 889–896.

Crank J (1975). *The Mathematics of Diffusion*, 2nd Edn. (Clarendon Press, Oxford).

FDA Guidance for Industry (2011). Residual drug in transdermal and related drug delivery systems. http://www.fda.gov/downloads/Drugs/GuidanceComplianceRegulatoryInformation/Guidances/UCM220796.pdf

Flynn GL, Yalkowsky SH and Roseman TJ (1974). Mass transport phenomena and models: theoretical concepts. *J Pharm Sci*, 63, pp. 479–510.

Gu F, Younes HM, El-Kadi AOS, Neufeld RJ and Amsden BG (2005). Sustained interferon-gamma delivery from a photocrosslinked biodegradable elastomer. *J Control Release*, 102, pp. 607–617.

Hasimi A, Stavropoulou A, Papadokostaki KG and Sanopoulou M (2008). Transport of water in polyvinyl alcohol films: effect of thermal treatment and chemical crosslinking. *Eur Polym J*, 44, pp. 4098–4107.

Higuchi T (1961). Rate of release of medicaments from ointment bases containing drugs in suspension. *J Pharm Sci*, 50, pp. 874–875.

Higuchi T (1963). Mechanisms of sustained action medication. Theoretical analysis of rate of release of solid drugs dispersed in solid matrices. *J Pharm Sci*, 52, pp. 1145–1149.

Hoffman AS (2008). The origins and evolution of "controlled" drug delivery systems. *J Control Release*, 132, pp. 153–163.

Hopfenberg HB (1976). Controlled release polymeric formulations. ACS Symp. Ser. No. 33. In Paul DR and Harris FW, Eds., *Controlled Release from Erodible Slabs, Cylinders, and Spheres*. (American Chemical Society, Washington), pp. 26–32.

Hopfenberg HB and Hsu KC (1978). Swelling-controlled, constant rate delivery systems. *Polym Eng Sci*, 18, pp. 1186–1191.

Huang X, Chestang BL and Brazel CS (2002). Minimization of initial burst in poly(vinyl alcohol) hydrogels by surface extraction and surface-preferential crosslinking. *Int J Pharm*, 248, pp. 183–192.

Khan W, Farah S and Domb AJ (2012). Drug eluting stents: developments and current status. *J Control Release*, 161, pp. 703–712.

Kim C-J and Lee PI (1992). Composite poly(vinyl alcohol) beads for controlled drug delivery. *Pharm Res*, 9, pp. 10–16.

Lee PI (1986). Initial concentration distribution as a mechanism for regulating drug release from diffusion controlled and surface erosion controlled matrix systems. *J Control Release*, 4, pp. 1–7.

Lu S and Anseth KS (1999). Photopolymerization of multilaminated poly(HEMA) hydrogels for controlled release. *J Control Release*, 57, pp. 291–300.

Malcolm RK, Edwards K-L, Kiser P, Romano J and Smith TJ (2010). Advances in microbicide vaginal rings. *Antiv Res*, 88S, pp. S30–S39.

Malcolm RK, McCullagh SD, Woolfson AD, Gorman SP, Jones DS and Cuddy J (2004). Controlled release of a model antibacterial drug from a novel self-lubricating silicone biomaterial. *J Control Release*, 97, pp. 313–320.

Mandal AS, Biswas N, Karim KM, Guha A, Chatterjee S, Behera M and Kuotsu K (2010). Drug delivery system based on chronobiology — a review. *J Control Release*, 147, pp. 314–325.

Nokhodchi A, Raja S, Patel P and Asare-Addo K (2012). The role of oral controlled release matrix tablets in drug delivery systems. *BioImpacts*, 2, pp. 175–187.

Panou AI, Papadokostaki KG and Sanopoulou M (2014). Release mechanisms of semipolar solutes from poly(dimethylsiloxane) elastomers: effect of a hydrophilic additive. *J Appl Polym Sci*, 131, pp. 9381–9388.

Papadokostaki KG, Sanopoulou M and Petropoulos JH (2009). An advanced model for composite planar three-layer matrix-controlled release devices, part II. Devices with non-uniform material properties and a practical example. *J Membrane Sci*, 343, pp. 128–136.

Papadokostaki KG, Stavropoulou A, Sanopoulou M and Petropoulos JH (2008). An advanced model for composite planar three-layer matrix-controlled release devices, part I. Devices of uniform material properties and non-uniform solute load. *J Membrane Sci*, 312, pp. 193–206.

Paudel KS, Milewski M, Swadley CL, Brogden NK, Ghosh P and Stinchcomb AL (2010). Challenges and opportunities in dermal/transdermal delivery. *Ther Deliv*, 1, pp. 109–131.

Paul DR (2011). Elaborations on the Higuchi model for drug delivery. *Int J Pharm*, 418, pp. 13–17.

Peppas NA and Narasimhan B (2014). Mathematical models in drug delivery: how modeling has shaped the way we design new drug delivery systems. *J Control Release*, 190, pp. 75–81.

Petropoulos JH, Papadokostaki KG and Amarantos SG (1992). A general model for the release of active agents incorporated in swellable polymeric matrices. *J Polym Sci Part B*, 30, pp. 717–725.

Petropoulos JH, Papadokostaki KG and Sanopoulou M (2012). Higuchi's equation and beyond: overview of the formulation and application of a generalized model of drug release from polymeric matrices. *Int J Pharm*, 437, pp. 178–191.

Puranik AS, Dawson ER and Peppas NA (2013). Recent advances in drug eluting stents. *Int J Pharm*, 441, pp. 665–679.

Ritger PL and Peppas NA (1987). A simple equation for description of solute release. II. Fickian and anomalous release from swellable devices. *J Control Release*, 5, pp. 37–42.

Robertson DN, Sivin I, Nash HA, Braun J and Dinh J (1983). Release rates of levonorgestrel from silastic[R] capsules, homogeneous rods and covered rods in humans. *Contraception*, 27, pp. 483–495.

Roseman TJ (1980). Controlled release technologies: methods, theory and applications. In Kydonieus AF, Ed., *Monolithic Polymer Devices*, Chapter 2 (CRC Press, Boca Raton, FL), pp. 21–54.

Sanopoulou M and Petropoulos JH (2001). Systematic analysis and model interpretation of micromolecular non-Fickian sorption kinetics in polymer films. *Macromolecules*, 34, pp. 1400–1410.

Scheuplein RJ, Blank IH, Brauner GJ and MacFarlane DJ (1969). Percutaneous absorption of steroids. *J Investig Dermatol*, 52, pp. 63–70.

Schirrer R, Thepin P and Torres G (1992). Water absorption, swelling, rupture and salt release in salt–silicone rubber compounds. *J Mater Sci*, 27, pp. 3424–3434.

Siegel RA (2014). Stimuli sensitive polymers and self-regulated drug delivery systems: a very partial review. *J Control Release*, 190, pp. 337–351.

Siegel RA and Rathbone MJ (2012). Fundamentals and applications of controlled release drug delivery. In Siepmann J, Siegel RA and Rathbone MJ, Eds., *Overview of Controlled Release Mechanisms*, Chapter 2 (Springer, New York), pp. 19–43.

Siepmann J and Siepmann F (2012). Modeling of diffusion controlled drug delivery. *J Control Release*, 161, pp. 351–362.

Soulas DN and Papadokostaki KG (2011a). Experimental investigation of the release mechanism of proxyphylline from silicone rubber matrices. *J Appl Polym Sci*, 120, pp. 821–830.

Soulas DN and Papadokostaki KG (2011b). Regulation of proxyphylline's release from silicone rubber matrices by the use of osmotically active excipients and a multilayer system. *Int J Pharm*, 408, pp. 120–129.

Soulas DN, Sanopoulou M and Papadokostaki KG (2009). A comparative study on the release kinetics of osmotically active solutes from hydrophobic elastomeric matrices, combined with the characterization of the depleted matrices. *J Appl Polym Sci*, 113, pp. 936–949.

Stamatialis DF, Papaenburg BJ, Girones M, Saiful S, Bettahalli SNM, Schmitmeier S and Wessling M (2008). Medical applications of membranes: drug delivery, artificial organs and tissue engineering. *J Membrane Sci*, 308, pp. 1–34.

Vrentas JS, Jarzebski CM and Duda JL (1975). Deborah number for diffusion in polymer–solvent systems. *AIChE J*, 21, pp. 894–901.

Wang J, Jiang A, Joshi M and Christoforidis J (2013). Drug delivery implants in the treatment of vitreous inflammation. *Mediat Inflamm*, 2013, p. 780634.

Wiedersberg S and Guy RH (2014). Transdermal drug delivery: 30+ years of war and still fighting! *J Control Release*, 190, pp. 150–156.

Wu JC and Peppas NA (1993). Modeling of penetrant diffusion in glassy polymers with an integral sorption Deborah number. *J Polym Sci Part B*, 31, pp. 1503–1518.

Chapter 2
Membranes for Artificial Kidneys

J. Vienken

University of Applied Sciences, Gießen, Germany
vienken.usingen@gmail.com

2.1 Prolog and Introduction

It was in the middle of the 19th century when Thomas Graham, the famous Scottish scientist, defined for the first time the term "dialyzer" [Graham, 1854]. At that time, dialysis was used *in vitro* for the separation or purification of molecules from aqueous solutions. Nobody imagined that this procedure would develop into a successful clinical therapy for the treatment of kidney patients. To date and without doubt, kidney dialysis represents a success story of the global medical device industry. To understand this statement in more detail, a few statistical data and a short historical retrospective of hemodialysis is given.

Since the first application of dialyzers at the onset of the 20th century by John Abel in the United States on dogs [Abel *et al.*, 1913] and by Georg Haas in Germany on patients [Haas, 1923], the development of this blood purification technique is remarkable and astounding. This holds true especially for the years 1920ff, when the contemporaries of Haas and Abel were extremely reluctant to accept the idea of dialysis as a treatment for chronically sick patients. At that time, the famous German clinician Franz Vollhardt (1872–1950) blocked the ongoing research on clinical dialysis of Haas by publicly commenting in the 1920s: "Dialysis is useless and even dangerous for the patient!" Obviously, the treatment of a patient with a chronic disease and without hope of a complete recovery was against the common understanding of medical intervention at that time. Despite these obstacles, the experimental procedure of hemodialysis, using an extracorporeal blood circuit for blood purification with membranes (Fig. 2.1), has become a routine therapy about a hundred years later and is applied currently to more than 2.5 million patients with end-stage renal failure (Fig. 2.2).

A major contribution to the development of kidney dialysis stems from research and manufacturing of dialysis membranes. It is interesting to note that in the early 1980s, when cellulosic membranes dominated the

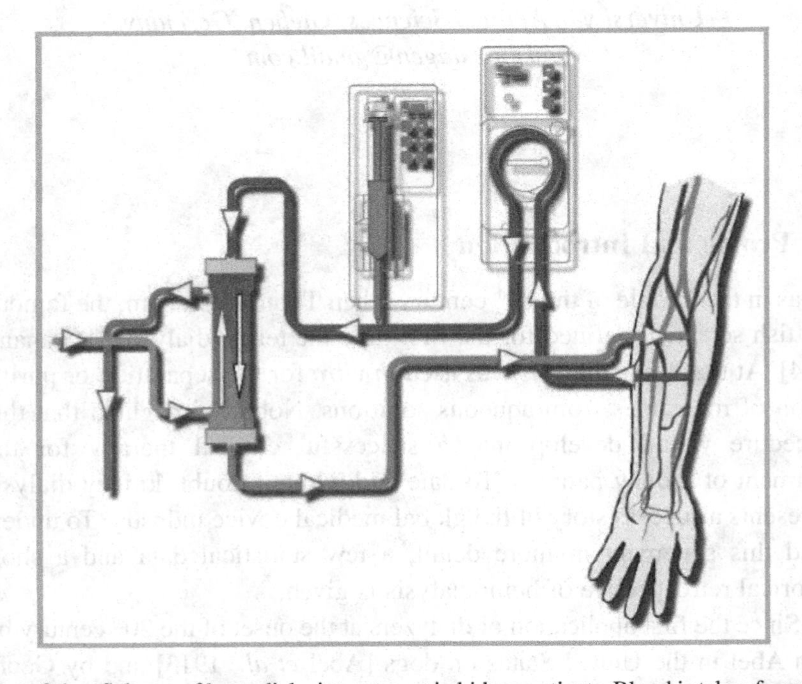

Figure 2.1. Scheme of hemodialysis treatment in kidney patients. Blood is taken from the forearm vein of a patient thrice per week and recirculated for about 4 h. It is guided extracorporeally through a dialyzer with the support of a peristaltic pump. Before the dialyzer, an anticoagulant, mostly consisting of heparin, is supplemented to the blood stream in order to avoid blood clotting within the circuit. Blood purification occurs, when toxins from the blood cross the dialysis membrane in the dialyzer. These toxins are removed by a dialysis fluid which is entering the dialyzer by countercurrent flow (© by the author).

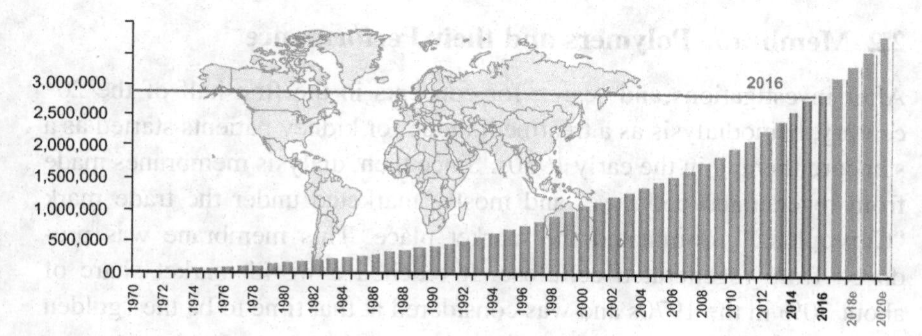

Figure 2.2. Recent years have shown a steady and exponential increase in hemodialysis patients, reaching a figure of more than 2.5 million patients in 2016 worldwide. This number is expected to grow further with an annual growth rate of 5–6%. In the light of the increase of the world population (1.1% annually), the prevalence of kidney patients on hemodialysis is growing faster. Reasons for this observation are demographic alterations with an increase in the elderly population with more comorbidities, the increase in the prevalence of diabetes type II as one of the reasons for kidney failure, a better survival of patients on dialysis therapy and an increased available budget for dialysis treatments in many countries (© by the author).

dialysis market, the global increase in patient numbers paralleled the increase in membrane availability.

Thus, at that time, the decision of industrial managers to promote a higher membrane production capacity in their facilities had a direct impact on the realization of clinical therapies. Assuming further that to date the average hemodialysis patient is subjected to a hemodialysis treatment thrice per week, a total of around 250 million filters is needed annually worldwide, while neglecting a minor dialyzer reuse in some countries. Thus, a weekly need of about 5 million dialyzers has to be realized by manufacturers and their worldwide logistic network. Given that today a standard dialyzer contains on average 2.5 km of capillary membranes, an overall length of about 600 million km of capillary membrane has to be produced annually. This figure is equivalent to four times the distance between the Earth and the Sun. It also reflects the success story of hemodialysis technology, the associated skill of engineers in industrial production and the enormous need for pure, medical grade polymers in recent years.

2.2 Membrane Polymers and their Performance

After investigations and search for concepts in the first half of the 20th century, hemodialysis as a treatment mode for kidney patients started as a standard therapy in the early 1950s. Since then, dialysis membranes made from regenerated cellulose, and mostly marketed under the trade mark "Cuprophan®", dominated the market place. This membrane was produced from regenerated cellulose. It reached a world market share of about 70% in the 1970s and was considered at that time to be the "golden standard" for dialysis membranes.

Its later fate in the dialysis market may serve as an example for the economic failure of such a medical device. Concerns of the medical community about the alleged lack of blood compatibility of Cuprophan® and a famous publication from 1985 entitled "Cellulose membranes, time for a change?" have successfully challenged the ongoing success of this membrane polymer [Henderson & Chenoweth, 1985]. As a consequence of intense biochemical and physiological investigations during *in vitro* and clinical use of Cuprophan®, its disadvantageous results on blood compatibility together with the increasing hesitance of nephrologists to use this biomaterial, its main producer Akzo Nobel/Membrana GmbH, Germany decided to cease the production of dialyzers with this membrane polymer in 2006.

What are the current consequences of this observation? Many scientific publications compared the properties and outcomes of Cuprophan® membrane application with results in favor or disfavor of other membrane polymers. These publications have lost their validity, because this cellulosic membrane polymer is now unavailable in the market. The search for a new polymer to serve as a negative standard is ongoing. An adequate negative standard is still lacking.

On the other hand, investigations on performance and blood compatibility of Cuprophan® membranes since then have not been performed in vain: the knowledge gained by means of such investigations which refers to the *in vitro* and *in vivo* behavior of membrane polymers and the effects of polymer composition to clinical sequelae can now be successfully applied for new polymer developments. This also includes the appropriate *in vitro* testing in the laboratories of manufacturers, which allow to predict the subsequent *in vivo* performance later.

Recent years have seen two major changes in the global market for dialysis membranes. First, synthetic membrane polymers, such as polysulfone (PSu) polyethersulfone (PES), polyacrylonitrile (PAN), polymethylmethacrylate (PMMA) and ethyl-vinyl-copolymer (EVAL), have continuously replaced the classical membranes made from regenerated cellulose. Synthetic dialysis membranes have proven to be more biocompatible and are now preferred by the majority of nephrologists. A survey on the development of worldwide market figures for dialysis membrane polymers is given in Fig. 2.3.

Besides, membrane performance has become a first-choice property. This refers predominantly to the membrane's ultrafiltration properties. So-called low-flux and high-flux membranes differ in their capacity to have a lower or higher hydraulic permeability, a property that can be described by their ultrafiltration coefficient (see Table 2.1). The worldwide market shares of low- and high-flux membranes are given in Fig. 2.4.

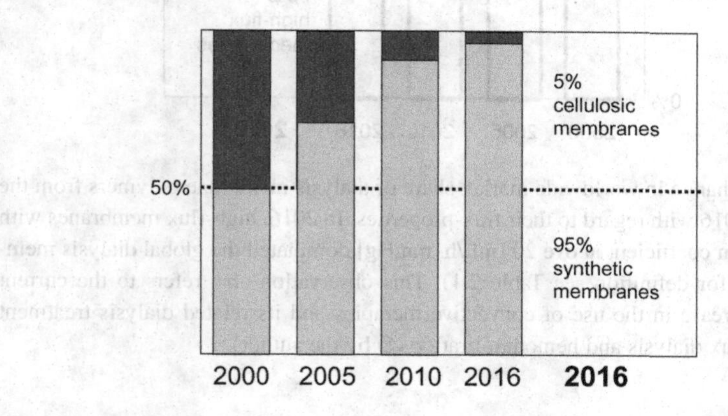

Figure 2.3. Change in worldwide market share of dialysis membrane polymers. The previously dominating cellulosic dialysis membranes have lost their importance and cover only a marginal 5% market share in 2016. The only remaining cellulosic membrane in the market is cellulose-tri-acetate (CTA). Synthetic membranes, such as PSu, PES, PMMA and PAN have replaced their cellulosic counterparts. As a consequence, published data on comparisons between cellulose and synthetic membranes from the last decades for performance and biocompatibility are not representative any more (© by the author).

Table 2.1: Definition of ultrafiltration coefficients for currently available dialysis membranes. High-efficiency membranes obtain their higher UF-coefficient by a larger membrane surface area and not by larger membrane pores.

Membrane type	UFC [mL/h · mmHg]	Membrane surface area [m^2]
Low flux	<20	<1.5
High efficiency	>10	>1.5
High flux	>20	
Hemofilter	>40	

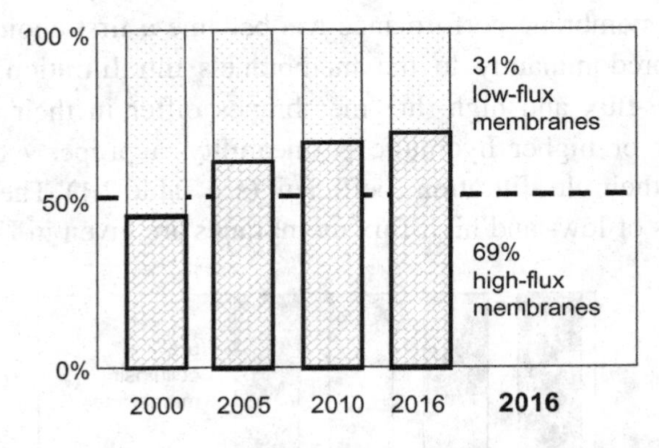

Figure 2.4. Change in worldwide market share of dialysis membrane polymers from the year 2000 to 2016 with regard to their flux-properties. In 2016, high-flux membranes with an ultrafiltration coefficient above 20 [mL/h · mmHg] dominated the global dialysis membrane market (for definition see Table 2.1). This observation also refers to the current continuous increase in the use of convective therapies and its related dialysis treatment modes, high-flux dialysis and hemodiafiltration (© by the author).

2.3 Five Polymer Families are Characteristic for Dialysis Membranes

The first group is represented by the PSu family and consists of a variety of PSu membrane types. Since about 20 years, the PSu-polymer has overtaken the previous role of Cuprophan® as a "Golden Standard" for dialysis membranes all around the world. All major international manufacturers of dialysis membranes now offer dialyzers with a PSu-type of membrane.

This observation proves the general acceptance by both, the medical and the industrial community. This can be explained by the versatility of the membrane PSu-polymer both, in terms of clinical performance and biocompatibility, as well as in production and sterilization technology.

Among them are (related meaningful publications in brackets):

1. Polysulfone (PSu, Fresenius Medical Care D-GmbH, Germany) [Streicher & Schneider, 1983].
2. Polyethersulfone (PES, Membrana/3M, Germany/USA) [Krieter & Lemke, 2011].
3. Polyethersulfone (PES-Elisio, Nipro Medical Corporation, Japan) [Martinez-Miguel *et al.*, 2015].
4. Toraysulfone (PSu, Toray Industries Inc., Japan) [Fournier *et al.*, 2015],
5. Polysulfone (APS, ASAHI Kasei Medical Corporation, Japan) [Linnenweber & Lonnemann, 2000].
6. Polyesterpolymer-Alloy (PEPA, Nikkiso Corporation, Japan) [Igoshi *et al.*, 2011].
7. Polyamide/Polysulfone mixtures (Polyamix, PA/PES, Gambro-Baxter, Sweden/USA) [Schindler *et al.*, 2000].

Many clinicians and scientists use "polysulfone", "polyethersulfone" and "polyarylethersulfone" as synonyms for the same polymer due to their great similarity in performance and chemical stability. Therefore, a short explanation on differences is needed. Generally speaking, PSus are a group of polymers that contain sulfone- (-SO_2-) and alkyl- or aryl-groups. According to the chemical nomenclature, only those polymers belong to the PSu family, which contain an additional isopropylidene group. Polymers without the isopropylidene group are called "polyarylethersulfones (PAES) or in short PES. In order to better understand the chemical difference between PSu and PAES/PES dialysis membranes, the detailed chemical formula of the involved polymers is shown in Fig. 2.5.

Hydrophilicity and wall structure of PSu membranes

The majority of membrane manufacturers from Europe and Asia produce membranes as a blend made of PSu or PES with

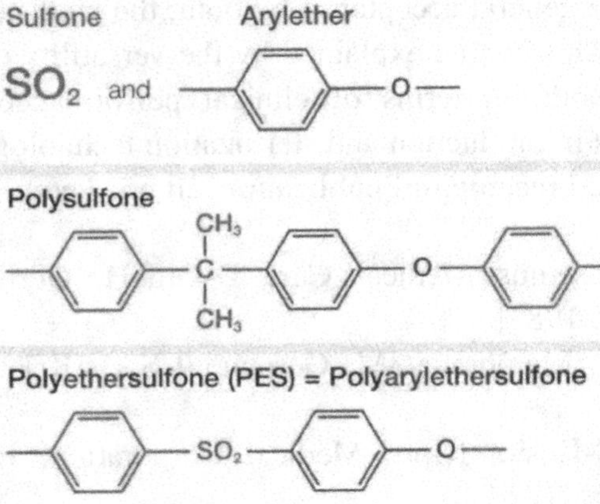

Figure 2.5. The chemical formula of PSu and PES differ in details of their chemical composition. In contrast to PES, PSu membranes contain a Bisphenol A (BPA) component, which is not present in PES membranes (© by the author).

polyvinylpyrrolidone (PVP). PVP is used as a hydrophilizing agent. Crude PSu membranes are hydrophobic and have to be rendered partially hydrophilic by blending with PVP, otherwise an increased transmembrane pressure has to be applied for an easy ultrafiltration during dialysis treatment.

As an example, the first membranes made from a PSu polymer were applied as a hemofilter membrane by the Amicon company in the USA. This membrane did not contain PVP (Fig. 2.6). Careful investigations have shown that its blood compatibility was meager and membranes could only be used as hemofilters due to their large pore sizes.

In contrast to Amicon, the first high-flux membrane for standard clinical hemodialysis came from Fresenius Medical Care in Germany. Its membrane polymer was blended for the first time with PVP [Streicher & Schneider, 1983; Heilmann & Keller, 2011] and serves since then as a membrane prototype with excellent biocompatibility properties. A further advantage turned out to be its high adsorptive capacity for endotoxins. Bacterial contaminants which might possibly be present in the dialysis fluid are, thus, unable to cross the membrane. The PSu membrane, therefore, acts as an efficient barrier for biological contaminants of water (see below). The membrane had an ultrafiltration coefficient of above

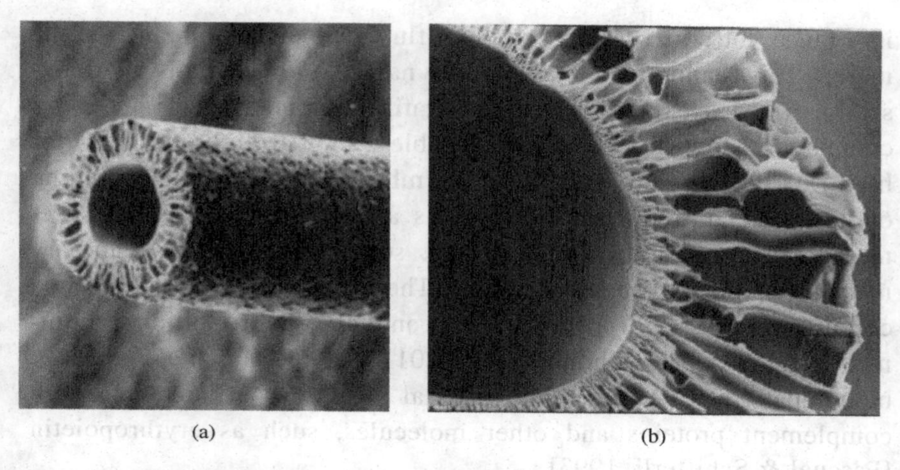

Figure 2.6. Electron-micrograph of a capillary membrane for hemofiltration provided by the Amicon company (a) and its cross-section (b) in the late 1970s (© by the author).

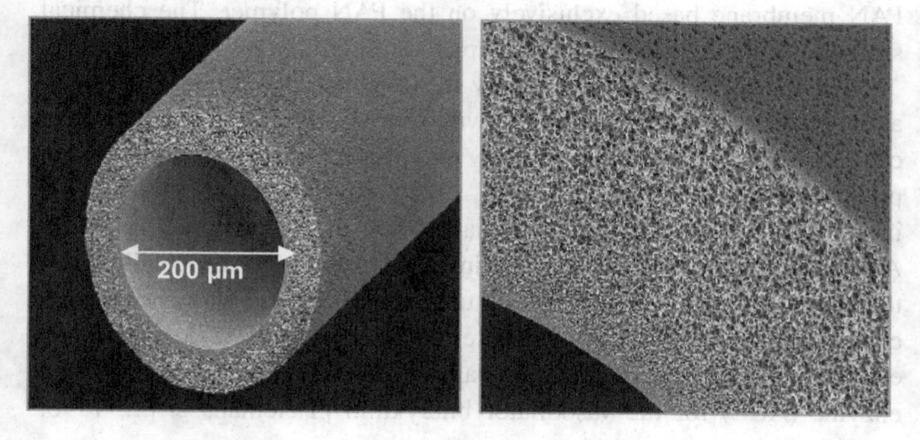

Figure 2.7. Electron-micrograph of a capillary membrane from Fresenius-Polysulfone®. The inner diameter of the hollow fiber is 200 μm, the wall thickness 40 μm. The rather dense support structure of this membrane contains less open voids as compared to its Amicon counterpart (© by the author).

40 [mL/h · mmHg] and was available as the first high-flux membrane (Table 2.1) sterilized by steam (Fig. 2.7).

The second group of synthetic membrane polymers consists of polymers, such as PAN. Already in 1972, the Rhone-Poulenc company in France introduced the first high-flux dialysis membrane to the market. It was annotated to the famous name "AN69". High-flux dialysis membranes exhibit a higher ultrafiltration-coefficient (UFC) as compared to low-flux membranes (Table 2.1). Currently, the UFC for high-flux is generally defined as >20 [mL/h · mmHg]. At the beginning of its market introduction, AN69 was available only in a flat sheet membrane configuration and it took some time until its capillary membrane version became available. The membrane was made from a copolymer, the hydrophobic PAN and the hydrophilic sodium-meth-allyl-sulfonate [Thomas *et al.*, 2011]. AN69 had an alleged high biocompatibility, because this material is able to efficiently adsorb complement proteins and other molecules, such as erythropoietin [Pascual & Schifferli, 1993].

Years later, the Japanese corporation ASAHI Kasei wanted to profit also from the excellent image of the AN69 membrane and introduced a PAN membrane based exclusively on the PAN polymer. The chemical structure of the AN69 polymer is depicted in Fig. 2.8.

The meth-allyl-sulfonate moiety in AN69 exhibits a negative charge at its surface. It is generally known from the literature that negative charges with a defined charge density provoke the activation of the contact phase system [Rollason & Sefton, 1992]. Several reports and clinical investigations, thus, confirmed the activation of the contact phase with AN69 including a series of severe clinical adverse events, especially given that this membrane material was simultaneously applied with the pharmaceutical drug ACE-inhibitor. The latter obviously amplified the membrane effect by blocking the degradation capacity of the angiotensin-converting enzyme (ACE) for the vasodilator bradykinin [Tielemans *et al.*, 1990;

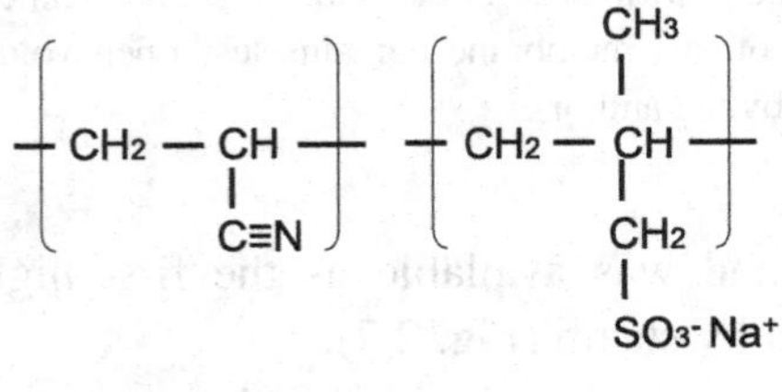

$$\left[CH_2 - \underset{\underset{C\equiv N}{|}}{CH} \right] \left[CH_2 - \overset{\overset{CH_3}{|}}{\underset{\underset{\underset{SO_3^- Na^+}{|}}{\underset{CH_2}{|}}}{C}H} \right]$$

Figure 2.8. The AN69 membrane represents a polymer blend made of PAN and sodium-meth-allyl sulfonate as shown by its chemical structure. Due to the sulfonate group, the molecule bears a negative charge.

Brunet *et al.*, 1992; Désormeaux *et al.*, 2008]. This effect, however, could be prevented by modifying the type of buffer solution with the use of bicarbonate buffer during dialysis therapy [Renaux *et al.*, 1999].

The third group of membrane polymers for hemodialysis is represented by the PMMA family. It is exclusively provided by Toray Industries from Japan. PMMA membranes are now available in all configurations and were the first in the market to be sterilized by gamma rays in 1977 [Sugaya & Sakai, 1998]. Obviously, the release of the sterilization gas ethylene oxide (ETO) from dialyzers containing PMMA membranes, which was standardly used at that time, was extremely long. Suspicions on ETO as a cause for allergic reactions in patients became true, and so alternative sterilization methods had to be developed.

Dialysis membranes from PMMA exhibit specific adsorptive features at their surface. The middle molecule β_2-microglobulin is effectively removed by adsorption both, at the inner surface of the PMMA capillary membrane and within the capillary wall. This also holds true for serum free κ and λ light chains [Fabbrini *et al.*, 2013].

Some PMMA membranes exhibit negative charges at their surface, similar to the PAN ones. Consequently, reports on anaphylactoid reactions in dialysis patients related to contact phase activation can also be found in the literature [Schwarzbeck *et al.*, 1993]. The adsorptive capacity of PMMA membranes is also considered as an explanation for improvements in adverse itching events (*psoriasis, prurigo nodularis*) in dialysis patients, although careful analyses about the detailed nature of adsorbed molecules is still lacking [Goeksel *et al.*, 2013].

The fourth group of currently available dialysis membranes represents membranes made from EVAL and EVOH. These membranes are provided by the Japanese company Kuraray Laboratories. EVAL is a strongly hydrophilic synthetic membrane material [Nakano, 2011]. It is known for its excellent blood compatibility with medium ultrafiltration coefficients. This can be explained by its comparably high numbers of small membrane pores which allow for an adequate water permeability. EVAL membranes have a very smooth surface and retain structural water. As a consequence, they adsorb only a few plasma proteins and membrane fouling due to protein adsorption during hemodialysis is rare.

The fifth group refers to the classical cellulosic membranes. As indicated above, the membranes from regenerated cellulose, such as

Cuprophan®, are not available any more in the dialysis market since 2006. The only member of that group with reasonable world market share (5%) is CTA [Sunohara *et al.*, 2011]. CTA is a rather hydrophilic membrane with slight hydrophobic properties due to its total three acetyl ester groups. It is currently provided by the Japanese Corporation Nipro Medical. Due to the ester groups and the associated lack of OH-groups there, the membrane exhibits an excellent blood compatibility. Complement activation, which was the major reason for the withdrawal of Cuprophan® from the market is markedly reduced. This can be explained by the blockage of hydroxyl groups in cellulose by the esterification with acetyl groups. We currently know that OH-groups offer binding sites for the C3b moiety of the complement protein, which is the initial event of the complement activation cascade [Kinoshita, 1991; Johnson *et al.*, 1990]. Analysis of the protein adsorption capacity of CTA membranes with the help of proteomics has shown that CTA binds more proteins than its PSu counterpart (PSu Helixone, Fresenius Medical Care). This is in contrast to many earlier reports that cellulose acetate membranes show only a low binding capacity for peptides/proteins [Urbani *et al.*, 2012].

2.4 Some Equations to Explain Membrane Transport

Blood purification with hemodialysis can be controlled by two transport mechanisms, convection and diffusion. Peptides or small proteins are removed more efficiently by convective transport mechanisms, due to their larger dimensions (molecular weights). Convective transport is facilitated by increased ultrafiltration rates. The term "solvent drag" is currently being used to describe this phenomenon (see below).

Small uremic toxins, such as urea, creatinine or phosphate ions are transported across the membrane by diffusion. Adolph Fick, a professor in Zürich, Switzerland published his famous law on diffusion already in 1855, [Fick, 1855]. According to his law, the movement of molecules across a membrane in a defined time dn/dt can be described as follows:

$$\frac{dn}{dt} = -D_k \cdot A \frac{dc}{dx}, \tag{2.1}$$

where *Dk* stands for the diffusion coefficient, A for the membrane surface area and *dc/dx* the concentration gradient across the membrane with the thickness *dx*.

D_k can be assessed according to the famous Stokes–Einstein equation as follows:

$$D_k = \frac{k_B \cdot T}{6\eta \cdot \pi \cdot r_0}, \tag{2.2}$$

where k_B — Boltzmann constant, T — temperature, h-dynamic viscosity of the solvent and r_0 hydrodynamic radius of the molecular entity.

A rough and less complicated estimation of "*D*" can be obtained by

$$D = \frac{1}{\sqrt[3]{\text{molecular weight}}}. \tag{2.3}$$

It is often neglected, that *dn/dt* refers to all affected individual molecules independently. Thus, each molecule has its own concentration gradient. Because the diffusion coefficient D_k is inversely proportional to the molecular radius, D_k is small for large molecules, so those are not transported by diffusional processes and this diffusive mechanism refers most exclusively to small molecules. An increase of diffusive transport can be achieved under two conditions: having a larger membrane surface area and a larger concentration gradient. The medical need for larger membrane surface is currently met by many membrane manufacturers; they offer dialyzers with membrane surface areas of up to 2.2 m^2.

During hemodialysis, dialysis fluids are guided in a countercurrent flow through the device which keeps the concentration gradient between the blood and the dialysate compartment "*dc*" as large as possible. As can be seen from Fig. 2.7, the membrane wall of PSu capillaries has an asymmetric structure of 40 μm thickness. A dense layer on the lumen side with a thickness of about 1 μm represents the layer with membrane function, whereas the rest of the 39 μm is used for its mechanic stability. The capillary wall has finally a funnel-like structure with pores sizes of 1–2 μm at its outer layer, their size is reduced down to around 3 nm at the blood contacting side and determines the sieving coefficient of the membrane there.

Table 2.2: Capillary membranes made from synthetic polymers differ in their ultrastructure and geometric dimensions. For an optimal diffusional transport, the wall thickness should be as small as possible.

Membrane polymer	Name	Inner diameter capillary [μm]	Wall thickness capillary [μm]	Wall ultrastructure	Manufacturer
PSu	APS	200	40	Asymmetric	ASAHI Kasei
PSu	Helixone	185	35	Asymmetric	Fresenius Medical Care
PSu	Toraysulfone	200	40	Asymmetric	Toray Industries
PA/PSu	Revaclear	190	35	Three layer structure	Gambro/Baxter
PES	DiaPES	200	30	Asymmetric	Membrana/3M
PES	Polynephron	200	40	Asymmetric	Nipro Ltd
PEPA		210	30	Three layer structure	Nikkiso Co
EVAL		175	60	Homogeneous	Kuraray Co
PMMA		200	20/30	Homogeneous	Toray Industries
CTA	Sureflux	200	15	Homogeneous	Nipro Ltd

Membrane manufacturers have successfully reduced the thickness of the membrane wall in a capillary membrane, thereby considerably achieving high membrane fluxes for a better diffusional process. Table 2.2 provides the wall thicknesses of some representative capillary membranes.

Nephrologists have discussed for years about the target of dialysis therapy, in other words regarding the question of which molecules should be removed from the blood of patients with kidney failure. With a precise identification of retention solutes, though sometimes these are also wrongly referred to as "uremic toxins", one would be able to determine and improve the optimal treatment modality. Under controversy are, in this context, treatment modalities and the related dialyzer membranes such as low-flux dialysis, high-flux dialysis or hemodiafiltration.

According to intense investigations of the EuTox group [Vanholder *et al.*, 2003], an individual molecule cannot yet be identified which has shown a proven toxicity and consequently can be made responsible for kidney failure. Of course, exceptions for this statement are “water”, “potassium” and “phosphate ions”. Due to this uncertainty, one follows an empirical approach and postulates as a major target that a large spectrum of molecules including retention solutes with small and large molecular weights should be removed during dialysis therapy.

It’s interesting to note, that the focus of dialysis therapy moves to a lesser extent to the removal of individual molecules rather than to molecule families or groups. Diffusive mechanism of transport is restricted to the removal of small molecules, and thus is insufficient. For instance, complement proteins, cytokines, advanced-glycation end-products (AGEs) or metabolic waste products, which are considered to cause oxidative stress, cannot be removed by diffusive transport mechanisms. Additional transport mechanisms, such as convection, are needed. For this purpose, membranes with large ultrafiltration-coefficients (UFC) are needed (Table 2.1). They are known today under the prefix “high-flux”. In fact, already in the early years of hemodialysis, nephrologists tried to use high ultrafiltration rates as a vehicle for the transport of large molecules across the dialysis membrane.

Ultrafiltration is determined by transmembrane pressure (TMP). The higher the TMP, the more water can be moved across the membrane. While the increase in ultrafiltration is linear in low-flux membranes and directly dependent on TMP, high-flux membranes show an exponential rise in UF with increasing TMP. This is why high ultrafiltration rates can be achieved with high-flux membranes with moderate TMPs.

Which factor determines the UF-rate?

The ultrafiltration volume “V_{UF}” depends on both, the hydrostatic and the osmotic pressure exerted by impermeable peptides and proteins in the blood compartment of the dialyzer. It reads:

$$V_{UF} = L \cdot A\,(P_{TMP} - P_{osm}), \tag{2.4}$$

where V_{UF} — ultrafiltration volume, L — hydraulic permeability, A — membrane surface area, P_{TMP} — transmembrane pressure and P_{osm} — osmotic pressure.

An increased membrane surface area and an increased trans membrane pressure difference consequently leads to a higher ultrafiltration rate and can be achieved by technical means. In case, a nephrologist prefers to remove larger molecules in addition to small molecules during dialysis treatment, he will have to apply convective therapies in addition to diffusive therapies. This is feasible with the help of large ultrafiltration rates and the associated "solvent drag". The related convective clearance of molecules can be assessed by Eq. (2.5):

$$C_{\text{convective}} = SC \cdot V_{\text{UF}}, \tag{2.5}$$

where SC is the individual sieving coefficient of a molecule applied to a specific membrane, and V_{UF} the filtrate flow.

The sieving coefficient of a membrane can be defined as:

$$SC = \frac{2C_{\text{dialysate}}}{C_{\text{blood in}} - C_{\text{blood out}}}, \tag{2.6}$$

where $C_{\text{dialysate}}$ — concentration of a molecule in the filtrate, $C_{\text{blood in}}$ — concentration of a molecule at dialyzer inlet and $C_{\text{blood out}}$ — concentration of a molecule at dialyzer outlet.

Filtrate flow to be used for the removal of large molecules and its related solvent drag will increase, if the pressure gradient across the membrane increases. This can be described by the law of Hagen–Poiseuille:

$$\Delta P = (V_{\text{blood}} \cdot 8\eta) \cdot \left(\frac{L}{N \cdot \pi \cdot r^4} \right), \tag{2.7}$$

where ΔP — pressure difference along the length of the dialyzer, η — blood viscosity, N — number of capillary membranes in a dialyzer and r — hollow fiber radius.

A pressure drop in a dialyzer which finally determines ultrafiltration depends on the length of a dialyzer, the inner radius of the capillary membrane (power of 4), blood flow and blood viscosity (influence of erythropoietin (EPO) administration). The right-hand side of Eq. (2.7) is deliberately separated by two parentheses, because they reflect the individual responsibility of both, nephrologist and membrane manufacturer.

Nephrologists may vary the blood flow rate during treatment and affect *via* the administration of (EPO) also blood viscosity (η). The manufacturer of dialyzers can modify dialyzer length (L), the number of capillaries (N) and the hollow fiber radius (r). Following Hagen–Poiseuille's law, both expert groups are, thus, able to modify ultrafiltration and the related solvent drag.

Convective therapies, such as hemodiafiltration and high-volume hemodiafiltration with an exchange rate of >20 L of substitution fluid are increasingly used in many dialysis centers. Clinical trials have confirmed that the application of this treatment mode improves patient survival and patient quality of life [Maduell *et al.*, 2013].

2.5 Conditions for an Optimal Use of Dialysis Membranes

Blood and dialysis fluid are guided through a dialyzer in a counter-current flow in order to achieve the highest possible concentration gradient at all sites of the dialyzer. This involves, of course, pressure differences between the blood and the dialysate compartment. As a consequence, ultrafiltration from blood to the dialysate compartment is present preferentially in the first part of the dialyzer, whereas in the second part backfiltration from the dialysate compartment to the blood compartment occurs. Simultaneously, we have to accept a process of back diffusion, if molecules on the dialysate side are present in higher concentration than at the blood side. Fick's law is valid for each molecule independently. Along that line, the terms "back transport" and "internal filtration" have been introduced.

The dialysis membrane is not a one-way-street!

This notion is extremely valid under the premises of a dialysis fluid, which may be contaminated with biological contaminants, i.e. microorganisms, endotoxins and viruses. In order to exclude pathological consequences for dialysis patients, enormous efforts have to be realized in order to guarantee the provision of a clean dialysis fluid or as in the case of hemodiafiltration, an ultrapure substitution fluid. New International Standard Organization (ISO) norms such as ISO 13959 have addressed this problem in high detail [International Standard Organization, 2014].

The choice of polymers for dialysis membranes also impacts the possible transport of biological contaminants across the membrane. The use of polymers with aromatic compounds have proven to give rise to endotoxin adsorption in the membrane wall [Henrie *et al*., 2008; Nakatani *et al*., 2003; Hayama *et al*., 2002; Weber *et al*., 2004]. Among them are membranes made of PSu and polyamide. Especially long-term dialysis patients will profit from these membrane properties.

2.6 New Approaches for Membrane Application in Dialysis

Currently used membrane polymers in hemodialysis have to satisfy a series of rather heterogeneous needs. Requirements differ according to both, technical production and clinical application. Polymers for dialysis membranes should be suitable for a reproducible membrane manufacturing, allow an easy sterilization and show long-term stability, at least along the time line of the expiry date of the final product.

Clinical parameters related to polymers applied in dialyzers refer to blood compatibility and biostability. Membrane polymers should have adsorptive capacity for specific uremic retention products, even when these are unknown yet [Goeksel *et al*., 2013]. Adsorption features, e.g. for endotoxins [Henrie *et al*., 2008; Nakatani *et al*., 2003; Hayama *et al*., 2002; Weber *et al*., 2004] or for anaphylatoxins, such as complement factor D, C3a and C5a [Pascual & Schifferli, 1993] have considerably contributed to the safety and biocompatibility of dialysis treatments.

Extractables and leachables, which may be released from polymers, have become an additional important parameter of polymer characteristics and performance. Body fluids, such as blood, serum or interstitial fluids are able to wet all surfaces independent of their chemical composition. This can be explained by the rather heterogeneous composition of these fluids, it relates to their water, lipid, electrolyte and enzyme content. As a consequence, leachables from polymers might be continuously extracted by blood or other body fluids, and accumulate in the patient's organism with deleterious consequences.

Due to the actual increasing number of elderly dialysis patients and of patients on long-term hemodialysis or peritoneal dialysis, leachables from medical devices and especially from dialyzer membranes are of paramount interest. This holds true for all polymers which are applied for medical disposables, from tubing, solution bags, dialyzer housing to dialysis membranes. Prominent components for leachables from medical devices are phthalate plasticizers (DEHP, DBP), found in PVC tubing or "bisphenol A" found in polycarbonate housing, some potting materials and some PSu membranes, as shown, in *in vitro* studies [Bosch-Panadero *et al.*, 2016, Fig. 2.9]. These compounds are known either as "endocrine disruptors" or "endogenous hormones", because they are able to interfere with estrogen receptors and induce hormone-like signals on a cellular level.

Dialysis patients with comorbid conditions, such as diabetes type II, show higher blood levels of BPA in the clinical setting. It is still a matter of debate whether BPA originating from membranes and dialyzers might act as a culprit molecule for diabetes in these patients [Turgut *et al.*, 2016].

The dialysis industry currently invests much effort to improve this situation by selecting optimal polymers, avoiding mal-performing types or applying specific rinsing procedures.

Further investigations on membrane development focus on membranes with biologically active surfaces. PSu membranes which contain Vitamin E at their luminal surface are already available. They show a reduced capacity for oxidative stress and a slight improvement of anemia in dialysis patients. Apart from possible clinical advantages, the

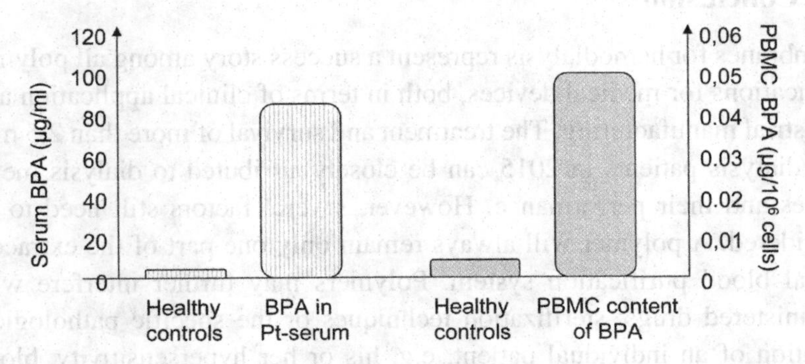

Figure 2.9. The exposure of patient blood to some PSu dialysis membranes may lead to the presence of extractable BPA both in serum (left panel) and in the cytoplasm of polymorphonuclear cells (PBMCs), the latter shown in *in vitro* experiments (adapted from Bosch-Panadero *et al.*, 2016).

development of Vitamin-E coated membranes prove further that even rather inert materials can be modified with biological compounds and that a subsequent sterilization is without effect on membrane functionality [D'Arrigo *et al.*, 2017].

The notion, that molecular weights of some uremic retention solutes are too large to be removed with the actual membrane types due to their moderate cut-off, has led to another concept: filtration should be accompanied by adsorption, e.g. of endotoxins or molecules with pathological properties. So-called "mixed matrix membranes" where the membrane wall contains resins or charcoal particles contribute to these challenges [Tijink *et al.*, 2014; Pavlenko *et al.*, 2016]. They currently wait for clinical application.

Further investigations on membrane performance might address the question whether one of the current dogmata of membrane permeability is correct. It reads that a dialysis membrane should be impermeable for the protein albumin. Recent investigations have shown, however, that the conformation of albumin changes during kidney and liver disease [Varshney *et al.*, 2011; Klammt *et al.*, 2012]. As a consequence, the binding capacity of albumin for uremic retention solutes or for medicinal drugs is reduced and the original property of albumin as a detoxifying protein in patient blood is hampered. Whether these observations stimulate new concepts, e.g. albumin removal, is also still a matter of debate.

2.7 Conclusion

Membranes for hemodialysis represent a success story among all polymer applications for medical devices, both in terms of clinical application and industrial manufacturing. The treatment and survival of more than 2.5 million dialysis patients in 2015 can be closely attributed to dialysis membranes and their performance. However, several factors still need to be considered. A polymer will always remain only one part of the extracorporeal blood purification system. Polymers may further interfere with administered drugs, sterilization techniques or the specific pathological situation of an individual patient, e.g. his or her hypersensitivity, blood composition (uremia, diabetes) or even an individual circadian rhythm that may affect physiological parameters. Obviously, open questions in the realm of dialysis membranes still remain and require answers.

List of Abbreviations

ACE	Angiotensin-converting enzyme
AGE	Advanced glycation end-product
APS	Asahi polysulfone
BBP	Benzylbutylphthalate
BPA	Bisphenol A
CTA	Cellulose-tri-acetate
DEHP/DOP	Di-ethyl-hexyl phthalate / di-octylphthalate
EVAL	Ethyl-vinyl-acetate copolymer
ETO	Ethylene oxide
L	Hydraulic permeability of a membrane
N	Number of capillary membranes per dialyzer
PAN	Polyacrylonitrile
PAES	Polyarylethersulfone
PBMC	Polymorphonuclear cells, white blood cells
PES	Polyethersulfone
PEPA	Polyester polymer alloy
PMMA	Polymethylmethacrylate
PSu	Polysulfone
PVP	Polyvinylpyrrolidone
SC	Sieving coefficient
TMP	Transmembrane pressure
UFC	Ultrafiltration coefficient
V_{UF}	Ultrafiltration volume

References

Abel J, Rowntree L, Turner B (1913). On the removal of diffusible substances from the circulating blood of living animals by means of dialysis. *J Pharmacol Exp*, 5, pp. 275–293.

Bosch-Panadero E, Mas S, Sanchez-Ospina D, Camarero V, Pérez-Gómez Saez-Calero I, Abaigar P, Ortiz A, Egidoi J, González-Parra E (2016). The choice of hemodialysis membrane affects Bisphenol A levels in blood. *J Am Soc Nephrol*, 27, pp. 1566–1574.

Brunet P, Jaber K, Berland Y, Baz M (1992). Anaphylactoid reactions during hemodialysis and hemofiltration: role of associating AN69 membrane and angiotensin I converting enzyme inhibitors. *Am J Kidney Dis*, 9, pp. 444–447.

D'Arrigo G, Baggetta R, Tripepi G, Galli F, Bolignano D (2017). Effects of Vitamin E-coated versus conventional membranes in chronic hemodialysis patients: A systematic review and meta analysis. *Blood Purif*, 43, pp. 101–122.

Désormeaux A, Moreau ME, Lepage Y, Chanard J, Adam A (2008). The effect of electronegativity and angiotensin-converting enzyme inhibition on the kinin-forming capacity of polyacrylonitrile dialysis membranes. *Biomaterials*, 29, pp. 1139–1146.

Fabbrini P, Sirtori S, Casiraghi E, Pieruzzi F, Genovesi S, Corti D, Brivio R, Gregorini G, Como G, Carati M, Vignano M, Stella A (2013). Polymethylmethacrylate membrane and serum free light chain removal enhancing adsorption properties. *Blood Purif*, 35 (Suppl. 2), pp. 52–58.

Fick A (1855). Über Diffusion. *Ann Phys*, 170, pp. 59–86.

Fournier A, Birmelé B, Francois M, Prat L, Halimi JM (2015). Factors associated with albumin loss in post-dilution hemodiafiltration and nutritional considerations. *Int J Artif Organs*, 38, pp. 76–82.

Goeksel T, Xie, W, Ritzerfeld M, Heidenreich S, Mann H (2013). Prurigo nodularis and dialyzer membrane. *Blood Purif*, 35(2), pp. 26–27.

Graham T (1854). The Bakerian lecture: on osmotic force. *Philos Trans Roy Soc Lond*, 144, pp. 177–228.

Haas G (1923). Dialysieren des strömenden Bluts am Lebenden. *Klin Wochenschr*, 2, pp. 1888.

Henrie M, Ford C, Andersen M, Stroup E, Diaz-Buxo J, Madsen B, Britt D, Ho C (2008). *In vitro* assessment of dialysis membrane as an endotoxin transfer barrier: geometry, morphology and permeability. *Artif Organs*, 32 pp. 701–710.

Hayama M, Miyasaka T, Mochizuki S, Asahara H, Tsujiika K, Kohori F, Sakai K, Jinbo Y, Yoshida M (2002). Visualization of distribution of endotoxin trapped in an endotoxin-blocking filtration membrane. *J Membr Sci*, 210, pp. 45–53.

Heilmann K, Keller T (2011). Polysulfone: the development of a membrane for convective therapies. *Contrib Nephrol*, 175, pp. 15–26.

Henderson L, Chenoweth D (1985). Cellulosic membranes — time for a change? *Contrib Nephrol*, 44, pp. 112–126.

Igoshi T, Tomisawa N, Hori Y, Jinbo Y (2011). Polyesterpolymer-alloy, as a high performance membrane. *Contrib Nephrol*, 173, pp. 48–155.

International Standard Organization (2014), ISO 13959 *Water for Hemodialysis and related therapies*, 3rd Edn. c: ISO 2014.

Johnson R, Lelah N, Sutliff T, Boggs D (1990). A modification of cellulose that facilitates the control of complement activation. *Blood Purif*, 8, pp. 318–328.

Klammt S, Wojak HJ, Mitzner A, Koball S, Rychly J, Reisinger E, Mitzner S (2012). Albumin-binding capacity (ABiC) is reduced in patients with chronic kidney disease along with an accumulation of protein-bound uraemic toxins. *Nephrol Dial Transplant*, 27, pp. 2377–2383.

Kinoshita T, (1991). Overview of complement biology. *Immunol Today*, 12, pp. 291–294.

Krieter D, Lemke HD (2011). Polyethersulphone as a high performance membrane. *Contrib Nephrol*, 173, pp. 130–136.

Linnenweber S, Lonnemann G (2000). Pyrogen retention by the ASAHI APS-650 polysulfone dialyzer during *in vitro* dialysis with whole human donor blood. *ASAIO J*, 46, pp. 444–447.

Maduell F, Moreso F, Pons M and the Catalunya dialysis group (2013). High-efficiency post-dilution online hemodiafiltration reduces all-cause mortality in hemodialysis patients. *J Am Soc Nephrol*, 24, pp. 487–497.

Martinez-Miguel P, de Sequera P, Albalate M, Medrano D, Sanchez-Villanueva R, Molina A, Sousa F, Benito J, Nunez J, Vozmediano C, Barril G, Rodriguez-Puyol D, Perez-Garcia R, López-Ongil S (2015). Evaluation of a polynephron dialysis membrane considering new aspects of biocompatibility. *Int J Artif Organs*, 38, pp. 45–53.

Nakano A (2011). Ethylene vinyl alcohol co-polymer as a high-performance membrane. An EVOH membrane with excellent biocompatibility. *Contrib Nephrol*, 173, pp. 164–171.

Nakatani T, Tsuchida K, Sugimura K, Yoshimura R, Takemoto Y (2003). Investigation of endotoxin adsorption with polyether polymer alloy dialysis membranes. *Int J Mol Med*, 11, pp. 195–197.

Pascual M, Schifferli J (1993). Adsorption of complement factor D by polyacrylonitrile membranes. *Kidney Int*, 43, pp. 903–911.

Pavlenko D, van Geffen E, van Steenbergen, MJ, Glorieux G, Vanholder R, Gerritsen KGF, Stamatialis D (2016). New low-flux mixed matrix membranes that offer superior removal of protein-bound toxins from human plasma. *Sci Rep*, 6, 34429.

Renaux J, Thomas M, Crost T, Loughraieb N, Vantard G (1999). Activation of the kallikrein-kinin system in hemodialysis: role of membrane electronegativity, blood dilution and pH. *Kidney Int*, 55, pp. 1097–1103.

Rollason G, Sefton M (1992). Measurement of the rate of thrombin production in human plasma in contact with different materials. *J Biomed Mat Res*, 26, pp. 675–693.

Schindler R, Boenisch O, Fischer C, Frei U (2000). Effect of the hemodialysis membrane on inflammatory reaction *in vivo*. *Clin Nephrol*, 53, pp. 452–459.

Schwarzbeck A, Wittenmeier KW, Hällfritzsch U, Frank J (1993). Anaphylactoid reactions ACE inhibitors and extracorporeal haemotherapy. *Nephron*, 65, pp. 499–500.

Streicher E, Schneider H (1983). Polysulphone membrane mimicking human glomerular basement membrane. *Lancet*, 322, pp. 1136.

Sugaya H, Sakai Y (1998). Polymethylmethacrylate: from polymer to dialyzer. *Contrib Nephrol*, 125, pp. 1–8.

Sunohara T, Masuda T (2011). Cellulose Triacetate as a high performance membrane. *Contrib Nephrol*, 173, pp. 156–163.

Thomas M, Moriyama K, Ledebo I (2011). AN69, the evolution of the world's first high permeability membrane. *Contrib Nephrol*, 173, pp. 11–129.

Tijink M, Kooman J, Wester M, Sun J, Saiful S, Joles J, Borneman Z, Wessling M, Stamatialis D (2014). Mixed matrix membranes: a new asset for blood purification therapies. *Blood Purif*, 37, pp. 1–3.

Tielemans C, Madhoun P, Lenaers M, Schandene L, Goldman M, Vanherweghem JL (1990). Anaphylactoid reactions during hemodialysis on AN69 membranes in patients receiving ACE inhibitors. *Kidney Int*, 38, pp. 982–16.

Turgut F, Sungur S, Okur R, Yaprak M, Ozsan M, Ustun I, Gokce C (2016). Higher serum bisphenol A levels in diabetic hemodialysis patients. *Blood Purif*, 42, pp. 77–82.

Urbani A, Louisell S, Sirolli V, Bucci S, Amoroso L, Pavone B, Pieroni L, Sacchetta P, Bonomini M (2012). Proteomic analysis of protein adsorption capacity of different haemodialysis membranes. *Mol Biosyst*, 8, pp. 1029–1039.

Vanholder R, DeSmet G, Glorieux G and the Eutox group (2003). Review on uremic toxins: classification, concentration and interindividual variability. *Kidney Int*, 63, pp. 461–470.

Varshney A, Rehan M, Subbarao N, Rabbani G, Khan H (2011). Elimination of endogenous toxin, creatinine from blood plasma depends on albumin conformation: site specific uremic toxicity & impaired drug binding. *PloS ONE*, 6, pp. e17230.

Weber V, Linsberger I, Rossmanith E, Weber C, Falkenhagen D (2004). Pyrogen transfer across high-flux dialysis and low-flux hemodialysis membranes. *Artif Organs*, 28, pp. 210–217.

Chapter 3
Advanced Blood Purification Therapies

O. ter Beek, I. Geremia, D. Pavlenko and D. Stamatialis*

MIRA Institute, Faculty of Science and Technology, Bioartifical Organs Group, Biomaterials Science and Technology Department, University of Twente, Enschede, The Netherlands
**d.stamatialis@ utwente.nl*

3.1 Introduction

Every day, blood purification therapies save the life of many patients suffering from, for example, renal failure, liver failure or poisoning. All therapies aim to improve the health and quality of life of patients by removing the toxins from their blood. These therapies can be generally divided into two main categories:

(1) those based on diffusion or convection, such as hemodialysis, hemofiltration, hemodiafiltration (HDF) and plasmapheresis;
(2) those which combine different toxin removal strategies; in this chapter, we will refer to them as "advanced therapies". One can distinguish two types: the artificial systems with no biological cells used and the bioartificial systems, where biological cells, for example, kidney cells, are used.

The artificial blood purification systems include physics- and chemistry-based techniques, and the bioartificial systems combine technology with liver or renal cells. The artificial systems focus primarily on detoxification and purification, whereas the bioartificial systems could also address the synthetic and regulatory functions of, for example, the liver or kidney [Rozga, 2006]. This chapter focuses on artificial systems, whereas the bioartificial systems are described in Chapters 5 and 6. In the next section, we will briefly describe hemodialysis, hemofiltration, HDF and plasmapheresis because these therapies lay the foundation of the advanced systems. The reader can find more details on hemodialysis or hemofiltration in Chapter 2.

3.2 Filtration-Based Therapies

3.2.1 *Hemodialysis*

The EUTox work group of the European Society for Artificial Organs (ESAO) divided all blood toxins into three main categories: water-soluble, small-molecular-weight toxins, middle molecules and protein-bound toxins [Eloot *et al.*, 2012b]. In the past, it was assumed that only small-molecular-weight toxins needed to be removed from patients' blood. Therefore, hemodialysis was the extracorporeal blood purification system of choice [Rozga, 2006]. Now, we know that each type of toxin has its unique removal pattern and can be addressed with a different degree of success by hemodialysis [Eloot *et al.*, 2012a].

Hemodialysis is based on the diffusion principle: the transport of solutes across a semi-permeable membrane takes place due to a concentration gradient. In other words, the osmolar gradient between blood and dialysis solution allows the water-soluble, small-molecular-weight toxins to diffuse through the membrane, whereas larger molecules and blood cells are retained in the blood. In contrast, middle molecules and cytokines are only partially removed. Moreover, hemodialysis cannot address the removal of the protein-bound toxins [Eloot *et al.*, 2012b]. The adequacy of the dialysis treatment is constantly developed to improve the removal of the water-soluble, small-molecular-weight toxins [Vanholder *et al.*, 2015].

3.2.2 *Hemofiltration and Hemodiafiltration*

Hemofiltration is based on the convection principle: the transport of fluid and solutes across a semi-permeable membrane occurs due to a pressure gradient across the membrane, allowing the transport of larger solutes through the membrane [Bello *et al.*, 2012].

HDF combines diffusion with convective transport (see Fig. 3.1).

The combination of diffusion and convection leads to an increase in the filtration rate, which enhances the removal of water-soluble solutes compared to what can be obtained with diffusion alone; this is reflected in an improvement of the performance of the HDF in terms of morbidity and mortality [Eloot *et al.*, 2014].

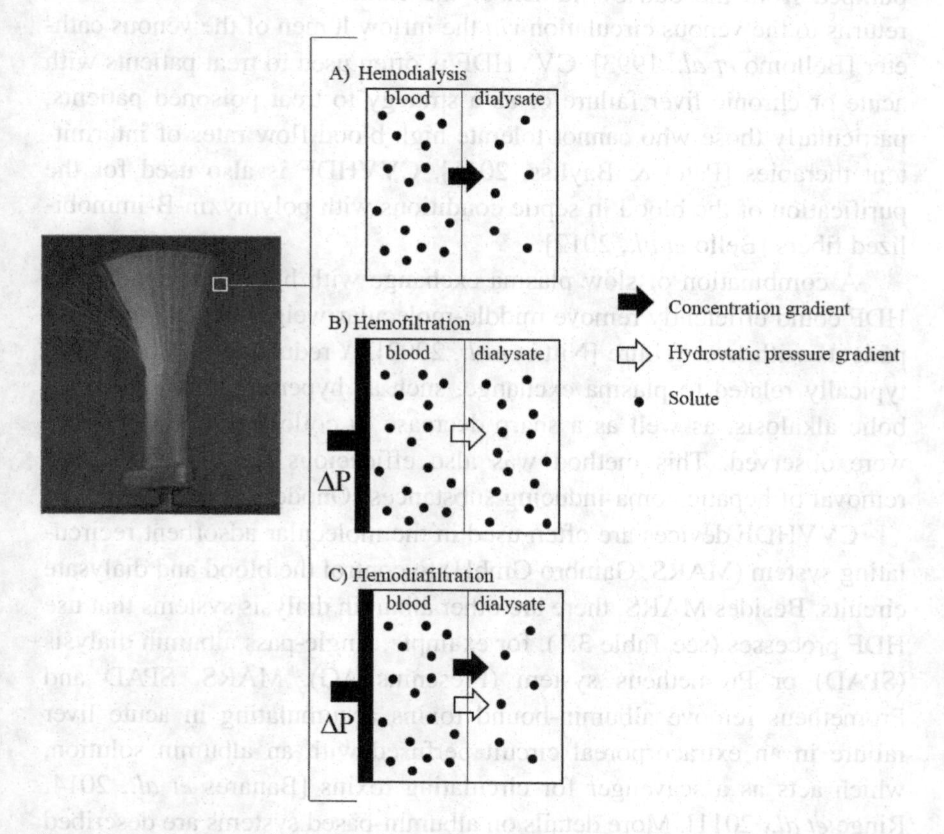

Figure 3.1. Schemes of the mechanisms of hemodialysis, hemofiltration and HDF. Image of dialysis module reprinted from Stamatialis *et al.* [2008], with permission from Elsevier.

In hemofiltration and HDF, the fluid removal exceeds that gained by the patient, contrary to hemodialysis where the fluid removal is equivalent to the fluid gained by the patient between the treatments. Thus, in hemofiltration and HDF, a suitable substitution liquid has to be infused to the patient. The electrolyte replacement solution can be delivered to the extracorporeal blood stream before the filtration process ("pre-dilution HDF"), during the filtration process ("mid-dilution HDF") or downstream from the hemofilter ("post-dilution HDF") [Stamatialis *et al.*, 2008].

Continuous veno-venous HDF (CVVHDF), amongst others, is a variant of traditional HDF where a double-lumen hemodialysis catheter is inserted into one of the large veins (subclavian or femoral). The blood is pumped from the outflow lumen of the catheter into a hemofilter and returns to the venous circulation *via* the inflow lumen of the venous catheter [Bellomo *et al.*, 1993]. CVVHDF is often used to treat patients with acute or chronic liver failure or as a strategy to treat poisoned patients, particularly those who cannot tolerate high blood flow rates of intermittent therapies [Patel & Bayliss, 2015]. CVVHDF is also used for the purification of the blood in septic conditions with polymyxin-B-immobilized fibers [Bello *et al.*, 2012].

A combination of slow plasma exchange with high-flow continuous HDF could efficiently remove middle-molecular-weight hepatic toxins in patients with liver failure [Nitta *et al.*, 2002]. A reduction of side effects typically related to plasma exchange, such as hypernatremia and metabolic alkalosis, as well as a sharp decrease in colloid osmotic pressure were observed. This method was also efficacious for the continuous removal of hepatic coma-inducing substances [Onodera *et al.*, 2006].

CVVHDF devices are often used in the molecular adsorbent recirculating system (MARS, Gambro GmbH) to control the blood and dialysate circuits. Besides MARS, there are other albumin dialysis systems that use HDF processes (see Table 3.1), for example, single-pass albumin dialysis (SPAD) or Prometheus system (Fresenius AG). MARS, SPAD and Prometheus remove albumin-bound toxins accumulating in acute liver failure in an extracorporeal circuit perfused with an albumin solution, which acts as a scavenger for circulating toxins [Banares *et al.*, 2014; Ringe *et al.*, 2011]. More details on albumin-based systems are described later in this chapter.

Table 3.1: Main applications of HDF in hepatic pathologic conditions.

Pathological condition	HDF involvement	Advantages
Liver failure	MARS	Removal of albumin-bound toxins
	Prometheus	
	SPAD	
	HDF combined with slow plasma exchange	Reduction of side effects typically related to plasma exchange
Poisoned patients	Often in the form of CVVHDF	Continuous therapy, no problems related to intermittent therapy
Septic conditions	HDF using antibiotics immobilized fibers	Removal of circulating cytokines and other inflammatory mediators

3.2.3 *Wearable Devices*

Wearable or portable dialysis devices could prolong the dialysis time, thus eliminating the problem of having intermittent dialysis treatments. This could improve the quality of life of patients as well as reduce hospital length stay and care unit utilization [Fissell *et al.*, 2013]. In general, long and slow hemodialysis have been reported to be associated with better survival, improvements of quality of life, better intradialytic hemodynamic stability, better control of blood pressure, a reduced need for stimulating agents for red blood cell production and a decrease in arterial stiffness and cardiovascular morbidity and mortality [Eloot *et al.*, 2014].

The development of a wearable artificial kidney (WAK) is really challenging, since it needs to satisfy a lot of different technical and clinical aspects (Fig. 3.2):

- proper vascular access (easy to connect and disconnect) in order to have a continuous therapy and to reduce as much as possible the risk of infections and clotting;
- adequate safety measures in the circuit including air detection, pressure sensors, visual and audible alarms;
- remote control to allow the patient to accurately program and deliver the scheduled therapy together with a regular control of the physiological state of the patient;

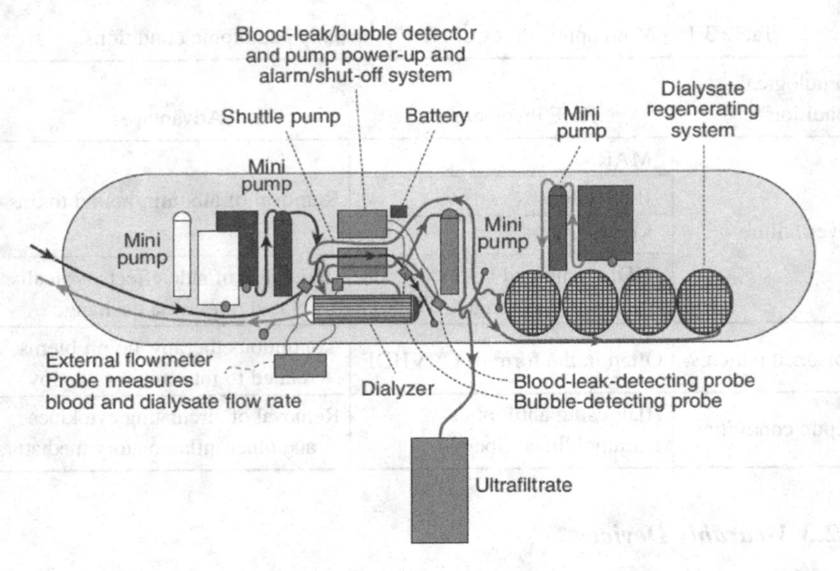

Figure 3.2. Scheme of the configuration of a wearable artificial kidney. Reprinted from Fissell *et al.* [2013], with permission from Elsevier.

- independence from the electrical outlet;
- minimal volume of dialysate (lower than 500 cm^3) that must be continuously regenerated;
- lightweight and ergonomic design that would be adapted to the body.

The first idea of wearable artificial systems for hemodialysis was reported in the 1970s by the team of Kolff [Friedman, 2009; Stephens *et al.*, 1976]. Recently, new research has been published, showing interesting and promising results on the application of the WAK. Some of them use extra-corporeal hemodialysis [Gura *et al.*, 2005], whereas others use peritoneal dialysis as a treatment modality (ViWAK and AWAK) [Lee & Roberts, 2008; Ronco & Fecondini, 2007]. One of the main problems related to the development of the WAK is the need to dramatically reduce the amount of the dialysate to be independent on a fixed water supply. There are also reports of applications of nanotechnology for wearable or implantable hemodialysis devices without dialysate [Nissenson *et al.*, 2005] or to develop a system for the regeneration of the dialysate using mixtures of different nanosorbents (Nanodialysis, Oirschot, The Netherlands) [Fissell *et al.*, 2013].

The WAK devices have the potential to become a real practice for the treatment of patients with chronic kidney disease. Although, at the moment, larger clinical trials are needed to confirm their safety and efficacy, the continuous treatment due to the miniaturization and wearability of these systems would enormously impact the society, not only improving the quality of life of the patients, but also reducing the utilization of nursing resources and the medical care costs.

3.3 Plasmapheresis

Plasmapheresis is a procedure where plasma is removed from the cellular components and replaced by albumin or fresh frozen plasma (see Fig. 3.3). In plasmapheresis, plasma separation is performed by centrifugation or by membrane filtration. An earlier study showed that both membrane- and centrifugal-based approaches are similar with regard to efficiency and safety [Gurland *et al.*, 1984].

Plasmapheresis is widely used for the treatment of variety of disorders. The American Society for Apheresis Guidelines describe the use of plasma exchange in 100 clinical situations which cover 65 types of diseases [Reeves & Winters, 2014; Schwartz *et al.*, 2013].

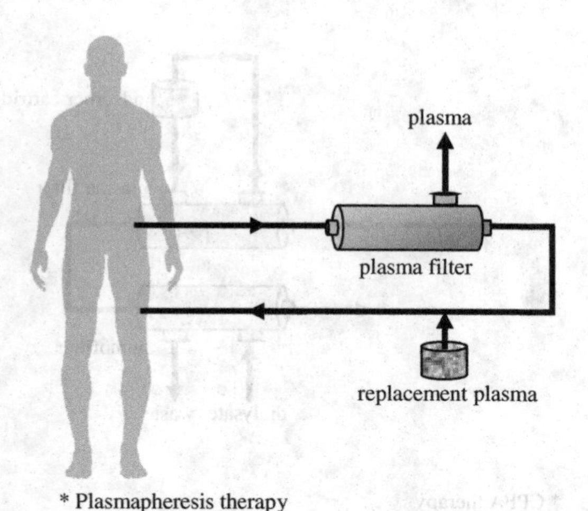

Figure 3.3. Scheme of plasmapheresis. Fresh plasma is infused after separation of the plasma from the blood.

3.4 Advanced Therapies for Treatment of Kidney Failure

3.4.1 *Coupled Plasma Filtration Adsorption*

The lack of commercially available sorbents that combine excellent blood compatibility with high removal of inflammatory mediators led to the development of coupled plasma filtration adsorption (CPFA) therapies [Formica *et al.*, 2007]. There, plasma is separated from the blood by the means of plasma-filtration membrane (see Fig. 3.4).

It is then passed through the cartridge with the sorbent and is reinfused into the blood. In this way, only the human plasma is directly exposed to the sorbent, making it possible to avoid hemocompatibility complications of the sorbent–blood contact. The advantage of this technique, compared to plasmapheresis, is that patients' plasma can be regenerated. In this way, the risks related to the infusion of fresh plasma may be eliminated [Tetta *et al.*, 1998].

The first CPFA *in vitro* studies highlighted that the removal rates of inflammatory mediators are dependent on the type of the adsorbent used [Tetta *et al.*, 1998]. A follow-up study by the same group [Tetta *et al.*, 2000], using a rabbit model with the septic shock, indicated improved survival of the rabbits. In more recent clinical studies, CPFA showed

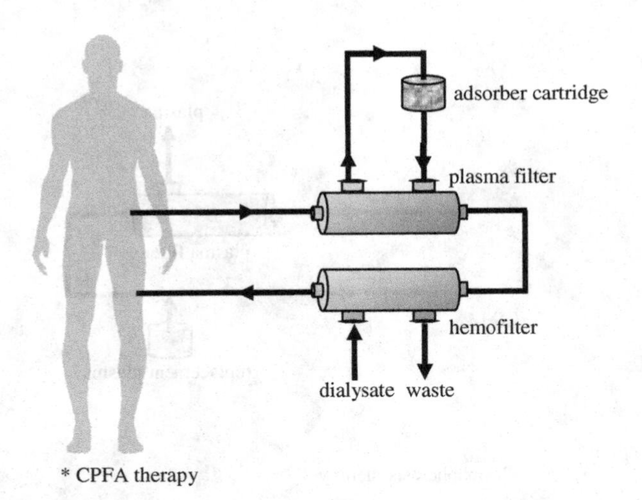

Figure 3.4. Scheme of CPFA. This system separates the plasma from the blood and filters the plasma before blood purification by a hemofilter.

results of superior removal of solutes for patients with sepsis in comparison to high-volume hemofiltration [Hu *et al.*, 2012; Mao *et al.*, 2009]. Table 3.2 gives an overview of all the benefits of filtration-, plasma- and sorption-based therapies.

3.5 Sorption-based Therapies

Many researchers drew the conclusion that more sophisticated purification therapies were necessary to overcome the problems of toxin removal [Denis *et al.*, 1978]. In 1982, Gimson *et al.* [1982] removed the water-soluble toxins in hepatic failure patients with Haemocol 100, a 100-g charcoal column. The utilization of sorption-based techniques led to new types of advanced therapies for blood purification as explained below.

3.5.1 *Hemosorption/Hemoperfusion*

Hemoperfusion was introduced for the first time by Yatzidis in the early 1960s. He described a new extracorporeal apparatus for the effective removal of toxins (such as creatinine, uric acid, phenolic compounds, guanidine bases, etc.) directly from the recirculating, heparinized blood of patients with end-stage renal disease by perfusion over charcoal [Yatzidis, 1964]. Nowadays, the number of hemoperfusion therapies is exponentially increasing, not only for renal and hepatic failure but also in the treatment of other disease states, such as sepsis, cardiopulmonary bypass, drug overdoses and multi-organ failure [Mikhalovsky, 2003]. Hemoperfusion, in contrast to the hemodialysis treatment, seems better for removing middle molecules, cytokines and protein-bound toxins from patients' blood. However, the inability to correct the fluid balance, to remove urea and to eliminate frequent hemocompatibility complications noticeably lowered its use in US hospitals [Tyagi *et al.*, 2008].

Adsorption is solute-specific rather than size-specific, and the binding depends on the chemical affinity between the solute and the sorbent and on the accessible surface area of the sorbent for the adsorbate which determines the availability of binding sites. Moreover, to have effective adsorption, various other parameters should also be taken into account including insolubility of the sorbent in water, stability for processing, pressure drop,

Table 3.2: Comparison of the benefits of filtration-, plasma- and sorption-based therapies.

Function	Hemodialysis	Hemoperfusion	Hemofiltration	Hemodiafiltration	Plasmapheresis	CPFA
Corrects electrolyte balance	YES	NO	YES	YES	YES	YES
Corrects volume status	YES	NO	YES	YES	YES	YES
Removes small molecules	YES	Partly	YES	YES	YES	YES
Removes middle molecules	Partly	Partly	Partly	Partly	YES	YES
Removes protein-bound toxins	Partly	YES	Partly	Partly	YES	YES

resistance to sterilization and biocompatibility (when the sorbent has to be in direct contact with the blood). Sorbents can be developed in different formulations: particles, resins and membranes, but the most common forms are beads and microparticles which combine a large surface area with high porosity.

Sorbents used in hemoperfusion can be natural or synthetic. Among the natural sorbents, activated carbon is the most commonly used. It is a broad-spectrum adsorbent that can remove different kind of substances, such as organic metabolic wastes, drugs and other undesirable components from the blood [Xue *et al.*, 2002]. Although activated carbon can adsorb many of the uremic toxins in the middle-molecule-weight range, it does not remove urea or acidic solutes. Because of this, when the blood of uremic patients needs to be purified, hemoperfusion and hemodialysis need to be combined. Despite its great adsorption capacity, activated carbon has rather poor biocompatibility. In fact, high affinity of activated carbon to blood components such as platelets might lead to the formation of emboli. For this reason, the direct contact of activated carbon with blood in a hemoperfusion circuit should be avoided. The hemocompatibility of different kinds of sorbents can be improved by the addition of hemocompatible coatings or by chemical modifications of the starting materials [Bello *et al.*, 2012].

Synthetic sorbents are usually in the form of uncharged or ion-exchange resins. These resins are particularly important in hepatic treatment since, although often their adsorption capacity is lower than that of activated carbon, they have a higher clearance rate toward lipophilic and hydrophobic substances, such as bile acid, bilirubin, free fatty acids and amines [Duan *et al.*, 2006].

The great success of hemoperfusion has also led to a growing interest toward new sorbent formulations. Many efforts have been and are still being focused on developing smart adsorbents able to bind one or more desired target molecules. Not only can the chemistry of the sorbents be tuned, their porosity can also be engineered.

3.5.2 *Hemodiabsorption*

Hemodiabsorption is a combination of dialysis and hemoperfusion where blood is passed through the hemodialyzer which contains adsorption particles at the dialysate side. Such approach allows for the use of small adsorptive particles, which is almost impossible to achieve in standard hemoperfusion, due to high pressure drop there. Smaller particle size improves the overall adsorption capacity of the sorbent used in the device in comparison to hemoperfusion columns [Ash *et al.*, 1992]. Nevertheless, the first clinical studies of this system were quite encouraging [Ellis *et al.*, 1999; Hughes *et al.*, 1994], although they did not show improved survival of the patients. Therefore, hemodiabsorption systems are not available commercially [Cerda *et al.*, 2011].

3.5.3 *Mixed Matrix Membranes*

Recently, a potential alternative to hemosorption for the removal of protein-bound toxins is being developed: the so-called mixed matrix membrane (MMM) [Tijink *et al.*, 2013]. These membranes consist of two layers: a polymeric, porous layer with embedded activated carbon particles (the MMM layer) and a layer consisting of a porous, polymeric particle-free layer (see Fig. 3.5(a)). Incorporation of activated carbon particles into the macroporous MMM makes it possible to combine the benefits of filtration and adsorption in one membrane. The particle-free polymeric layer prevents direct contact between patient's blood and the activated carbon particles. Additionally, this layer is responsible for the selectivity of the whole membrane.

In later studies, MMM hollow fibers were fabricated too [Pavlenko *et al.*, 2016; Tijink *et al.*, 2013] (see Fig. 3.5(b)). The MMMs pose a number of advantages compared to conventional therapies. First, it is possible to use relatively small adsorptive particles. Use of small particles increases the available surface area for the adsorption of the uremic toxins without the high pressure drops that can be observed in the adsorption columns. Second, the use of adsorptive particles inside the outer layer of the membrane increases the removal of the toxins by keeping the concentration gradient of the toxin at the maximum level, as most of the toxins that reach the outer layer are adsorbed. Finally, the presence of the outer layer can protect the blood from possible impurities that are sometimes present in the dialysate water.

The additive effect of the adsorption inside the membrane has been recently demonstrated for the removal of the protein-bound uremic toxins

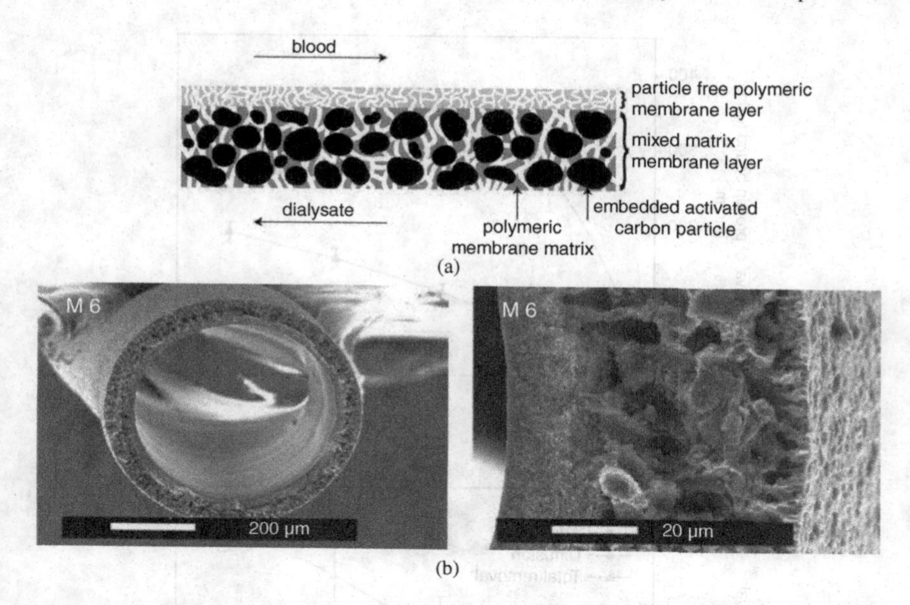

Figure 3.5. (a) Concept of MMMs which combines filtration and adsorption in one step. Reprinted from Tijink *et al.* [2013], with permission from Elsevier. (b) Scanning electron microscopic image of dual-layer hollow fiber MMM. Magnifications 100× and 500×. Reprinted from Pavlenko *et al.* [2016], with permission from Scientific Reports.

in comparison to industrial Fresenius F8HPS membranes. Fig. 3.6(a) compares the removal of indoxyl sulfate from human plasma by the hollow fiber MMMs and the F8HPS membrane. The removal rate of indoxyl sulfate of the hollow fiber MMMs is higher in comparison to the Fresenius hemodialysis fibers (367 and 187 mg/m^2, respectively). Fig. 3.6(b) shows that for the hollow fiber MMMs, creatinine is removed by the combination of diffusion and adsorption [Pavlenko *et al.*, 2016].

3.6 Advanced Therapies for Treatment of Liver Failure

Advanced therapies for treatment of liver failure are also based on hemodialysis, hemofiltration and adsorption. They should be able to remove large and/or protein-bound toxins such as bilirubin, bile acids, aromatic amino acids and medium-chain fatty acids [Rademacher *et al.*, 2011]. The most important carrier of these toxins in human blood is albumin (MW: 66.5 kDa). Several advanced therapies like MARS, SPAD, Prometheus

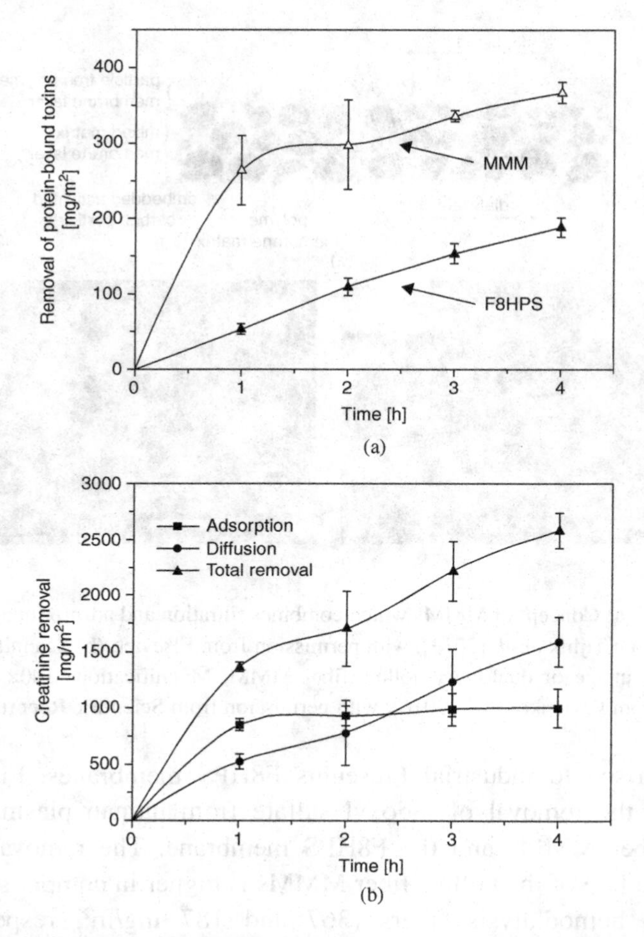

Figure 3.6. (a) Removal of the protein-bound uremic toxin indoxyl sulfate by Fresenius F8HPS (solid line) vs MMMs (dotted line). (b) Creatinine removal by the MMMs. Total creatinine removal is achieved by the combined effect of adsorption and diffusion. Reprinted from Pavlenko *et al.* [2016], with permission from Scientific Reports.

and selective plasma filtration therapy (SEPET) actually use albumin for the removal of the protein-bound toxins [Marieb & Hoehn, 2007; Rademacher *et al.*, 2011]. Albumin can be temporarily filtered from patients' blood in order to be purified by, for example, resins, or extra albumin (exogenous) is used to remove toxins that are bound to patients' own albumin (endogenous) [Podoll *et al.*, 2012].

3.7 Molecular Adsorbent Recirculating System

The MARS (Gambro), sometimes called the molecular adsorbent recycling system, has been developed by Stange *et al.* [1993]. The system (Fig. 3.7) is based on dialysis, filtration and adsorption, and it was first used in a clinical setting in 1993.

It is one of the most frequently used methods for blood purification in liver failure. The patients are linked up to the system *via* a dialysis catheter for 6–8 h/day to remove the protein-bound and water-soluble toxins from their blood [Faybik & Krenn, 2013; Podoll *et al.*, 2012; Rademacher *et al.*, 2011; Stadlbauer *et al.*, 2009]. The patients' blood flows *via* the catheter toward a high-flux, albumin-coated polysulfone hemodialyzer with a molecular weight cutoff of 50 kDa, the MARS-flux filter, thus not allowing albumin to pass (see Fig. 3.8). Toxins that dissociate from the plasma albumin cross the membrane because of a concentration gradient and bind to the albumin of a 20% albumin-enriched dialysate solution.

In a second circuit, the "used" albumin solution is filtered first by a high-flux hemodialysis filter in order to remove the water-soluble toxins,

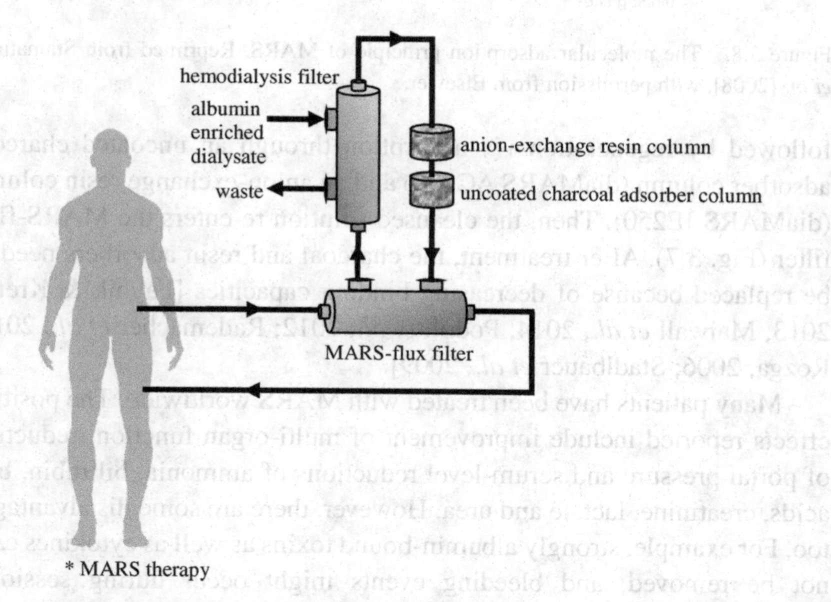

Figure 3.7. Scheme of MARS. A blood purification system based on dialysis, filtration and adsorption, which makes use of an albumin-based dialysate solution.

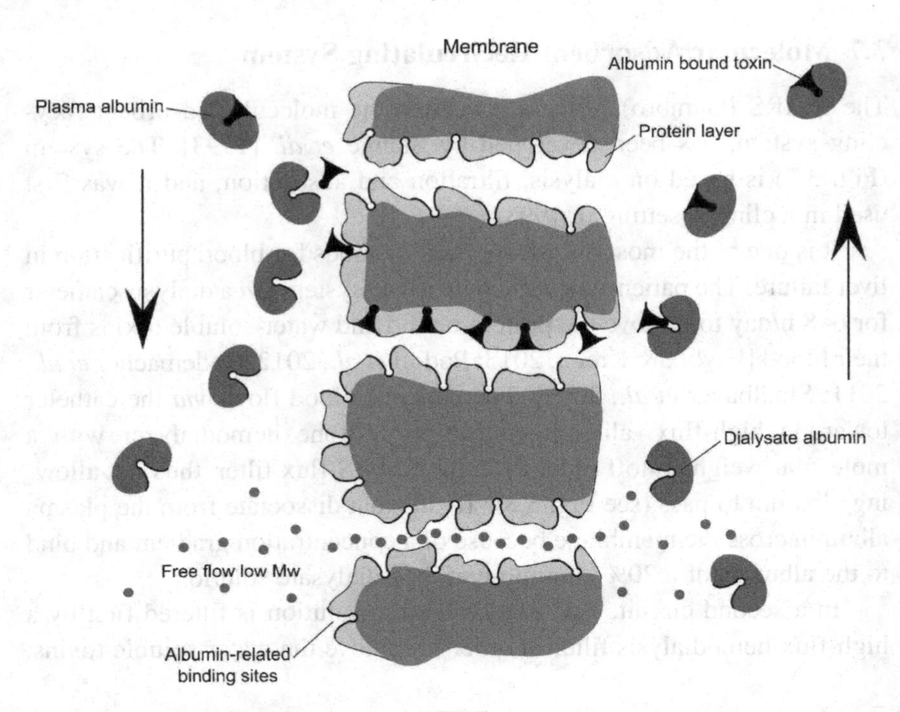

Figure 3.8. The molecular adsorption principle of MARS. Reprinted from Stamatialis *et al.* [2008], with permission from Elsevier.

followed by regeneration *via* adsorption through an uncoated charcoal adsorber column (diaMARS AC250) and an anion-exchange resin column (diaMARS IE250). Then, the cleansed solution re-enters the MARS-flux filter (Fig. 3.7). After treatment, the charcoal and resin adsorbers need to be replaced because of decreasing binding capacities [Faybik & Krenn, 2013; Maiwall *et al.*, 2014; Podoll *et al.*, 2012; Rademacher *et al.*, 2011; Rozga, 2006; Stadlbauer *et al.*, 2009].

Many patients have been treated with MARS worldwide. The positive effects reported include improvement of multi-organ function, reduction of portal pressure and serum-level reductions of ammonia, bilirubin, bile acids, creatinine, lactate and urea. However, there are some disadvantages too. For example, strongly albumin-bound toxins as well as cytokines cannot be removed, and bleeding events might occur during sessions. Nevertheless, MARS has an acceptable safety profile [Drolz *et al.*, 2011; Podoll *et al.*, 2012; Rademacher *et al.*, 2011].

3.8 Single-Pass Albumin Dialysis

SPAD is another therapy where albumin is used to remove the protein-bound toxins (see Fig. 3.9).

This therapy makes use of one circuit which consists of an albumin-impermeable, high-flux dialyzer. Human serum albumin is added to a conventional dialysate solution and acts as a binding agent for solutes. The albumin dialysate solution flows in counter-current direction to the bloodstream. The albumin concentration of the dialysate is much lower compared to MARS, namely 2–5%. Besides, in contrast to the MARS therapy, the dialysate is disposed after one treatment cycle of 6–10 h each day [Faybik & Krenn, 2013; Maiwall *et al.*, 2014; Podoll *et al.*, 2012; Rademacher *et al.*, 2011; Rozga, 2006; Stadlbauer *et al.*, 2009].

3.9 Prometheus

Prometheus (Fresenius) combines the fractionated plasma separation and adsorption (FPSA) technique with high-flux dialysis (see Fig. 3.10). FPSA is a combined membrane and adsorbent system (a polysulfone filter which is able to separate albumin from blood up to 90%, a dialysis

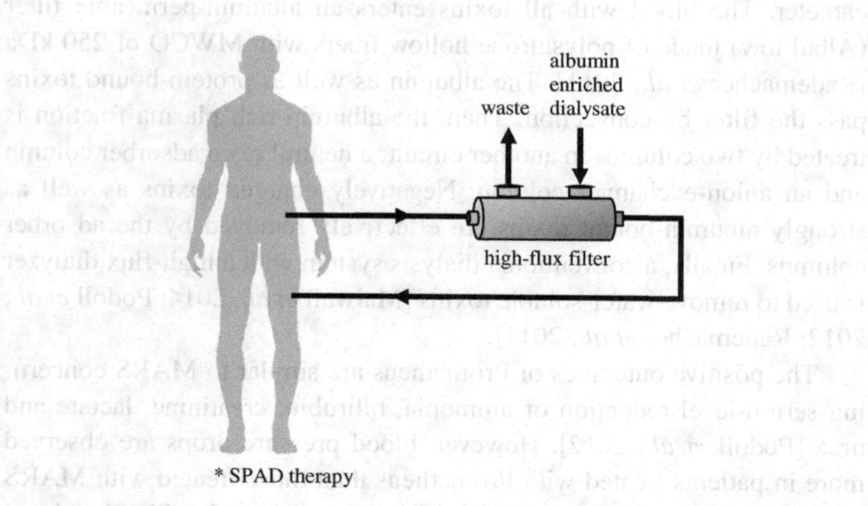

Figure 3.9. Scheme of SPAD. Hemodialysis device containing albumin-impermeable high-flux dialyzer.

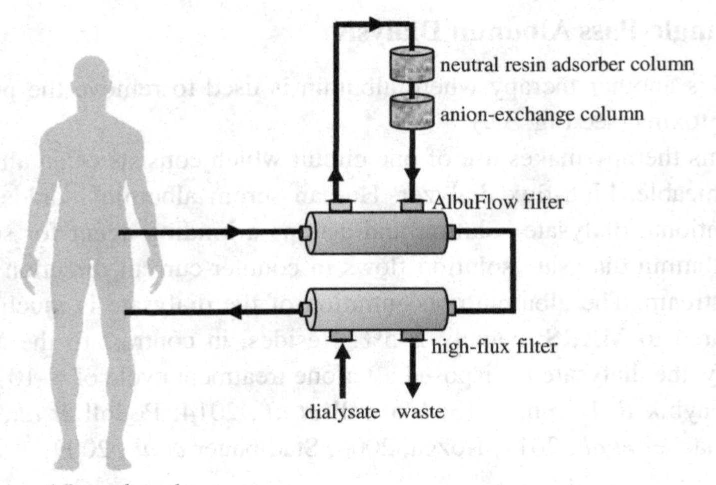

Figure 3.10. Scheme of Prometheus. Hybrid blood purification system which combines FPSA.

high-flux dialyzer, an uncoated activated charcoal column and an anionic exchange column) [Falkenhagen *et al.*, 1999].

The patient is connected to Prometheus *via* a standard dialysis catheter. The blood with all toxins enters an albumin-permeable filter (AlbuFlow) made of polysulfone hollow fibers with MWCO of 250 kDa [Rademacher *et al.*, 2011]. The albumin as well as protein-bound toxins pass the filter by convection. Then, the albumin-rich plasma fraction is treated by two columns in another circuit: a neutral resin adsorber column and an anion-exchanger column. Negatively charged toxins as well as strongly albumin-bound toxins are effectively removed by the adsorber columns. Finally, a conventional dialysis system with a high-flux dialyzer is used to remove water-soluble toxins [Maiwall *et al.*, 2014; Podoll *et al.*, 2012; Rademacher *et al.*, 2011].

The positive outcomes of Prometheus are similar to MARS concerning serum-level reduction of ammonia, bilirubin, creatinine, lactate and urea [Podoll *et al.*, 2012]. However, blood pressure drops are observed more in patients treated with Prometheus than those treated with MARS or SPAD. There is an acute reduction of intravascular blood volume because the extracorporeal circuit needs to be filled. In general, no other clinically relevant changes in hemodynamic, systemic and coagulation parameters were observed, and Prometheus could be considered as a safe extracorporeal liver therapy [Rademacher *et al.*, 2011].

3.10 Selective Plasma Filtration Therapy

SEPET is another therapy for liver failure patients and was developed by Cedars Sinai Medical Center and Arbios Systems (California) [Rozga, 2006] (see Fig. 3.11).

This system contains one dialyzer with a molecular-weight cutoff of 100 kDa which allows albumin, hepatic toxins, hepatic regeneration inhibitors and inflammation mediators to go through. Immunoglobulins, blood clotting factors, complement system proteins and liver regeneration factors remain in the blood. The filtered blood plasma is disposed and needs to be replaced by electrolyte solution, 5% albumin solution and fresh frozen plasma to maintain hemodynamic, systemic and coagulation parameters. SEPET could be considered a hybrid system, because of the blood purification step and the fluid replacement therapy [Rozga, 2006; Stadlbauer *et al.*, 2009].

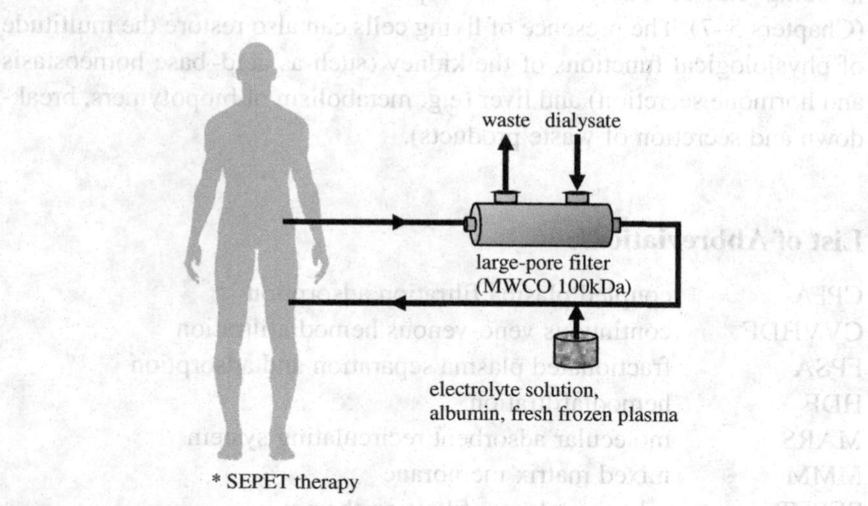

Figure 3.11. Scheme of SEPET. Electrolyte solution, albumin and fresh frozen plasma are infused after blood purification.

3.11 Conclusion and Outlook

The advanced blood purification therapies described in this chapter are promising in terms of reduction of the morbidity and mortality of the patients, but a lot of research still needs to be done to improve their benefits. One main drawback is related to the intermittence of the treatment which leads to the accumulation of toxins between consecutive sessions of therapy, thus not mimicking the normal physiological function of the organ (kidney or liver). Wearable artificial devices would assure a continuous (24/7) purification of the blood. These could also improve the quality of the life of patients as well as reduce the length of hospital stay and medical care costs. However, development of wearable artificial system is really challenging since it needs to satisfy a lot of different technical aspects. The amount of the dialysate needs to be drastically reduced in order to be independent on fixed water supply (continuous recycling of the dialysate). The hemocompatibility of the membranes together with that of the sorbent materials has to be improved because of the long-term contact with blood and so on.

Finally, all therapies described in this chapter, although beneficial for the removal of most of the toxins from patients' blood, do not mimic completely the function of the damaged organ. For this reason, lots of research is being carried out on the development of the bioartificial systems (Chapters 5–7). The presence of living cells can also restore the multitude of physiological functions of the kidney (such as acid–base homeostasis and hormone secretion) and liver (e.g. metabolism of biopolymers, breakdown and secretion of waste products).

List of Abbreviations

CPFA	coupled plasma filtration adsorption
CVVHDF	continuous veno-venous hemodiafiltration
FPSA	fractionated plasma separation and adsorption
HDF	hemodiafiltration
MARS	molecular adsorbent recirculating system
MMM	mixed matrix membrane
SEPET	selective plasma filtration therapy
SPAD	single-pass albumin dialysis

References

Ash SR, Blake DE, Carr DJ, Carter C, Howard T and Makowka L (1992). Clinical effects of a sorbent suspension dialysis system in treatment of hepatic-coma (the biologic-dt). *Int J Artif Organs*, 15, pp. 151–161.

Banares R, Catalina MV and Vaquero J (2014). Molecular adsorbent recirculating system and bioartificial devices for liver failure. *Clin Liver Dis*, 18, pp. 945–956.

Bello G, Di Muzio F, Maviglia R and Antonelli M (2012). New membranes for extracorporeal blood purification in septic conditions. *Minerva Anestesiol*, 78, pp. 1265–1281.

Bellomo R, Tipping P and Boyce N (1993). Continuous venovenous hemofiltration with dialysis removes cytokines from the circulation of septic patients. *Crit Care Med*, 21, pp. 522–526.

Cerda J, Tolwani A, Gibney N and Tiranathanagul K (2011). Renal replacement therapy in special settings: extracorporeal support devices in liver failure. *Semin Dial*, 24, pp. 197–202.

Denis J, Opolon P, Nusinovici V, Granger A and Darnis F (1978). Treatment of encephalopathy during fulminant hepatic-failure by hemodialysis with high permeability membrane. *Gut*, 19, pp. 787–793.

Drolz A, Saxa R, Scherzer T and Fuhrmann V (2011). Extracorporeal artificial liver support in hypoxic liver injury. *Liver Int*, 31(Suppl 3), pp. 19–23.

Duan ZJ, Li LL, Ju J, Gao ZH and He GH (2006). Treatment of hyperbilirubinemia with blood purification in china. *World J Gastroenterol*, 12, pp. 7467–7471.

Ellis AJ, Hughes RD, Nicholl D, Langley PG, Wendon JA, O'Grady JG and Williams R (1999). Temporary extracorporeal liver support for severe acute alcoholic hepatitis using the biologic-dt. *Int J Artif Organs*, 22, pp. 27–34.

Eloot S, Dhondt A, Van Landschoot M, Waterloos MA and Vanholder R (2012a). Removal of water-soluble and protein-bound solutes with reversed mid-dilution versus post-dilution haemodiafiltration. *Nephrol Dial Transpl*, 27, pp. 3278–3283.

Eloot S, Van Biesen W and Vanholder R (2012b). A sad but forgotten truth: the story of slow-moving solutes in fast hemodialysis. *Semin Dial*, 25, pp. 505–509.

Eloot S, Ledebo I and Ward RA (2014). Extracorporeal removal of uremic toxins: Can we still do better? *Semin Nephrol*, 34, pp. 209–227.

Falkenhagen D, Strobl W, Vogt G, Schrefl A, Linsberger I, Gerner FJ and Schoenhofen M (1999). Fractionated plasma separation and adsorption system: a novel system for blood purification to remove albumin bound substances. *Artif Organs*, 23, pp. 81–86.

Faybik P and Krenn CG (2013). Extracorporeal liver support. *Curr Opin Crit Care*, 19, pp. 149–153.

Fissell WH, Roy S and Davenport A (2013). Achieving more frequent and longer dialysis for the majority: wearable dialysis and implantable artificial kidney devices. *Kidney Int*, 84, pp. 256–264.

Formica M, Inguaggiato P, Bainotti S and Wratten ML (2007). Coupled plasma filtration adsorption. *Acute Kidney Injury*, 156, pp. 405–410.

Friedman EA (2009). Will nephrologists use a wearable artificial kidney? *Clin J Am Soc Nephrol*, 4, pp. 1401–1402.

Gimson AES, Mellon PJ, Braude S, Canalese J and Williams R (1982). Earlier charcoal hemoperfusion in fulminant hepatic failure. *Lancet*, 2, pp. 681–683.

Gura V, Beizai M, Ezon C and Polaschegg HD (2005). Continuous renal replacement therapy for end-stage renal disease — The wearable artificial kidney (wak). *Cardiovasc Disord Hemodial*, 149, pp. 325–333.

Gurland HJ, Lysaght MJ, Samtleben W and Schmidt B (1984). A comparison of centrifugal and membrane-based apheresis formats. *Int J Artif Organs*, 7, pp. 35–38.

Hu DL, Sun S, Zhu B, Mei Z, Wang L, Zhu SZ and Zhao WH (2012). Effects of coupled plasma filtration adsorption on septic patients with multiple organ dysfunction syndrome. *Renal Failure*, 34, pp. 834–839.

Hughes RD, Pucknell A, Routley D, Langley PG, Wendon JA and Williams R (1994). Evaluation of the biologic-dt sorbent-suspension dialyzer in patients with fulminant hepatic failure. *Int J Artif Organs*, 17, pp. 657–662.

Lee DBN and Roberts M (2008). A peritoneal-based automated wearable artificial kidney. *Clin Exp Nephrol*, 12, pp. 171–180.

Maiwall R, Maras JS, Nayak SL and Sarin SK (2014). Liver dialysis in acute-on-chronic liver failure: current and future perspectives. *Hepatol Int*, 8, pp. S505–S513.

Mao HJ, Yu S, Yu XB, Zhang B, Zhang L, Xu XR, Wang XY and Xing CY (2009). Effects of coupled plasma filtration adsorption on immune function of patients with multiple organ dysfunction syndrome. *Int J Artif Organs*, 32, pp. 31–38.

Marieb EN and Hoehn K (2007) *Human Anatomy & Physiology* (Pearson Benjamin Cummings, San Francisco, CA).

Mikhalovsky SV (2003). Emerging technologies in extracorporeal treatment: focus on adsorption. *Perfusion-UK*, 18, pp. 47–54.

Nissenson AR, Ronco C, Pergamit G, Edelstein M and Watts R (2005). Continuously functioning artificial nephron system: the promise of nanotechnology. *Hemodial Int Int Symp Home Hemodial*, 9, pp. 210–217.

Nitta M, Hirasawa H, Oda S, Shiga H, Nakanishi K, Matsuda K, Nakamura M, Yokohari K, Hirano T, Hirayama Y, Moriguchi T and Watanabe E (2002).

Long-term survivors with artificial liver support in fulminant hepatic failure. *Therapeut Apheresis*, 6, pp. 208–212.

Onodera K, Sakata H, Yonekawa M and Kawamura A (2006). Artificial liver support at present and in the future. *J Artif Organs*, 9, pp. 17–28.

Patel N and Bayliss GP (2015). Developments in extracorporeal therapy for the poisoned patient. *Adv Drug Deliver Rev*, 90, pp. 3–11.

Pavlenko D, van Geffen E, van Steenbergen MJ, Glorieux G, Vanholder R, Gerritsen KG and Stamatialis D (2016). New low-flux mixed matrix membranes that offer superior removal of protein-bound toxins from human plasma. *Sci Rep*, 6, p. 34429.

Podoll AS, DeGolovine A and Finkel KW (2012). Liver support systems — a review. *ASAIO J*, 58, pp. 443–449.

Rademacher S, Oppert M and Jorres A (2011). Artificial extracorporeal liver support therapy in patients with severe liver failure. *Expert Rev Gastroenterol Hepatol*, 5, pp. 591–599.

Reeves HM and Winters JL (2014). The mechanisms of action of plasma exchange. *Br J Haematol*, 164, pp. 342–351.

Ringe H, Varnholt V, Zimmering M, Luck W, Gratopp A, Konig K, Reich S, Sauer IM, Gaedicke G and Querfeld U (2011). Continuous veno-venous single-pass albumin hemodiafiltration in children with acute liver failure. *Pediatr Crit Care Mem*, 12, pp. 257–264.

Ronco C and Fecondini L (2007). The vicenza wearable artificial kidney for peritoneal dialysis (viwak pd). *Blood Purif*, 25, pp. 383–388.

Rozga J (2006). Liver support technology — an update. *Xenotransplantation*, 13, pp. 380–389.

Schwartz J, Winters JL, Padmanabhan A, Balogun RA, Delaney M, Linenberger ML, Szczepiorkowski ZM, Williams ME, Wu YY and Shaz BH (2013). Guidelines on the use of therapeutic apheresis in clinical practiceevidence-based approach from the writing committee of the American Society for Apheresis: the sixth special issue. *J Clin Apheresis*, 28, pp. 145–284.

Stadlbauer V, Wright GAK and Jalan R (2009). Role of artificial liver support in hepatic encephalopathy. *Metab Brain Dis*, 24, pp. 15–26.

Stamatialis DF, Papenburg BJ, Girones M, Saiful S, Bettahalli SNM, Schmitmeier S and Wessling M (2008). Medical applications of membranes: drug delivery, artificial organs and tissue engineering. *J Membrane Sci*, 308, pp. 1–34.

Stange J, Ramlow W, Mitzner S, Schmidt R and Klinkmann H (1993). Dialysis against a recycled albumin solution enables the removal of albumin-bound toxins. *Artif Organs*, 17, pp. 809–813.

Stephens RL, Jacobsen SC, Atkin-Thor E and Kolff W (1976). Portable/wearable artificial kidney (wak) — initial evaluation. *Proc Eur Dial Transplant Assoc*, 12, pp. 511–518.

Tetta C, Cavaillon JM, Schulze M, Ronco C, Ghezzi PM, Camussi G, Serra AM, Curti F and Lonnemann G (1998). Removal of cytokines and activated complement components in an experimental model of continuous plasma filtration coupled with sorbent adsorption. *Nephrol Dial Transpl*, 13, pp. 1458–1464.

Tetta C, Gianotti L, Cavaillon JM, Wratten ML, Fini M, Braga M, Bisagni P, Giavaresi G, Bolzani R and Giardino R (2000). Coupled plasma filtration–adsorption in a rabbit model of endotoxic shock. *Crit Care Med*, 28, pp. 1526–1533.

Tijink MSL, Wester M, Glorieux G, Gerritsen KGF, Sun JF, Swart PC, Borneman Z, Wessling M, Vanholder R, Joles JA and Stamatialis D (2013). Mixed matrix hollow fiber membranes for removal of protein-bound toxins from human plasma. *Biomaterials*, 34, pp. 7819–7828.

Tyagi PK, Winchester JF and Feinfeld DA (2008). Extracorporeal removal of toxins. *Kidney Int*, 74, pp. 1231–1233.

Vanholder R, Glorieux G and Eloot S (2015). Once upon a time in dialysis: the last days of kt/v? *Kidney Int*, 88, pp. 460–465.

Xue J, Wang Y and Weng Y (2002). An experimental study on protective effects of blood infusion on organs postoperatively in obstructive hyperbilirubinemia. *Chin J Hepatobiliary Surg*, 8, pp. 232–234.

Yatzidis H (1964). A convenient haemoperfusion micro-apparatus over charcoal for the treatment of endogenous and exogenous intoxications. It’s use as an effective artificial kidney. *Proc Eur Dial Transplant Assoc*, 1, pp. 83–87.

Chapter 4
Membranes for Artificial Lung and Gas Exchange Applications

F. Wiese

Consulting Membrane Technology,
Starenstr. 100, 42389 Wuppertal, Germany
wiesef@web.de

4.1 Introduction

Membranes for gas exchange are used in several medical, biotechnological and technical applications. Membrane oxygenators are used inside heart–lung machines during open heart surgeries or for lung support systems. Around 1.5 million open heart surgeries per year are carried out with the aid of a heart–lung machine.

In the natural lung, oxygen and carbon dioxide are exchanged between blood and body environment. Oxygen is needed in the body tissues to sustain life. Carbon dioxide produced during metabolism has to be removed. Oxygenators are used in surgical interventions during which the heart–lung function is interrupted, e.g. for cardiovascular bypass, heart valve replacement or when repairing congestive heart failure [Lauterbach, 2002; Taylor, 1986; Tschaut, 1999]. Such a procedure takes 1–10 h. Furthermore, extracorporeal membrane oxygenation (ECMO) is used in several configurations for long-term lung support, e.g. in the case of multi-organ failure

(MOF) and in different pulmonary diseases [Philipp *et al.*, 2003; Schmid *et al.*, 2002; Zwischenberger & Alpard, 2002; Zwischenberger *et al.*, 2001]. These procedures last several days up to several weeks. Special membranes are required for long-term applications.

Implantable membrane devices for long-term lung support are under development since many years [Mallabiabarrena Ormaetxea, 2004; Mortensen, 1992], but not in a commercial stage up to now. Gas-exchange membranes are an important component also in membrane bioreactors for biotechnology applications and in hybrid bioartificial organs to take over the respiratory function. Furthermore, such membranes are used for degassing of fluids, e.g. of infusion solutions.

4.2 History

Milestones in the history of the development of blood membrane oxygenators are summarized in several papers [Dierickx, 2001; Lauterbach, 2002; Wodetzki *et al.*, 2000]. The first suggestion of extracorporeal circulation was made by César Julian Jean Le Gallois (1770–1814). He proposed that a part of the body might be preserved by a mechanical heart replacement and some kind of external perfusion device. His important monograph "Experiences sur le principe de la vie" was published in 1812/1813 [Le Gallois *et al.*, 1812, 1813]. Alexander Schmidt was the first to perfuse an isolated dog kidney with oxygenated blood in 1876 [Schmidt, 1867]. Many different types of disk, film and bubble oxygenators were developed for extracorporeal circulation experiments. All these early oxygenators exposed blood directly to gas mixtures or oxygen to provide oxygenation and remove CO_2. The developments started in the 1930s, resulted in disposable single-use bubble oxygenators and opened the area of cardiac surgery in the early 1950s. A pioneer in this development was John Gibbon [Clowes *et al.*, 1956; Gibbon, 1937; Lauterbach, 2002]. In 1955, the De Wall–Lillehei bubble oxygenator was a major breakthrough [De Wall & Lillehei, 1957; Lillehei, 1955]. The simplicity of the basic concept was linked to simple construction and disposability.

The principle: venous blood is pumped into an oxygenation chamber where oxygen bubbles are dispersed. Gas exchange occurs on the surface of the bubbles. The mixture of blood and gas which emerges from the bubble chamber has to be de-foamed in a de-foaming compartment.

The main disadvantage of bubble oxygenators was its poor biocompatibility. The blood–gas interface also represents a non-physiological state resulting, for example, in hemolysis, coagulopathy and so on.

Already in 1944, Kolff and Berk had observed that the blood during dialysis in a rotating drum turned to a brighter red color during treatment. They found out that venous blood was oxygenated while flowing through a cellophane dialyzer and being in contact with oxygen from air and air-containing dialysate. Oxygenation was done through the regenerated cellulose-based membrane [Kolff *et al.*, 1944]. This discovery stimulated the development of using gas-permeable membranes in order to separate the blood phase from the gas phase in an artificial lung. The first membrane oxygenator was reported by Kolff in 1955 [Kolff *et al.*, 1955, 1956] (Fig. 4.1). At this time, the available membrane materials were relatively impermeable to the respiratory gases.

The first membrane oxygenator built and used clinically is reported by Clowes *et al.* [1956]. It was constructed of ethylcellulose multi-layer flat-sheet membranes and had a membrane area of 25 m^2. These factors limited their clinical applications till 1970s and early 1980s. The development of polydimethylsiloxane with high permeability for oxygen and carbon dioxide brought a major advance to establish the technical feasibility of membrane oxygenators in the 1960s and 1970s. The required membrane area could be optimized up to lower than 6 m^2.

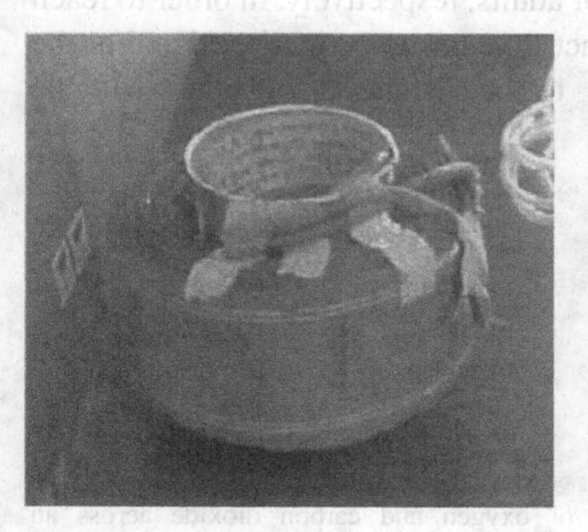

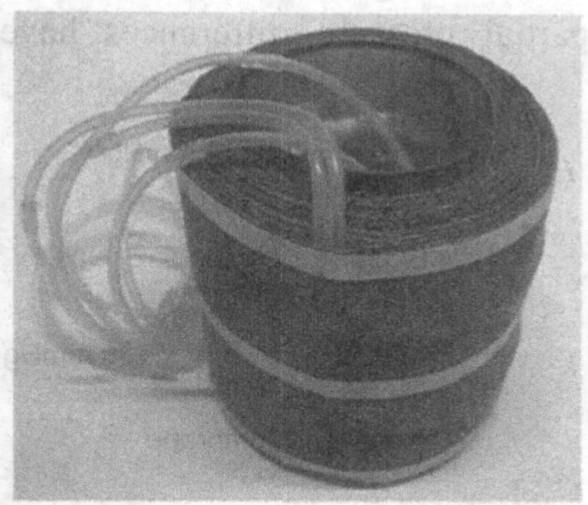

Figure 4.1. Prof. Kolff's artificial coil kidney, and the coil oxygenator from 60 years ago (Museum ICMT, Huston, TX).

A major advancement was the development of microporous hydrophobic flat-sheet membranes with pore sizes <0.1 μm. Because of the open pores, the resistance for gas transport was minimized. The real breakthrough, however, came sometime later in 1980s, when microporous hollow fiber membranes became commercially available. With the introduction of extraluminal flow oxygenators [Alpha *et al.*, 1986; Gassmann *et al.*, 1987], membrane areas of less than 2 m^2 were required to treat an adult patient.

4.3 Basics of Gas Transfer

The transport of gas into the blood is a process of convection and diffusion *via* the membrane and the blood combined with O_2 and CO_2 reaction with the erythrocyte hemoglobin. The hemoglobin in the erythrocytes has a specific chemical gas binding capacity for O_2 and CO_2 and assures the adequate transport of both gases inside the body.

The driving force for the gas exchange is the partial pressure difference of these gases between the blood and gas side (O_2) of the membrane. According to the pressure differences, gas diffuses through the membrane wall from the side with high partial pressure to the side of low partial pressure (Fig. 4.2).

Nowadays, the active area of membrane oxygenators is between 0.25 m^2 for young children and 2.5 m^2 for adults. This is around 10% of the natural lung of young children or adults, respectively. In order to reach a sufficient gas exchange, the contact time has to be increased and/or the partial pressure differences have to be increased or other suitable

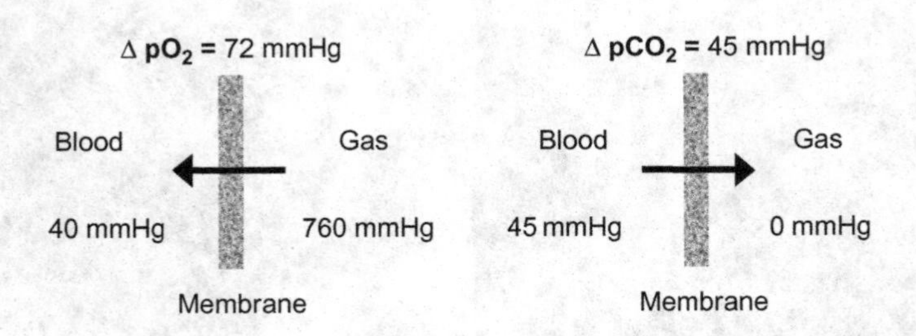

Figure 4.2. Partial pressure difference of oxygen and carbon dioxide across an oxygenation membrane.

conditions have to be adjusted, for example, decrease patient temperature, etc. The gas exchange efficiency can be influenced according to Fick's law [Lauterbach, 2002; Wodetzki *et al.*, 2000]:

$$V_{O_2} = \frac{P_1 - P_2}{L} KA\Delta t. \tag{4.1}$$

In Eq. (4.1), V_{O_2} is the amount of oxygen exchanged in a certain time, $P_1 - P_2$ is the partial pressure difference, K the diffusion factor (adsorption coefficient, turbulence), A the surface area, L the diffusion layer thickness and t the time.

The transfer of oxygen into the blood is hindered by three main resistances:

$$R_{\text{total}} = R_{\text{B}} + R_{\text{M}} + R_{\text{G}}. \tag{4.2}$$

The total resistance for the gas transport R_{total} is the sum of resistance on the blood side R_B, the resistance across the membrane R_M and the resistance on the gas side R_G (Fig. 4.3).

For a usual oxygenator type, with microporous capillary membranes as described in Section 4.4, the blood–boundary layer lies outside the capillaries. The resistance of the gas–boundary layer is infinitely small and can be neglected. The resistance of the membrane is about 1.25×10^{-4} cm² s cmHg/cm³. The resistance in the blood–boundary layer is approx. 100 times larger and should be minimized (see Section 4.6). Therefore, the mass transfer in relation to geometry flow pattern and the hydrodynamics

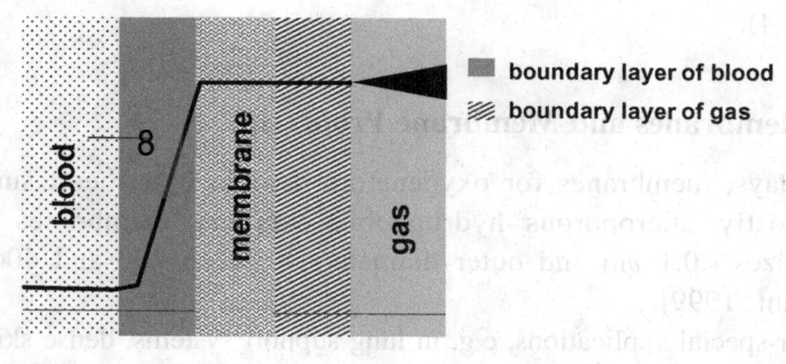

Figure 4.3. Mass-transfer model in an extraluminal flow oxygenator.

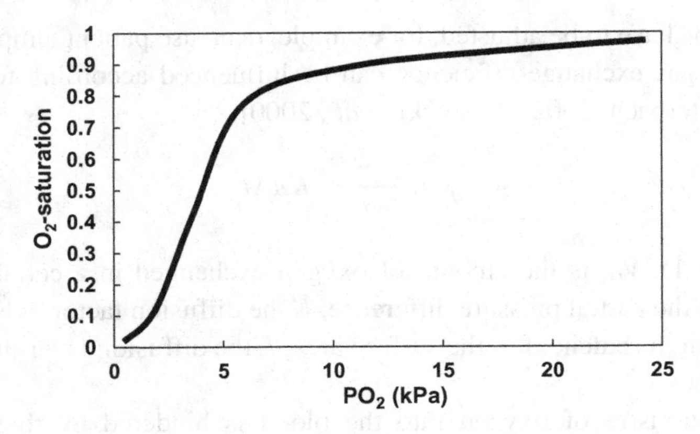

Figure 4.4. Blood saturation according to Hill.

of an artificial lung was investigated in hundreds of papers [Dierickx, 2001; Dierickx *et al.*, 2000; Mockros & Leonard, 1985; Vaslef *et al.*, 1994; Wicksramasinghe *et al.*, 1992].

The maximum concentration of chemically bound O_2, called the oxygen capacity, is calculated from the hemoglobin content of the blood and the binding capacity of hemoglobin for oxygen. For a mean hemoglobin content of Hb = 0.12 kg/l and a binding capacity of Ha = 1.34 l/kg, the oxygen capacity will be 0.1608 l O_2/l blood. This value will be reached at an O_2 partial pressure of approx. 20 kPa = 150 mmHg, which is the ambient partial pressure of oxygen. An additional increase in the O_2 content is possible but non-physiological.

The oxyhemoglobin dissociation curve is usually calculated according to a mathematical model of Hill [Severinghaus, 1979] (Fig. 4.4).

4.4 Membranes and Membrane Properties

Nowadays, membranes for oxygenators used in open heart surgery are mostly microporous hydrophobic capillary membranes with pore sizes <0.1 μm and outer diameters between 200 and 400 μm [Tschaut, 1999].

For special applications, e.g. in lung support systems, dense skinned membranes are used because of long-term blood–plasma resistance.

Table 4.1: Dimensions and pore sizes of current blood oxygenation membranes.

	Inner diameter (μm)	Outer diameter (μm)	Wall thickness (μm)	Pore size (μm)
OXYPHAN®	200, 280	300, 380	50	≤0.2
OXYPLUS®	200	380	90	n/a
CELGARD®	150, 240	200, 300	25, 40	0.04×0.1
Terumo	280	380	50	0.05

The main polymers used are polyolefins such as polypropylene (PP), polyethylene (PE) and poly-4-methylpentene (PMP). Further polymers used in small scale are polyvinylidene fluoride (PVDF) and silicone rubber (SR).

Around 75% of worldwide-used oxygenation membranes are produced by Membrana, Wuppertal. Other oxygenation membrane producers are the companies Terumo and Dainippon Inc. (see Table 4.1).

4.4.1 *Microporous Membranes*

The gas exchange between the blood side and gas side in microporous membranes occurs by diffusion and convection of the respiratory gases *via* the open pores. Thus, the transport resistance of the membrane is very low for the gas exchange, as explained in Section 4.3. Due to the hydrophobicity of these membranes and the pore size (<0.1 μm), gas molecules can pass the membrane wall, whereas liquids and corpuscular components are retained.

Due to membrane hydrophobicity [Wiese *et al.*, 1990], no wetting of the membrane pores with aqueous solutions, e.g. blood, is possible. A water contact angle on the membrane surface should create a high contact angle $\gg 90°$.

Most microporous oxygenator membranes are made of PP by thermally induced phase separation (TIPS) process.

The sponge-like structure of this membrane is homogeneous and isotropic, with open surfaces on both wall sides (see Fig. 4.5). These membranes achieve reliable, sufficient performance, and the mechanical stability in terms of tensile strength and elongation at break is high

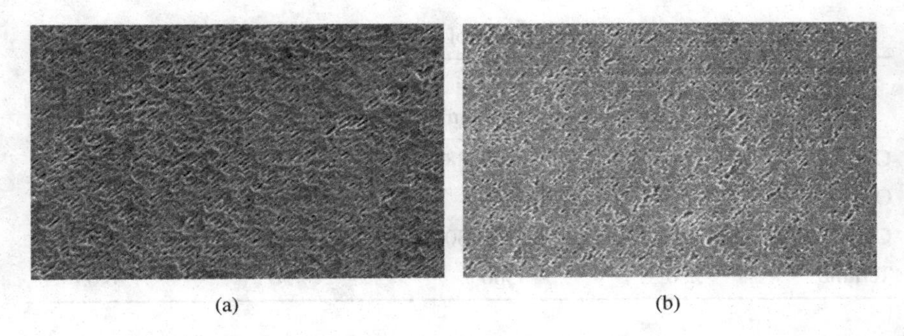

Figure 4.5. REM photograph of a microporous PP membrane: (a) outside wall; (b) inside wall (×2000).

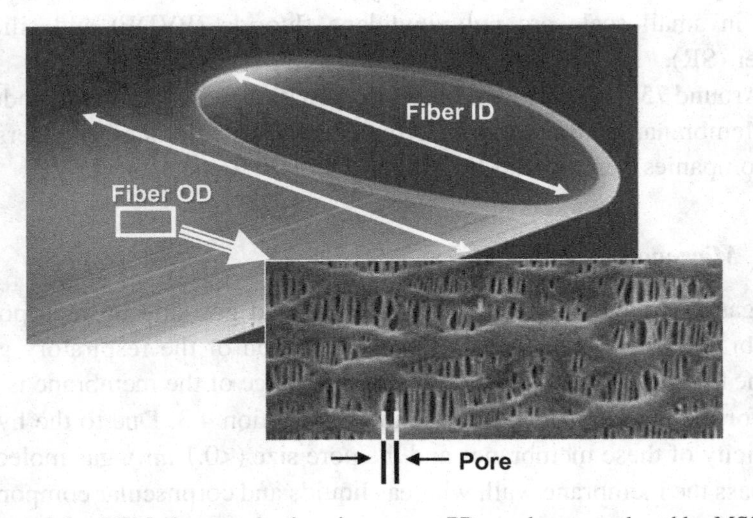

Figure 4.6. REM photograph of a microporous PP membrane produced by MSSP.

combined with high reliability and handling safety during the manufacturing process (see Section 4.5). Today, it is the most widely used oxygenation membrane.

Microporous membranes are also produced *via* melt spin stretch process (MSSP) (see Section 4.5), resulting in fibrillary polymer structures (see Fig. 4.6). Polyolefins are suitable for these processes, because only polymers with certain crystallinity are suitable to create such membrane structures. Performance concerning these membranes can reach a comparable level, as membranes prepared by TIPS.

For the duration time of an open heart surgery and up to several days, these open membranes are reliable and safe. However, during long-term treatment, plasma proteins are adsorbed first at the membrane surface and later on the membrane pores. As a result the surface energy the surface energy increases, the pores become wetted and plasma breakthrough from blood side to gas side is possible [Wiese *et al.*, 1990; Wiese, 2008].

4.4.2 *Dense Membranes*

Dense membranes, also called "diffusion" membranes, have no open pores [Baker, 2000; Breiter *et al.*, 2004; Krause *et al.*, 2006]. In long-term ECMO applications, such membranes are used to prevent the plasma breakthrough.

In a dense membrane, "solution diffusion" is the only transport mechanism. The permeance is determined by the intrinsic permeability (Barrer) of the polymer for the used gas and the path length [Nunes & Peinemann, 2001]. In the past, SR or silicon-skinned microporous membranes were used because of high permeability of this polymer. The disadvantage of these membranes, however, was the relatively high wall thicknesses because of mechanical requirements. Thus, large membrane areas were required to reach sufficient gas exchange. Very thin membranes made of PMP can overcome this problem. The membrane OXYPLUS® produced by ACCUREL® process is integral asymmetric, as it has a sponge-like microporous wall with a thin, dense outer skin (Fig. 4.7).

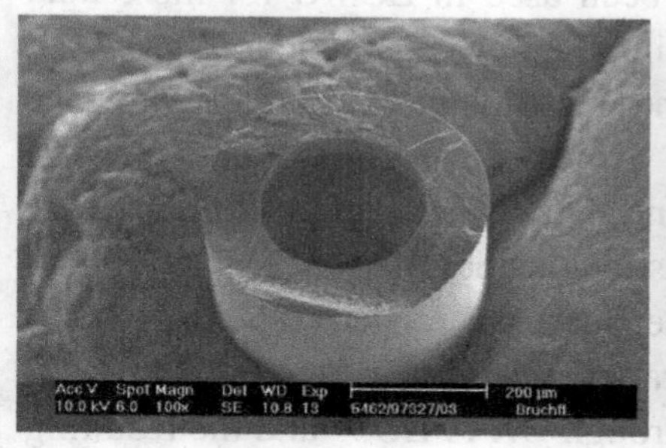

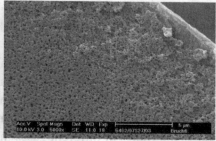

Figure 4.7. REM photograph of a microporous PMP membrane OXYPLUS® with dense outer skin.

Table 4.2: Gas permeability coefficients of PP and PMP for oxygen and carbon dioxide [Allen *et al.*, 1977].

Gas	PP	PMP
Oxygen	2.2	32.3
Carbon dioxide	9.2	92.6

Permeability (Barrer = 10–10 cm³ cm/(s cm² cmHg)).

Table 4.3: Gas permeabilities of OXYPLUS® for different gases and the resulting separation coefficients.

Gas	Flux l/(m² min bar)	Selectivity coefficient Related to N_2
Nitrogen	1.68	
Oxygen	5.90	3.53
Carbon dioxide	16.90	10.13

Due to relatively high specific permeability of PMP to O_2 and CO_2 (Table 4.2) and the very thin outer skin (<< = 1 μm), OXYPLUS® has gas-transfer capabilities comparable to common microporous membranes.

Related to plasma breakthrough, there is theoretically no time limit in using this membrane. In fact, it has been used in ECMO for more than 42 days without the need of exchanging the device [Bennett *et al.*, 2004; Philipp *et al.*, 2003]. Additionally, the dense outer skin largely prevents entry of gas into the blood and avoids direct blood–gas contact. Nonetheless, the transfer of volatile anesthetics is impaired [Philipp *et al.*, 2003], and the anesthetic protocol has to consider this.

The permeability of PMP is higher for O_2 as related to N_2, and therefore it is thus suitable for gas separation or enrichment, too. Table 4.3 shows the fluxes of different gases through OXYPLUS® and the resulting gas separation coefficients. With this membrane, the enrichment of O_2 is possible and effective in a single-step process as well.

4.5 Membrane Manufacture

Almost 70% of oxygenation membranes worldwide are produced by a special TIPS process called "Accurel" process [Castro, 1981; Henne *et al.*, 1983; Hiatt *et al.*, 1985] (Fig. 4.8(a)).

A suitable polymer and a solvent or solvent mixture such as natural seed oils (e.g. soybean and castor) are heated up together in an extruder to produce a homogeneously mixed polymer solution. This solution is

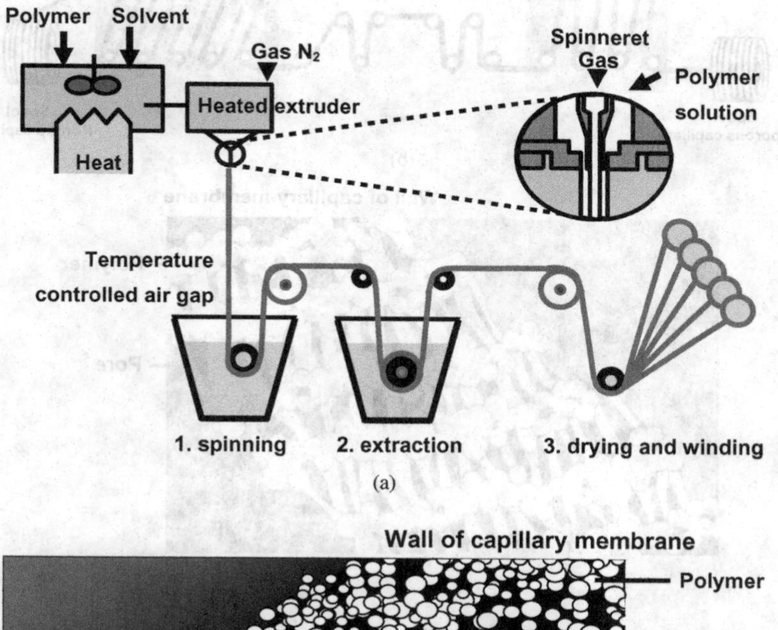

Figure 4.8. (a) Scheme of the ACCUREL® process for manufacturing of membranes by TIPS. (b) Schematic picture of ACCUREL® membrane wall, cross-section.

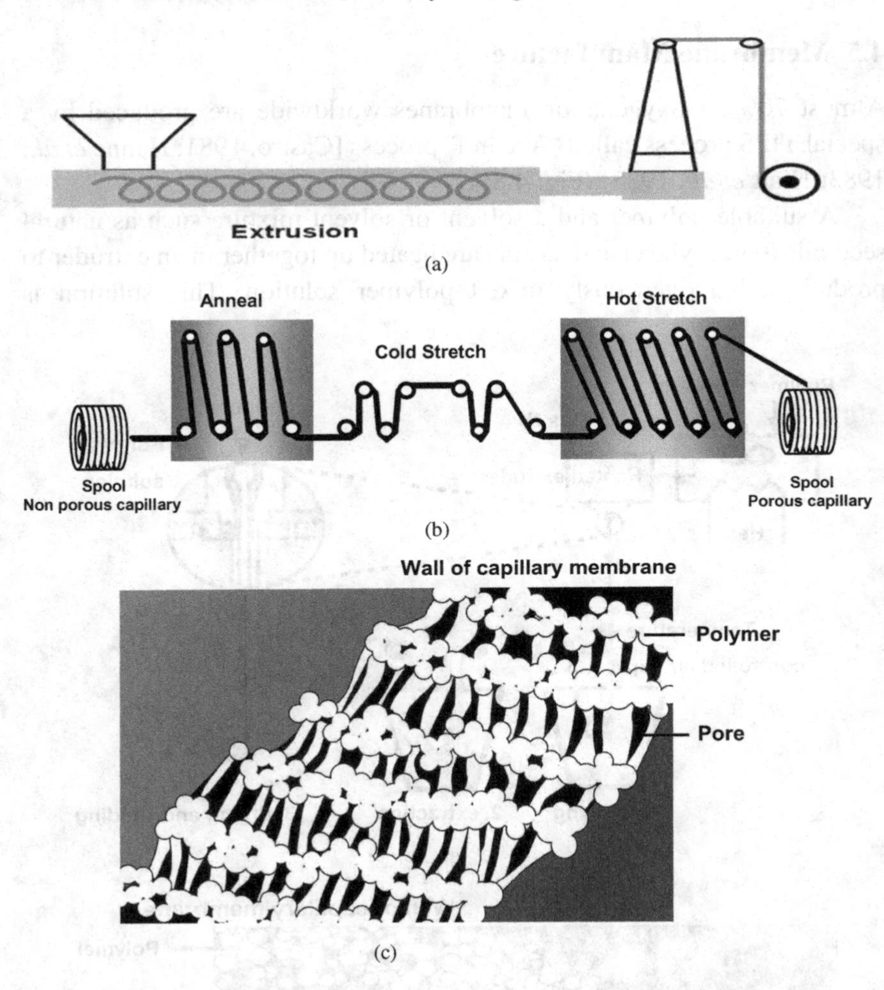

Figure 4.9. (a) Scheme of the stretching process to produce microporous membranes. (b) Scheme of the stretching process to produce microporous membranes. (c) Scheme of the microporous membrane produced by MSSP, cross-section.

pumped through a spinneret together with a gas as bore medium to create the right geometry of the hollow fiber. The pre-formed hollow fiber geometry is cooled down in an air gap and in cold spinning oil, initiating a phase separation of the solvent and the porous polymer matrix, with pores still being filled with oil.

After a washing step, e.g. with hot alcohol, to remove the solvent, the membrane is winded up on bobbins. The membrane structure is adjustable by composition of the polymer solution, the cooling speed and the different process temperatures during spinning and cooling.

A homogenous sponge-like structure can be formed as shown schematically in Fig. 4.8(b).

In the MSSP, the membrane pores are generated in a completely different way. At first, a suitable crystalline or semi-crystalline polymer is molten in an extruder. Then the polymer is pressed through a spinneret, and upon cooling a dense compact capillary or flat sheet is created. By annealing, cold stretching and hot stretching steps with a special temperature and tension profile in several repeating steps (see Figs. 4.9(a) and (b)), microporous membranes with completely different structures can be created. This process has advantages because no solvent and extraction are required, but it also has disadvantages due to its lower porosity, limited range of pore size and elongated pores (lower selectivity) of the membrane. The scheme of the structure of the membrane wall is shown in Fig. 4.9(c).

4.6 Operation and Construction of Oxygenators

The construction of the oxygenator and the arrangement of the membranes inside the oxygenator are as important as the performance of the oxygenation membrane itself. Oxygenators with blood flowing outside the capillaries (extraluminal flow) were developed in the mid-1980s [Alpha *et al.*, 1986; Catapano *et al.*, 2004; Wiese *et al.*, 1990; Wodetzki *et al.*, 2000]. More than 95% of the membrane oxygenators used in hospitals today are oxygenators with blood flow outside the capillaries.

The structure of these oxygenators with wound capillary membranes or with knitted mats provides good mixing of the blood and thus an improvement in the oxygen-transfer rates, especially in the reduced blood boundary layer. The used membrane surface can be minimized.

The most effective construction is using cross-laid knitted mats (Fig. 4.10(a)). The following advantages are achieved:

- "enhanced mass-transfer efficiency" with "local laminar mixing" (static mixer effect)

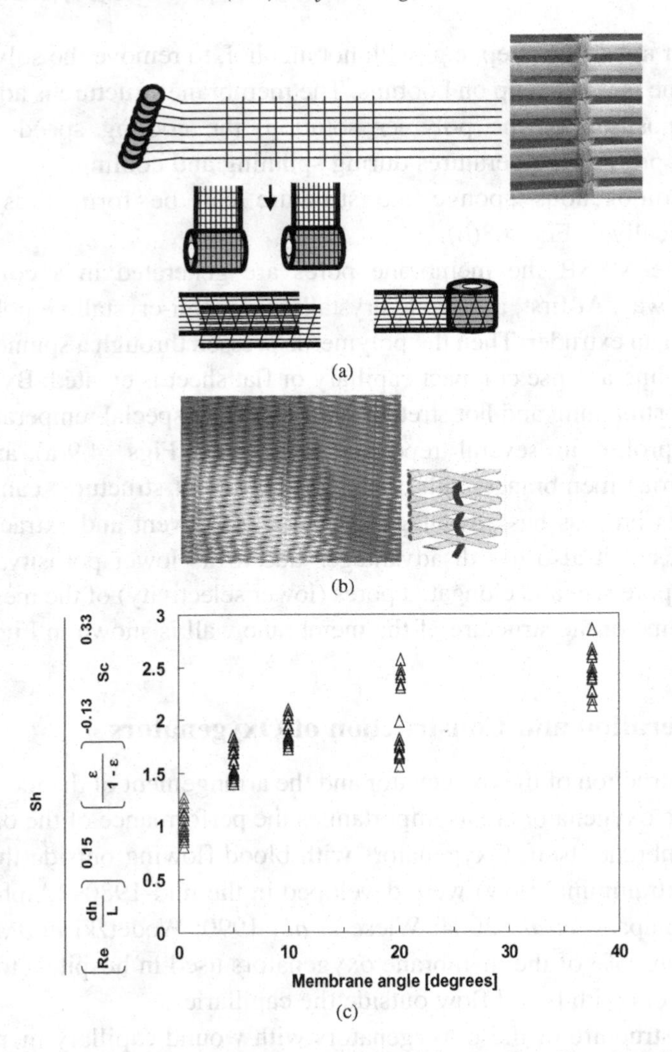

Figure 4.10. (a) Scheme of production of cross-laid knitted hollow fiber mats. (b) A cross-laid knitted membrane mat. (c) Mass-transfer coefficient vs membrane angle in a cross-wound mat device.

- repeated renewal of concentration boundary layers, therefore highest efficiency
- uniform distribution of capillaries
- capillaries fixed by warp threads (no movement)

- open for various oxygenator designs (axial, tangential, crossflow, etc.)
- blood film thickness (pressure drop) can be adjusted easily
- easy handling during manufacturing
- high production yield
- closed capillary ends for safe potting.

The process steps for production of cross-laid knitted mats are shown in Fig. 4.10(b). Several capillaries are continuously laid down in parallel at a knitting machine and connected with a warp thread in defined distances. During this step, multiple mats are cut, the membrane ends are closed and the mat spools are wounded up in parallel. In the next step, two mats are pulled in a defined angle each and wounded up together.

For each oxygenator set up, a special distance between the membranes, a special warp thread distance and an angle between the cross-wounded mats are possible and can be optimized. In this way, one can always create an optimal blood stream. The effects of design and operating variables on module performance were investigated with respect to oxygen transfer into water. It was found that the membrane angle with respect to the main direction of the liquid flow had a significant influence on oxygenator performance [Wiese, 2008; Wodetzki *et al.*, 2000]. The mass-transfer coefficient increased proportionally to the membrane angle up to about 10° and started leveling off at about 20–25° (Fig. 4.10(c)).

4.7 Extracorporeal Circulation

4.7.1 *Cardiopulmonary Bypass*

Figure 4.11 demonstrates an extracorporeal circuit called cardiopulmonary bypass (CPB) used during open heart surgery. Venous blood is removed from the patient using several cannulas and is then pumped directly or *via* a venous reservoir through the oxygenator. If applicable, it is mixed with a part of cardiotomic wound blood. Nowadays, a lot of surgeons do not recirculate this blood because it is highly activated (see Section 4.7.3). The blood flow through the oxygenator is between 3 and 6 l/min. Here, CO_2 is removed from the blood, and oxygen is transported into the blood. Figure 4.12 shows other examples of oxygenators with

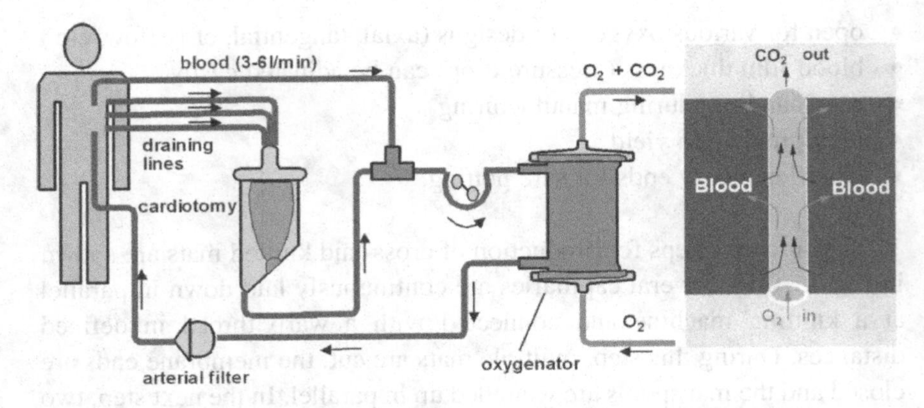

Figure 4.11. Scheme of an oxygenator in a heart–lung machine set up.

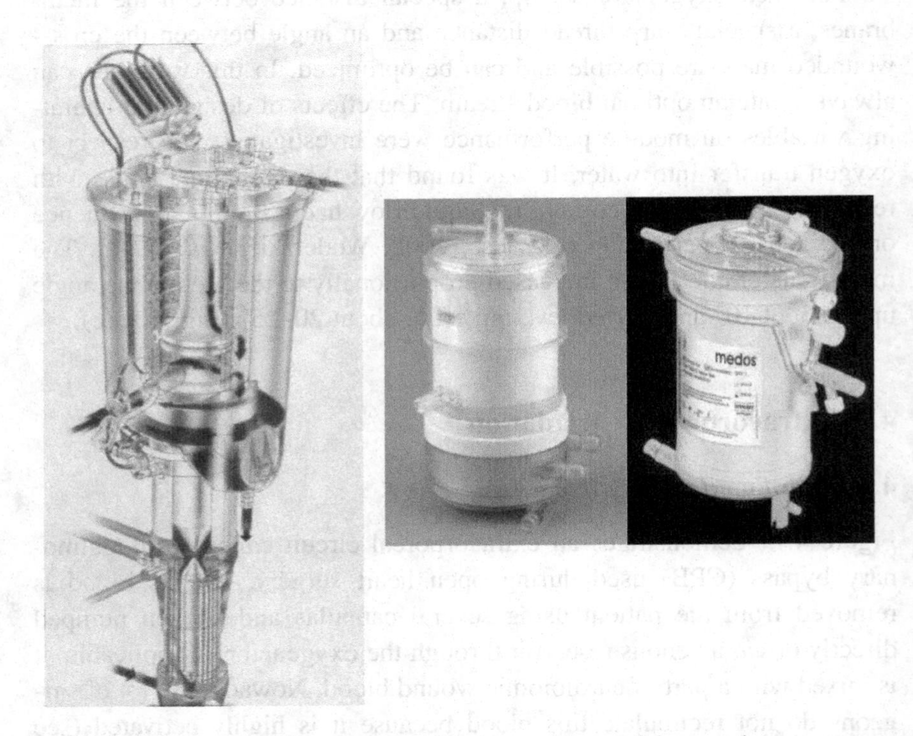

Figure 4.12. Example of an oxygenator set up with metal heat exchanger, venous reservoir, oxygenator and photos of an oxygenator with cross-laid knitted mats inside, heat exchanger bottom side and oxygenator polymer heat exchanger and arterial filter completely integrated.

metal heat exchanger, venous reservoir, oxygenator (left side) and photos of oxygenators with cross-laid knitted mats inside, heat exchanger bottom side (middle) and an oxygenator with polymer heat exchanger and arterial filter completely integrated. In fact, in the last decades, the oxygenators became more and more compact to reduce blood priming volume, pressure drop, contact area, piping, etc.

4.7.2 *Lung Support Systems*

If the native lung is diseased, e.g. by asthma, emphysema or acute respiratory distress syndrome (ARDS), or is injured and thus no longer able to supply the body with sufficient amounts of oxygen, two treatment options exist depending on severity and comorbidities: lung support with oxygen-enriched air or blood oxygenation (ECMO) [Raleigh *et al.*, 2015] or $ECCO_2R$ (extracorporeal CO_2 removal). For the first treatment option, there is need for a mobile oxygen-enriching device, whereas for the second option there is need for a gas exchange membrane suitable for long-term application (several days to weeks). Some membranes described in Section 4.4.2 are suitable for both tasks. In intensive care, ECMO or $ECCO_2R$ is used on acute lung failure (e.g. from virus pneumonia, after blunt trauma [Schmid *et al.*, 2002], following pancreatitis or in conjunction with sepsis or MOF) or for lung failure, e.g. post-transplant, post-OP or in pediatric cases.

An excellent example for a pumpless ECMO device is the Nova lung "membrane ventilator". Two cannulas are connected to big vessels of the patient and by the force of the patient's heart, the blood is pumped through the oxygenator to remove carbon dioxide and/or provide oxygen to the body [Jegger *et al.*, 2004] (see Fig. 4.13(a)). The membrane can even be suitable for use in long-term paracorporeal or implantable artificial lungs, e.g. inside vena cava [Zwischenberger & Alpard, 2002; Zwischenberger *et al.*, 2001]. Figure 4.13(b) shows an intravascular membrane oxygenator (IVOX®), the first venaitercaval device with membranes [Mallabiabarrena Ormaetxea, 2003; Mortensen, 1992].

Comparable devices and oxygenation membrane set ups as described in Sections 4.6 and 4.7 are used in biotechnology and bioartificial organs as "artificial liver" or perfusion in stem cell reactors [Gerlach, 1996; Gerlach *et al.*, 1990; Schmelzer *et al.*, 2015].

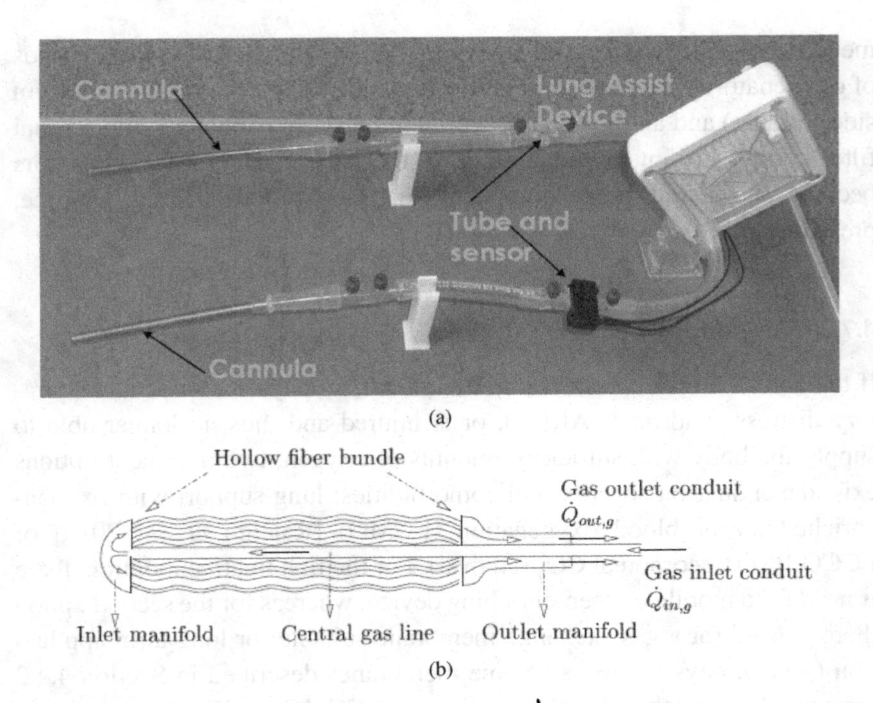

Figure 4.13. (a) Nova lung oxygenator for ECMO application. (b) Implantable lung support setup.

4.7.3 *Biocompatibility*

For the membranes used inside oxygenators in cardiac surgery, biocompatibility is not as such an issue as it is, e.g. in hemodialysis. The major surgical insult of a coronary artery bypass operation or valve replacement with opening of the chest and exposition of the heart undoubtedly has a larger impact to the patient that the biocompatibility of the membrane goes into the background.

Microporous membranes that are capable of providing a sufficient gas exchange performance need to be hydrophobic enough to avoid any plasma entrance into the pores and plasma breakthrough to the gas side. This hydrophobicity inevitably brings about contact phase activation and will lead to cell adhesion to the membrane, as shown in several investigations [Hsu, 1997; Janvier *et al.*, 1996]. Main concerns with the use of oxygenators are the activation of the coagulation cascade, thrombus formation, hemolysis and drops in cell counts. This is more related to the oxygenator set up (see Section 4.6) and the contribution of other components such as heat exchanger, housing, piping, etc. Manufacturers account for this problem by coating the whole circuit with biocompatible coatings like heparin. Every manufacturer has its own proprietary technology. All coatings seem to provide reduced cell adhesion, reduced coagulation and contact phase activation. However, the performance related to biocompatibility of an oxygenator is always a compromise [De Somer, 2013; Stanzel & Henderson, 2016; Stocker & Horton, 2015]. Biocompatibility is more of a concern for extracorporeal circuits used for longer term lung assistance [Marasco *et al.*, 2008].

References

Allen SM, Fujii M, Stannett V, Hopfenberg HB and Williams JL (1977). The barrier properties of polyacrylonitrile. *J Membr Sci*, 2, pp. 153–163.

Alpha D, King E and Bicknell DA (1986). *Proc Am Acad Clin Perform*, 7, pp. 32–34.

Baker RW (2000). *Membrane Technology and Applications* (McGraw-Hill, New York).

Bennett M, Horton S, Thuys C, Augustin S, Rosenberg M and Brizard C (2004). Pump-induced haemolysis: a comparison of short-term ventricular assist devices. *Perfusion-UK*, 19(2), pp. 107–111.

Breiter SM, Wiese F, Wodetzki A and Schuster O (2004). New gas exchange membrane for multiple lung support applications. *ASAIO J*, 50, p. 153.

Castro AJ (1981). US Patent No. 4,247,498.

Catapano G, Hornscheidt R, Wodetzki A and Baurmeister U (2004). Turbulent flow technique for the estimation of oxygen diffusive permeability of membranes for the oxygenation of blood and other cell suspensions. *J Membr Sci*, 230(1–2), pp. 131–139.

Clowes JJ, Hopkins AL and Neville WE (1956). An artificial lung dependent upun diffusion of oxygen and carbon dioxide through plastic membranes. *J Thoracic Surg*, 32(5), pp. 630–637.

De Somer F (2013). Does contemporary oxygenator design influence haemolysis? *Perfusion*, 28, pp. 280–285.

De Wall RA and Lillehei CW (1957). *Surg Gynecol Obstet*, 104, p. 699.

Dierickx PW (2001). Blood flow and gas transport in artificial lungs: *in numero* and *in vitro* analysis (Doctoral thesis). University of Gent.

Dierickx PW, De Somer F, De Wachter DS, Van Nooten G and Verdonck PR (2000). Hydrodynamic characteristics of artificial lungs. *ASAIO J*, 46(5), pp. 532–535.

Gassmann CJ, Galbraith GD and Smith RG (1987). Evaluation of three types of membrane oxygenators and their suitability for use with pulsatile flow. *J Extracorporeal Technol*, 19(3), pp. 297–304.

Gerlach JC (1996). Development of a hybrid liver support system: a review. *J Artif Org*, 19(11), pp. 645–654.

Gerlach JC, Kloppel K, Stoll P, Vienken J and Mulle C (1990). Gas supply across membranes in bioreactors for hepatic culture. *J Artif Org*, 14, pp. 328–222.

Gibbon JH (1937). Artificial maintenance of circulation during experimental occlusion of pulmonary artery. *Arch Surg*, 34(6), pp. 1105–1131.

Henne W, Pelger M, Gerlach K and Tretzel J (1983). Plasma separation and plasma fractionation, Lysaght MJ. (Boston, Mass.) and Gurland HJ. (Munich) (Ed.), In *Membrane technology for plasmapheresis* (Karger AG, Rottach-Egern), pp. 164–179.

Hiatt W, Vitzthum GH, Wagner KB, Gerlach K (1985). Materials science of synthetic membranes, In Douglas R. Lloyd (Ed.), *American Chemical Society*, Washington, DC., pp. 229–244.

Hsu L (1997). Biocompatibility in cardiopulmonary bypass. *J Cardiothoracic Vasc Anesthesia*, 11(3), pp. 376–382.

Janvier G, Baquey C, Roth C, Benillan N, Bélisle S and Hardy J (1996). Extracorporeal circulation, hemocompatibility, and biomaterials. *Ann Thoracic Surg*, 62(6), pp. 1926–1934.

Jegger D, Revelly JP, Horisberger J, Boone Y, Seigneul I, Jachertz M and Segesser von L (2004). *Ex vivo* evaluation of a new extracorporeal lung assist device: novalung membrane oxygenator. In *Paper presented at the ESAO*, Aachen.

Kolff WJ and Balzer BR (1955). *ASAIO Trans*.1, pp. 39–42.

Kolff WJ and Effler DB (1956). *Cleve Clin Q* 23, pp. 69–97.

Kolff WJ, Berk HTJ, Welle NM, van der Ley AJW, van Dijk EC and van Noordwijk J (1944). The artificial kidney: a dialyser with a great area. *Acta Med Scand*, 117(2), pp. 121–134.

Krause B, Göhl H and Wiese F (Eds.) (2006). Medizintechnik. In *Membranen* (Wiley-VCH Verlag GmbH & Co. KGaA, Weinheim), pp. 147–188.

Lauterbach G (2002). *Handbuch der Kardiotechnik* (Urban & Fischer, München).

Le Gallois JJC, Nancrede NC and Nancrede JG (1813). *Experiments on the principle of life and particularly on the principle of the motions of the heart, and on the seat of this principle: including the report made to the first class of the institute, upon the experiments relative to the motions of the heart* (M. Thomas, William Fry, Philadelphia, PA).

Le Gallois JJC, Nancrede JG, Nancrede NC and Percy P (1812). Expériences sur le principe de la vie, nottament sur celui des mouvements du coeur, et sur le siége de ce principe. *Suievies du Rapport fait à la première classe d l'Ínstitut sur celles relatives aux mouvemens du coeur* (D'Hautel, Paris), pp. 134–135.

Lillehei CW (1955). Controlled cross circulation for direct-vision intracardiac surgery: correction of ventricular septal defects, atrioventricularis communis, and tetralogy of Fallot. *Postgrad Med*, 17(5), pp. 388–396.

Mallabiabarrena Ormaetxea I (2003). Thèse École polytechnique fédérale de Lausanne EPFL. Retrieved from http://infoscience.epfl.ch/record/33348.

Mallabiabarrena Ormaetxea I (2004). Experimental set-up and numerical simulations of intravenous gas transfer devices. EPFL. Retrieved from http://infoscience.epfl.ch/record/33348.

Marasco SF, Lukas G, McDonald M, McMillan J and Ihle B (2008). Review of ECMO (extracorporeal membrane oxygenation) support in critically ill adult patients. *Heart Lung Circ*, 17, pp. S41–S47.

Mockros LF and Leonard R (1985). Compact cross-flow tubular oxygenators. *ASAIO J*, 31(1), pp. 628–633.

Mortensen JD (1992). Intravascular oxygenator: a new alternative method for augmenting blood gas transfer in patients with acute respiratory failure. *Artif Org*, 16(1), pp. 75–82.

Nunes SP and Peinemann KV (Eds.) (2001). Gas separation with membranes. In *Membrane technology* (Wiley-VCH Verlag GmbH), pp. 39–67.

Philipp A, Foltan M, Gietl M, Reng M, Liebold A, Kobuch R… Birnbaum D E. (2003). Interventionelle extrakorporale Lungenunterstützung (ILA) mittels arterio-venösem Shunt und einem neu entwickelten Low Resistance Lung Assistance Device (LAD). *Kardiotechnik*, 12(1), pp. 7–13.

Raleigh L, Ha R and Hill C (2015). Extracorporeal membrane oxygenation applications in cardiac critical care. *Sem Cardiothoracic Vasc Anesthesia*, 19(4), pp. 342–352.

Schmelzer E, Finoli A, Nettleship I and Gerlach JC (2015). Long-term three-dimensional perfusion culture of human adult bone marrow mononuclear cells in bioreactors. *Biotechnol Bioeng*, 112(4), pp. 801–810.

Schmid FX, Philipp A, Link J, Zimmermann M and Birnbaum DE (2002). Hybrid management of aortic rupture and lung failure: pumpless extracorporeal lung assist and endovascular stent-graft. *Ann Thoracic Surg*, 73(5), pp. 1618–1620.

Schmidt A (1867). Die Atmung innerhalb des Blutes. Zweite Abhandlung. aus dem physiologischen Institut zu Leipzig. *Berichte über die Verhandlungen der königlich sächsischen Gesellschaft der Wissenschaften zu Leipzig. Mathematisch–physische Classe*, 19, pp. 99–130, Leipzig.

Severinghaus JW (1979). Simple, accurate equations for human blood O_2 dissociation computations. *J Appl Physiol*, 46(3), pp. 599–602.

Stanzel RD and Henderson M (2016). Clinical evaluation of contemporary oxygenators. *Perfusion*, 31(1), pp. 15–25.

Stocker CF and Horton SB (2015). Anticoagulation strategies and difficulties in neonatal and paediatric extracorporeal membrane oxygenation (ECMO). *Perfusion*.

Taylor KM (1986). *Cardiopulmonary bypass: principles & management* (Lippincott Williams & Wilkins, Philadelphia, PA).

Tschaut RJ (1999). *Extrakorporale zirkulation in der theorie und praxis* (Pabst Science Publishers, Lengerich).

Vaslef SN, Mockros LF, Anderson RW and Leonard RJ (1994). Use of a mathematical model to predict oxygen transfer rates in hollow fiber membrane oxygenators. *ASAIO J*, 40(4), pp. 990–996.

Wicksramasinghe SR, Semmens MJ and Cussler EL (1992). *Hollow fiber for liquid–liquid extraction* (Elsevier, London).

Wiese F (2008). Membranes for artificial lungs. In *Membranes for the life sciences* KV, Peinemann, S, Nunes, publisher Wiley, ISBN: 978-3-527-31480-5, (Wiley-VCH Verlag GmbH & Co. KGaA, Weinheim), pp. 49–68.

Wiese F, Paul D, Possart W, Malsch G and Bossin E (1990). Grenzfläuchenenergie gequollener polymermembranen. *Acta Polym*, 41(2), pp. 95–98.

Wodetzki A, Breiter S, Scheuren J, Jeuck H and Wiese F (2000). OXYPHAN®, the world-wide leading oxygenation membrane. *Jpn Membr J*, 25(3), pp. 102–106.

Zwischenberger JB and Alpard SK (2002). Artificial lungs: a new inspiration. *Perfusion*, 17(4), pp. 253–268.

Zwischenberger JB, Anderson CM, Cook KE, Lick SD, Mockros LF and Bartlett RH (2001). Development of an implantable artificial lung: challenges and progress. *ASAIO J*, 47(4), pp. 316–320.

Chapter 5
Membranes for Bioartificial Kidney Devices

N. Chevtchik*, P. Caetano Pinto[†],
R. Masereeuw[†] and D. Stamatialis*,[‡]

** Faculty of Science and Technology,
Biomaterials Science and Technology Department,
MIRA Institute, University of Twente, The Netherlands*
*[†] Division Pharmacology, Department of Pharmaceutical Sciences,
Utrecht Institute for Pharmaceutical Sciences, Utrecht University,
Utrecht, The Netherlands*
[‡] d.stamatialis@ utwente.nl

5.1 Introduction

The kidneys play a fundamental role in maintaining whole-body homeostasis and are responsible for several physiological processes, including the production of hormones and the regulation of blood pressure, by controlling fluid volume in the body and keeping physiological pH by maintaining appropriate acid–base homeostasis. Kidneys are also responsible for nutrient re-absorption. At the heart of renal function are their excretory capabilities that account for the kidneys' blood purification function. Drugs, metabolic byproducts, endogenous wastes and environmental toxins, together named xenobiotics, are among the many compounds that are removed from systemic circulation by the kidneys, *via* urine production [Nigam *et al.*, 2015; Konig *et al.*, 2013; Hoenig & Zeidel, 2014]. In severe renal diseases, either chronic kidney disease (CKD) or end-stage renal disease (ESRD), a break-down in renal function leads to the accumulation of xenobiotics in the body, which subsequently results in disease progression. Moreover, sudden breakdown in renal function, termed acute kidney injury (AKI), is sometimes irreversible and can lead to the patient's death.

The current treatment for AKI, CKD and ESRD patients is mainly hemodialysis (described in Chapters 2 and 3). Hemodialysis only covers a fraction of the physiological renal function and its efficiency in waste removal is incomplete [Vanholder *et al.*, 2003a, 2003b]. Indeed, most of the large solutes and protein-bound toxins cannot be removed. Their accumulation is strongly linked to the fatal outcome of the patients [Vanholder *et al.*, 2014; Barreto *et al.*, 2009]. There is, therefore, a strong need for a device, extracorporeal or implantable, which could mimic and/or replace fully the kidney function.

In recent years, the research around bioartificial kidneys and bioengineered renal replacement therapies (RRTs) has brought together different disciplines, combining technical expertise with cellular and molecular biology. Different from organ regeneration, this research is focused on the creation of devices that can mimic (partially) the function of a healthy kidney. Such devices could be a hybrid combination of polymeric membranes and renal proximal tubule cells, called either the bioartificial kidney (BAK), renal assist device (RAD) or bioartificial renal tubule device (BTD). This chapter focusses on the role of artificial polymeric membranes for the development of these devices.

5.2 Renal Function

5.2.1 *Renal Tubular Function*

The kidney is composed of filtration units called nephrons (Fig. 5.1). In the nephron, blood initially passes through the glomerulus where its capillary network significantly increases pressure, causing filtration of small- and middle-size solutes and removing excess fluid out of the blood by convection. This glomerular filtrate is then transferred to the proximal tubules, which are responsible for re-absorbing essential components of

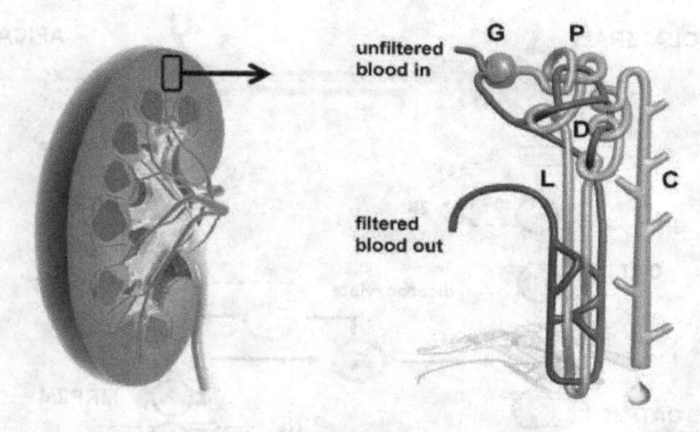

Figure 5.1. Renal physiology. A cross-section of the human kidney (left) which approximately consists of 1 million nephrons (right), the functional components of this organ. (Right) Unfiltered blood will enter the glomerulus (G) and small solutes and H_2O will be excreted *via* ultrafiltration into Bowman's space, which is contiguous with the lumen of the proximal tubule. Subsequently, PTECs (P) mediate re-absorption of H_2O and compounds such as amino acids, glucose and albumin from the filtered fraction, next to the active excretion of endo- and xenobiotics into the pro-urine. In addition, 65% of the total amount of electrolytes will be re-absorbed *via* paracellular pathways. Downstream of the proximal tubule segment, the loop of Henle (L), the distal convoluted tubule (D) and collecting tubule and duct cells (C) are localized. In brief, these cell types are equipped with specific water and ion channels involved in the homeostasis of water and electrolyte balance, finally contributing to homeostasis. Reproduced and adapted from Jansen *et al.* [2014a] with the permission of Elsevier.

the pre-urine but also for additional removal of a great variety of solutes and wastes from the blood stream, among which, the protein-bound toxins.

To this end, proximal tubule epithelial cells (PTECs) are equipped with highly specialized molecular machinery (Fig. 5.2). These polarized cells act as a barrier that compounds have to cross from the basolateral (capillary) side to the apical (pre-urine) side. The functional characteristics of PTECs are derived to a great extent from the presence of multiple, energy-dependent membrane transporters (carrier proteins) that mediate the transport of ions, small molecules, nucleotides, xenobiotics and other substances. These transporters can move solutes against steep concentration gradients and provide the cells their barrier-specific selectivity and high excretion capacity.

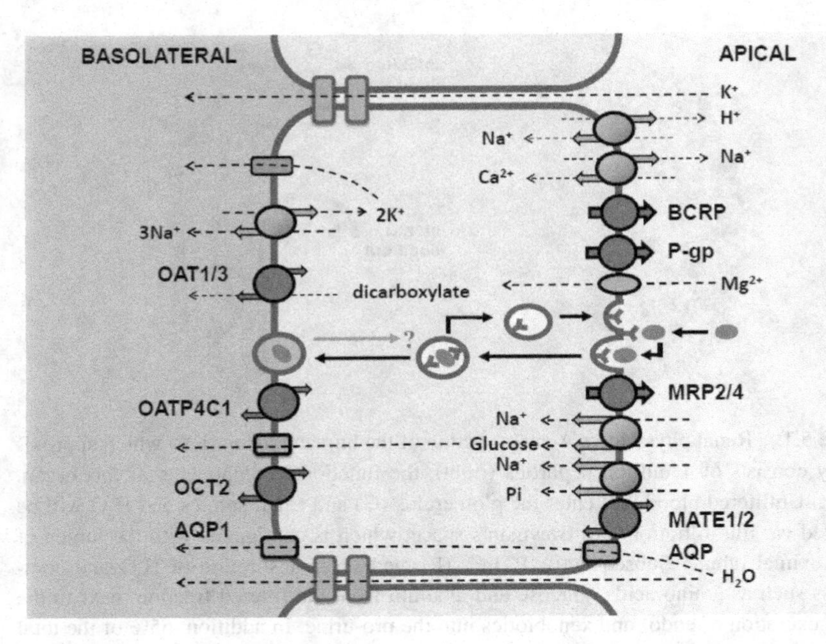

Figure 5.2. Schematic representation of the major basolateral and apical membrane transport systems in renal proximal tubule cells. Re-absorption mechanisms and drug transporters are presented.

The transporters of PTECs can be unidirectional efflux pumps, co-transporters, facilitated diffusion carriers and exchangers, belonging to either the adenosine triphosphate (ATP) binding cassette (ABC) [Vasiliou *et al.*, 2009] superfamily or the solute carrier family (SLC; www.slc.bioparadigms.org) of proteins [International Transporter *et al.*, 2010]. Function of ABC transporters requires ATP hydrolysis, a feature that has enabled PTECs to develop an increased mitochondrial activity to meet the energy demand. Activity of SLC transporters involves co-transport driven by the membrane potential, established by the basolaterally expressed Na/K-ATPase. Basolateral and apical transporters are complementary in substrate specificity to enable compounds that are taken up by the cells to be excreted subsequently [El-Sheikh *et al.*, 2013].

A comprehensive depiction of all major PTEC transporters is presented in Fig. 5.2. The most prominent uptake transporters are the organic anion transporter 1 (OAT1; *SLC22A6*), organic anion transporter 3 (OAT3; *SLC22A8*) [Hagos & Wolff, 2010] and organic cation transporter 2 (OCT2;

SLC22A2) [Motohashi & Inui, 2013]. The predominant efflux transporters are the breast cancer resistance protein (BCRP; *ABCG2*) [Huls *et al.*, 2008], P-glycoprotein (P-gp; *ABCB1*) and the multi-drug resistance proteins 2 and 4 (MRP2/4; *ABCC2/4*) [Russel *et al.*, 2008]. Other carriers, such as the transporter OAT polypeptide (OATP4C1; *SLCO4C1*), and the multi-drug and toxin extrusion 1 and 2 transporters (MATE1 and 2K; *SLC47A1-2K*) are also present at PTECs. These transporters share common regulatory pathways, and their functional expression can be influenced by drugs and external factors. After uptake, PTECs can also metabolize drugs and compounds *via* phase I and II enzymes, in a process that can increase the excretory efficacy of certain compounds [Lohr *et al.*, 1998]. An elegant example of the relevance of this process is the fact that glucuronidation augments substrate affinity for multi-drug resistance proteins (MRPs) and incidentally MRP4 is highly expressed in the apical membrane of PTECs [Gaganis *et al.*, 2007; El-Sheikh *et al.*, 2014]. Active membrane transport at the basolateral side also facilitates the removal of compounds that are bound to plasma proteins in blood. In fact, a great variety of toxins and drugs are transported in the blood stream coupled to plasma proteins, like albumin. Those protein-bound molecules can only be removed from the circulation *via* active membrane transport.

In addition to xenobiotic excretion, PTECs also play an extensive role in the re-absorption of nutrients and ions back into the blood stream, a process initiated from the apical (luminal) side (Fig. 5.2). An important re-uptake mechanism is receptor-mediated endocytosis. In this mechanism, proteins with different sizes, which initially pass through the glomerulus, can be shuttled back from the filtrate to circulation, mediated by three receptors expressed at the apical membrane, megalin, cubilin and amnionless [Nielsen *et al.*, 2016]. A number of key ions are also re-absorbed, although this process is not exclusive to PTECs, but can also take place along other segments of the nephrons and occurs passively with the high amount of water that diffuses back to the circulation or *via* a number of membrane carriers that handle, e.g. potassium (K^+), magnesium (Mg^{2+}), calcium (Ca^{2+}), phosphate (PO_4^{3-}) [Huang & Miller, 2007; Palmer & Sackin, 1988]. In addition, glucose is re-absorbed exclusively by PTECs *via* Na^{2+}-dependent co-transporters (*SLC5A* family members) [Rahmoune *et al.*, 2005]. Furthermore, the lumen of the proximal tubules is convoluted where the apical side of PTECs is organized into dense microvilli that form a brush border, a feature that provides an increased surface area of the membrane to enhance the re-absorption processes. Throughout the nephrons, continuous water re-absorption is facilitated by selective water channels known as aquaporins (AQP), with different channels expressed in the proximal tubules, loop of Henle and collecting duct [Xing *et al.*, 2014]. Although renal function derives from the actions of the different nephron segments, PTECs are key, since their activity account for a significant part of xenobiotic excretion.

5.2.2 *Renal Dysfunction*

More than 10% of the worldwide population is estimated to present a more or less severe form of kidney disease [Hill *et al.*, 2016; Mehta *et al.*, 2015; Zuk & Bonventre, 2016]. Population ageing and the combination of various factors such as genetic pre-disposition, diabetes or cardiovascular diseases lead to the deterioration of kidney function and the development or progression of CKD. In addition, the ingestion of nephrotoxic agents, such as recreational or medicinal drugs, and intravascular contrast-phase agents induces further progression of the disease, or can cause a brutal loss of kidney function [Hoste *et al.*, 2015; KDIGO, 2012]. Table 5.1 presents a classification of the stages of kidney disease based on KDIGO guidelines [KDIGO, 2013a].

The stage of kidney disease is expressed based on the glomerular filtration rate (GFR). The GFR is calculated from the concentration of serum creatinine and several other markers in urine and/or plasma. CKD or chronic renal failure (CRF) is diagnosed in case of a low GFR for a prolonged period of time. The kidney function in CKD patients progressively and irreversibly declines until total loss, or ESRD. In this case, the patients require a permanent RRT. According to Fresenius Medical Care report [Fresenius, 2013]: "The number of patients being treated for ESRD globally was estimated to be 3.2 million at the end of 2013 and, with a ~6% growth rate, continues to increase at higher rate than the world population". According to Hedgeman *et al.* [2015], "population prevalence estimates of CKD stages 3–5 in adults ranged from approximately 1 to 9%". For these patients, a palliative RRT is frequently proposed in developed countries.

Table 5.1: Classification of CKD progression, according to KDOQI CKD guidelines [KDIGO, 2013b].

Stages of CKD of all types		
Stage	Qualitative description	Renal function (mL/min/1.73 m^2)
1	Kidney damage — normal GFR	≥90
2	Kidney damage, mild ↓ GFR	60–89
3	Moderate ↓ GFR	30–59
4	Severe ↓ GFR	15–29
5	ESRD	<15 (or dialysis)

GFR: glomerular filtration rate.

A brutal loss of the kidney function is the AKI or acute renal failure (ARF). In this case, immediate renal therapy is urgently required [KDIGO, 2012]. AKI remains a major unmet medical need and a global public health concern impacting ~13.3 million patients per year [Mehta *et al.*, 2015]. AKI occurs in half of the intensive care patients. Although it is reversible most of the time, the patients have worse renal function at the time of hospital discharge, and 42% of them may develop CKD [Hoste *et al.*, 2015]. Moreover, although direct causality between AKI and death has been controversial, increasing AKI severity — classified based on the serum creatinine and the urine output [KDIGO, 2012] — is associated with morbidity, increased costs and mortality — about 1.7 million deaths per year.

5.2.3 *Existing RRTs and Their Limitations*

Figure 5.3 presents the schemes of the three current RRTs. The most popular therapy is kidney transplantation from deceased or living donors. Indeed, in the case of a successful transplantation, the kidney function is fully replaced and the quality of life of the patient is almost back to normal. More than 75,000 patients worldwide receive a kidney transplant yearly [GODT, 2014]. However, not all of the kidney patients are eligible, for example, in case of comorbidities a transplantation is not possible. Moreover, the success of the therapy is not total: after 10 years, about 50% of the transplanted kidneys are still functional [National Kidney

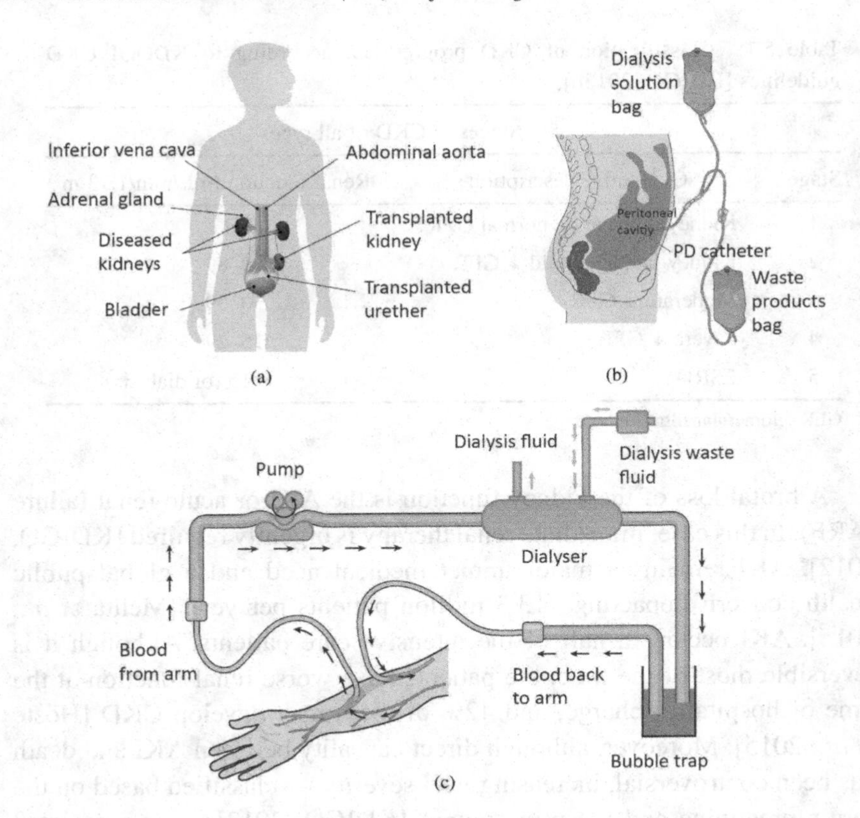

Figure 5.3. Schematic presentation of the three available RRTs. (a) Kidney transplant. The transplanted donor organ is implemented in the patient while both affected kidneys will remain in the body. A donor organ is the preferred treatment option for patients suffering from ESRD. (b) Peritoneal dialysis. During PD, a permanent tube will be connected to the patients' abdomen, and the peritoneum will be used as a membrane which allow for the removal of small waste products from the blood into the dialysis waste fluid. Peritoneal home-dialysis is possible as long as infections are suppressed and the quality of the peritoneum is maintained. (c) Hemodialysis. For hemodialysis, vascular access can be accomplished *via* three ways: (i) a central venous catheter; (ii) an arteriovenous fistula which is a surgical connection between an artery and a vein to achieve a suitable access point; or (iii) an arteriovenous graft which is a biocompatible tube surgically connected between an artery and a vein. The patients' blood will pass the dialyzer, which consists of numerous hollow fiber membranes, and ultrafiltration process occur. During dialysis, small waste products will be removed from the blood into the dialysis waste fluid and the filtered blood will return to the patient. In general, HD is performed three times a week and 4 h per session, often in a dialysis center or hospital. Reprinted and adapted from Jansen [2016] with the permission of the author.

Foundation, 2016b]. Besides, even after transplantation, patients have medical need for immunosuppressive therapy, which leads to a number of side effects.

The major limitation of transplantation remains the availability of organs. The waiting list varies per country and region, but is about 3–5 years. In 2016, the number of patients registered on the waiting list for receiving a kidney transplant was 10,900 in Europe [Eurotransplant, 2016] vs more than 100,000 in the USA [National Kidney Foundation, 2016a].

Patients who are not eligible for transplantations or registered on a waiting list for a transplant whose residual renal function (RRF) is insufficient — as well as AKI and ESRD patients — require other therapies such as peritoneal dialysis (PD) and/or hemodialysis (HD).

In PD, the peritoneum of the patient is used as a filtration membrane. This therapy can be used as ambulatory or home dialysis, which presents the advantage of a continuous filtration (in case of home-dialysis). Despite this, only 8.5% of the ESRD patients are treated with PD. HD is widely preferred [Fresenius, 2013] due to the high prevalence of catheter access problems and peritonitis episodes for the PD therapy. These complications often lead to ultrafiltration failure and volume overload of the patients. In addition, even in the absence of complications, the use of glucose as an osmotic agent in PD solutions damages the peritoneum quickly, after 1–2 years. For these reasons, more than 35% of the PD patients switch to HD within 2 years after the beginning of the treatment [Chaudhary, 2011]. More importantly, due to the intrinsic property of the peritoneum, only small-size solutes are being cleared.

HD remains the most common therapy, applied for 2.2 million patients worldwide [Fresenius, 2013]. They undergo HD 3–4 times a week, for a 3–4 h session in a hospital. Shorter dialysis times, chosen for budgetary and logistics reasons, have been associated with higher mortality among patients. In fact, dialysis sessions less than 4 h have been associated with a 42% increase in mortality [Brunelli *et al.*, 2010; Flythe *et al.*, 2013; Lacson & Brunelli, 2011]. To palliate this problem, home-HD is being developed for longer treatment sessions, preferably at night. However, the risk of infections and the fragility of the vascular access remain major issues, as well as the logistics for pure water production and storage of disposables [Karkar *et al.*, 2015].

For in center-HD as well as for home-HD, the size and range of toxins being removed are limited. Indeed, only small water-soluble molecules, <40 kDa, present in free fraction in the blood, can be eliminated [Vanholder *et al.*, 2015]. Research is ongoing to further improve existing techniques by varying parameters such as flow rates, membrane permeability and surface area, and combining diffusion, convection and/or adsorption mechanisms [Eloot *et al.*, 2014]. Molecules up to 200 kDa can be removed *via* adsorption, which is more solute-specific rather than size-specific. Protein-bound toxins can also be targeted *via* adsorption. For example, multi-layered mixed matrix membranes (MMMs) using activated carbon for the removal of protein-bound toxins have been developed in the recent years [Pavlenko *et al.*, 2016; Tijink *et al.*, 2012, 2013, 2014]. More details about the HD and MMMs are described in Chapters 2 and 3, respectively.

5.2.4 *The Need for a more Complete RRT — The BAK*

Several studies have established a direct link between the concentration of protein-bound toxins — namely indoxyl sulfate and paracresol sulfate — and cardiovascular events and/or mortality in ESRD patients [Barreto *et al.*, 2009; Meijers *et al.*, 2010]. These toxins are, in large part, handled by the proximal tubules [Schophuizen *et al.*, 2013] and, although traditional dialysis is able to remove small water-soluble toxins, the protein-bound solutes can only be removed through the biological processes inherent to PTECs [Masereeuw *et al.*, 2014; Vanholder *et al.*, 2015]. Besides, dialysis is removing a part of the toxin population but is not replacing the kidney endocrine and metabolic physiological functions. Therefore, the BAK, thanks to the use of PTECs, appears as a possible solution to bring a more complete kidney replacement therapy.

The requirements for a BAK should be the following:

(1) The cells used should be functional, from human origin, with a high availability and stability in time. These cells should form a tight monolayer to be functional and act as a barrier against the loss of components. The production of pro-inflammatory cytokines should be minimal and preferably oriented toward the waste compartment.

(2) The cells should be supported by a permeable membrane that is cytocompatible on one side and hemocompatible on the other. The membrane should allow, on the one hand, the passage of nutrients and toxins to the cells from the blood compartment, and, on the other hand, release of hormones, vitamins and other beneficial solutes into the patient's body fluid. It should also not evoke an immune response.
(3) The whole device has to be adequately designed to support cell growth and function. The device should allow gas exchange, and pH, pressure and temperature control. Moreover, it should remain stable in practice, including during transport and storage, as well as being cost-efficient.

The BAK is conceived to be used in combination with a classical hemofilter [Humes *et al.*, 1999; Song & Humes, 2009]. In this way, there is a direct similitude with the natural kidney. First, the glomerular function is replaced by the classical HD for removal of small-size, water-soluble molecules. Second, the glomerular filtrate, which comes out of the HD module, can be processed by the proximal tubules of the BAK. As explained in Section 5.2.1, the BAK should replace not only the excretory function to eliminate the protein-bound and larger-size toxins, but also the essential endocrine and metabolic functions of the kidney.

Figure 5.4 shows the composition of a BAK. It commonly has the configuration of a classical module for HD. The hollow fiber membrane (HFM) bioreactor presents the advantage of a three-dimensional configuration, close to the natural PTEC configuration within the kidney. This model has, therefore, the advantage of a simple extracorporeal circuit, but due to the presence of cells, its fabrication under conditions compliant to good manufacturing practice (GMP) conditions, storage and transport should be planned and organized carefully in case of clinical applications. The action of the system relies entirely on the integrity and function of the cell monolayer. It is, therefore, important to develop non-destructive testing for these devices and obviously to choose the appropriate cells (see Section 5.3).

5.3 Cells for Bioartificial Kidney

Renal cells can perform and regulate, with extreme efficiency, highly complex and specific chemical and physical processes simultaneously.

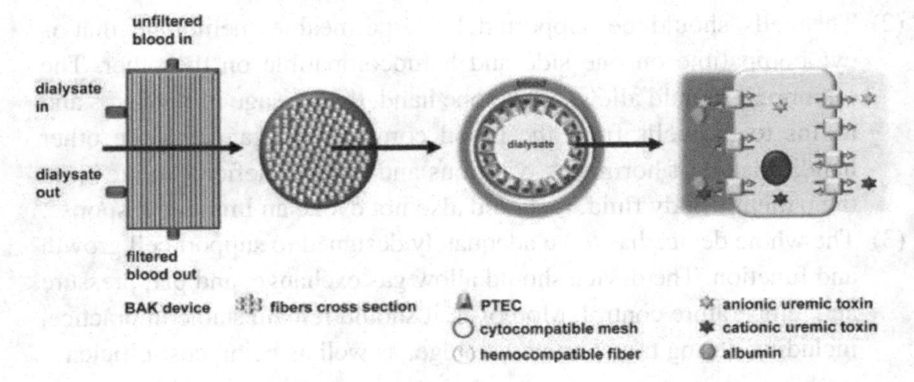

Figure 5.4. BAK composition and mechanism. Separated inlets and outlets for the patient's blood and the dialysate are incorporated in a BAK. The device will consist of numerous [hemocompatible HFM]. The inner surface of the HFM will be modified in order to induce cytocompatibility to stimulate monolayer integrity. A homogeneous and polarized cell monolayer will stimulate excretion of endo- and xenobiotics (e.g. protein-bound uremic toxins) and re-absorption of solutes (e.g. phosphate). Importantly, host albumin and IgG components will be retained due to appropriate molecular cut-off values of the membrane. Furthermore, potential metabolic and endocrine functions of the cells can contribute to an improved homeostasis of the patient. Preprinted from Jansen *et al.* [2014a] with the permission of Elsevier.

Harnessing and exploiting cells to study renal physiology and bioengineered kidneys is central in this line of investigation. Nowadays, a variety of renal-derived cell types are available from different sources and are used in fundamental bioengineered kidney research. A fundamental aspect of culturing cells *in vitro* is assuring that the cells retain a phenotype that closely resembles the *in vivo* situation.

Cells can drastically change their properties while being in culture, due to the artificial environment. Cellular plasticity allows cells to change their gene and protein expressions as well as their metabolic activity when confronted with an artificial environment. *In vitro*, cells are grown on flat plastic surfaces, fed with a cocktail of nutrients and factors (culture medium) and maintained in a humidified environment at physiological temperature. *In vivo*, cells are arranged in three-dimensional structures often containing multiple cell types that cross-talk and are nourished from the blood stream. Culture medium composition can be tailored to maintain tissue-specific phenotypes; however, the addition of growth factor and serum, often required to maintain proliferation, can influence chromosome stability and can lead to gene mutations, affecting the phenotype of the cells [Griffith & Swartz, 2006]. To monitor whether cells maintain their phenotype, an array of assays and techniques has to be performed.

When growing PTECs *in vitro*, it is key to determine whether the specific molecular machinery of this cell type is expressed at the gene and protein levels. It is also important to determine the proper morphology, capability of the cells to polarize, tight monolayer formation, generation of the appropriate membrane potential and selective barrier function. Subsequently, it is crucial to evaluate the functional activity of the cells, ensuring recapitulation of the activities of native PTECs.

5.3.1 *Primary Cells*

Primary cells are directly derived from renal tissue or urine, collected from healthy donors (either through a biopsy or from a discarded kidney transplant). The renal tissue is then disaggregated into a heterogeneous cell suspension that is purified further *via* flow cytometry or magnetic beads, making use of membrane markers in order to isolate PTECs from other cell types. Afterward, cells can be cultured and characterized to confirm the cell phenotype. These primary cells retain the PTEC phenotype only temporarily, losing their epithelial characteristics with each population doubling in culture and their use is limited to the availability of donors [Presnell *et al.*, 2011]. Due to these limitations, primary cells are not a preferred source for long-term applications and are mostly used for cellular and molecular research into the inner works of PTECs, as well as for drug efficacy and safety testing. An alternative source of PTEC cells also explored is urine [Jansen *et al.*, 2014b; Wilmer *et al.*, 2010b]. Being easily accessible, urine is an abundant source of cells, and incidentally PTECs are shed in reasonable numbers.

5.3.2 *Stem Cells*

Another primary cell source is stem or progenitor cells for which cells can be derived also from tissues other than the kidney. Stem cells are undifferentiated cells that can, on one hand, self-regenerate and, on the other, give rise to various terminally differentiated cell types [Vats *et al.*, 2002]. These cells are found in developing embryos, being pluripotent (able to generate any lineage) at earlier stages. As embryonic development progresses, stem cells differentiate into particular tissue lineages and gradually occupy specific niches. Stem cells can be isolated using specific membrane markers and cultured under defined conditions, they can be expanded without losing their properties or they can differentiate upon specific inducers [Klingemann *et al.*, 2008]. As with primary cells, stem cells are also limited by donor availability. They can be collected from embryos, which is directly associated with the additional challenge of being a highly controversial ethical issue and quite limited source. Alternatively, stem cells can be derived from adults, mainly from blood, bone marrow and adipose tissue. The latter source is the least invasive and relatively most abundant. However, the biggest bottleneck in the use of these cells is the differentiation *in vitro*, which is a time- and resource-consuming process for which adequate PTEC phenotype still needs to be demonstrated. Nonetheless, stem cells have the promise of providing an autologous cell source for biomedical research applications and can potentially be expanded in large quantities.

5.3.3 *Induced Pluripotent Stem Cells*

A cell type that was introduced less than a decade ago is induced pluripotent stem cell (iPS), which have now made their way to the spotlight of cellular research. The technique to produce this new type of cells bypasses the issues with limited sources since they can be derived from somatic cells [Freedman & Steinman, 2015]. Furthermore, the cells can differentiate into virtually any cell type in the body, hence subscribing their pluripotency. These iPS cells are generated by introducing a specific factor in adult cells (terminally differentiated) that will trigger the cells to re-arrange their genetic program and change their phenotype into undifferentiated stem-like cells, in a process labeled trans-differentiation. Several factors, namely pluripotency encoding genes, have been identified, and novel delivery vectors have been explored to prevent the use of viral transfection.

Human iPS cells have been obtained from fibroblasts and other sources, and kidney organoids grown from such cells formed functional

PTECs [Takasato *et al.*, 2015]. iPS cells are a potential source of autologous cells; however, their use and generation are still a laborious process. Cells trans-differentiated using viral vectors may not be appropriate for clinical use. The use of ectopic transcription factors can be potentially tumorigenic, and an incomplete re-programing compromises the cells pluripotency [Medvedev *et al.*, 2010; Pleniceanu *et al.*, 2010]. As renal-derived iPS cells become a reality, comprehensive validation is needed to confirm the cell function and determine the correct phenotype [Freedman & Steinman, 2015].

5.3.4 *Cell Lines*

Cell lines are also a prominent source of renal cells that usually originate from a primary cell culture that is transformed to enable prolonged culturing while maintaining the cell-type-specific phenotypical properties. These cells are widely used in research and can be obtained commercially or generated in an adequate facility, both for research or commercial uses. Drug screening and fundamental research into kidney pharmacology and physiology are important applications for kidney-derived cell lines. Two commonly used kidney cell lines, and examples of early developments in this area, are the Human embryonic kidney 293 (HEK293) and the Human kidney 2 (HK-2) cells.

HEK293 cells are derived from primary cultures of human embryonic kidney cells and transduced by adenovirus particles to achieve sustainable cell growth *in vitro* [Stepanenko & Dmitrenko, 2015]. Although originally derived from human renal tissue, these cells show abnormal chromosomes and lack a defined phenotype (namely the transport machinery characteristic of PTECs), while culture conditions for optimal proliferation are well established [Jenkinson *et al.*, 2012]. HEK293 cells are easy to transfect, stimulating their use in cellular research study protein expression on a molecular level.

HK-2 are derived from human primary PTEC cultures transfected with the human papilloma virus 16 E6/E7 genes (HPV) in order to obtain a stable cell line [Ryan *et al.*, 1994]. These cells express several enzymes present in primary PTECs along with certain functional aspects, such as glucose uptake. However, the HK-2 cells do not entirely resemble a PTEC phenotype and show, at most, residual active transport activity of xenobiotics [Jenkinson *et al.*, 2012; Sun *et al.*, 2011]. These early generations of renal cell lines underline the problems with generating a cell that is well defined in terms of phenotype and that retains key features of differentiated cells.

Non-human cell lines, isolated from mammals, are also widely applied. The Madin–Darby canine kidney (MDCK) cells retain a strong epithelial phenotype and are simple to culture [Dukes *et al.*, 2011]. Pig-derived LLC-PK1 cells also possess a well-characterized PTEC phenotype [Nielsen *et al.*, 1998]. Nevertheless, these cells have contributed to elucidate the cellular and molecular mechanisms involved in renal physiology and pathophysiology and also paved the way for more advanced and complex *in vitro* models that are becoming of increasing importance.

5.3.5 *Conditionally Immortalized Cell Lines*

In recent years, the amount of cell lines generated has increased as a consequence of improved molecular techniques, the need for more representative and well-defined cells and also in an attempt for refining or replacing the use of animals in research. A handful of cell lines has been developed relying on immortalization tools that reduce genetic variability, thereby improving the stability of the cells, largely for purposes of renal *in vitro* pathophysiology and drug safety testing.

The renal PTEC line (RPTEC) and NKi-2 cell lines were generated by overexpressing the human telomerase reverse transcriptase (hTERT) *via* viral transfection. This transformation allows the cells to maintain their intact chromosomes after every doubling, resulting in stable lines [DesRochers *et al.*, 2013; Simon-Friedt *et al.*, 2015; Wilmer *et al.*, 2016]. Functionally, the cells express metabolic enzymes, including esterase and glucuronidase [Mutsaers *et al.*, 2013], and are used as an *in vitro* model for kidney toxicity studies with emphasis on drug screening [Wilmes *et al.*, 2015]. These cells were non-invasively harvested and can be cultured *in vitro*. Subsequently, the cells are transformed to grow in a sustained way and characterized to confirm a PTEC phenotype. Conditionally immortalized human proximal tubule cells (ciPTEC) are a type of PTEC cells generated by overexpressing the simian virus 40 large T tsA58 antigen (SV40T) together with hTERT [Wilmer *et al.*, 2010b]. These transformations enable the cells to proliferate at a temperature of 33°C and subsequently mature at 37°C, inactivating the large T antigen and acquiring a differentiated PTEC phenotype. ciPTEC can be derived both from urine or adult renal tissue [Jansen *et al.*, 2014b; Wilmer *et al.*, 2010b] and functionally express OCT2, BCRP, P-gp and MRP4, key drug transporters that are native to PTECs. Consequently, the cells are sensitive to nephrotoxic drugs and can extrude protein-bound uremic toxins [Mutsaers *et al.*, 2015; Schophuizen *et al.*, 2013]. These cells can be grown abundantly and are functional after high population doublings. Arguably, cells derived from urine are different from cells derived from tissue; the fact they were shed from the proximal tubule epithelium can indicate a loss in functionality. Nonetheless, ciPTEC derived from both urine and kidney biopsies, and immortalized according to the same procedure, show similar gene expressions, membrane transport functions and enzyme activities, supporting the validity of urine-derived PTECs [Jansen *et al.*, 2014b].

5.3.6 *Cell Models — Challenges and Perspectives*

The concept of a bioartificial device that combines the properties of cells and membranes was pioneered by growing MDCK cells and pig kidney epithelial cells (LCC-PK1) on permeable membranes impregnated with matrigel (extracellular matrix extracted from mouse sarcoma) [Ip *et al.*, 1988]. This strategy proved that cells can confer selectivity and maintain transport function when grown on an artificial membrane. Further studies used human or porcine kidney cells seeded into modified hemofiltration cartridges to recover kidney function in uremic animals [Humes *et al.*, 2002]. These early approaches revealed that cellular properties can be harnessed to improve dialysis; however, the use of animal cells and/or animal-derived substrates hampers clinical applications. Therefore, human-derived cell sources have to be perused. Table 5.2 summarizes the human PTECs proposed for use in the development of BAK devices.

Despite all innovations in developing advanced cell models that recapitulate renal PTEC function, there are still considerable challenges on the

Table 5.2: Sources of human PTECs used or proposed for use in BAK.

Cell	Type	PTEC phenotype	Availability	References
HK-2	Cell line	Intermediate	High	Jenkinson *et al.* [2012]; Ryan *et al.* [1994]; Sun *et al.* [2011]
Primary	Primary	Strong	Low	Humes *et al.* [2002]; Oo *et al.* [2011]; Sanechika *et al.* [2011]; Saito *et al.* [2012]; Takahashi *et al.* [2013]
RPTEC	Cell line	Strong	Reasonable	Sanechika *et al.* [2011]; Simon-Friedt *et al.* [2015]
ciPTEC	Cell line	Strong	Reasonable	Jansen *et al.* [2016]; Schophuizen *et al.* 2015; Wilmer *et al.* [2010a]
Stem cells	Primary	Intermediate	Low	Klingemann *et al.* [2008]; Roberts *et al.* [2012]; Sciancalepore *et al.* [2015]
iPS	Primary	Intermediate	Reasonable	Freedman and Steinman [2015]; Yamanaka and Yokoo [2015]

road toward a BAK that incorporates living cells [Jansen *et al.*, 2014a]. A potential problem can arise from using PTECs to directly or indirectly remove solutes from the blood of patients with kidney disease due to differences in genetic background which can exert immune compatibility issues. The cells can excrete factors and express major histocompatibility complex (MHC) surface proteins, which can be recognized as foreign and trigger an immune response. Although this response may not affect the PTECs themselves, if MHC peptides are shed and end up in the patient's systemic circulation, immune cells can be activated leading to unwanted inflammatory events. Immunogenic responses can be avoided if the cells used are derived from stem cells or iPS cells, providing that the recipient is also the donor. In addition, the use of surfaces/materials that absorb such soluble factors and peptides can circumvent the issue as well [Jansen *et al.*, 2014a].

Immortalized PTEC lines form a tight monolayer, however implementation raises issues about monolayer stability and integrity. Cells can breakaway and compromise the barrier function and also be shed from any compartment that is not self-contained. Finally, the cell characteristics such as proliferation or function are strongly dependent on the culturing environment and especially the two-dimensional (2D) or three-dimensional (3D) configuration [Edmondson *et al.*, 2014; Li & Cui, 2014; Sanchez-Romero *et al.*, 2016]. Therefore, many PTEC cell models which were first studied in 2D may show a very different behavior when cultured on hollow fiber membranes for BAK applications. A recent work with ciPTEC grown on the outside of hollow fiber membranes has proven that these cells can form a tight monolayer around the fibers and actively take up and secrete substrates when perfused in dose-dependent manner [Chevtchik *et al.*, 2016; Jansen *et al.*, 2015, 2016].

5.4 Artificial Membranes for the Bioartificial Kidney

The requirements for artificial membranes for a BAK should be the following. First, one side of the membrane has to be in prolonged contact with blood or body fluid and has, therefore, to be hemocompatible and with low fouling, thus avoiding cell adhesion. The other side of the membrane should be highly cytocompatible and favor PTEC adhesion and function. The membrane should also provide high solute fluxes to allow the exchange of solutes between the PTEC and the patient fluid. Finally, it should act as an immunoprotective barrier to preserve the PTEC from an eventual immune attack.

The following paragraphs will summarize the membrane properties reported in literature which played an important role in the development of the BAK. Moreover, since the development of BAK began with commercially available membranes (presented more in detail in Section 5.5), surface modification was necessary in order to improve their cytocompatibility. These modifications will be discussed, as well.

5.4.1 *Membrane Materials*

The first BAK prototypes were build using the existing ultrafiltration or HD HFM, mostly from polysulfone (PSU) [Aebischer *et al.*, 1987; Humes *et al.*, 1999, 2002]. The reasons for this choice were the improved hemocompatibility, the high filtration rates and the high reproducibility and availability of the HFM. More recent work reported newer generations of

HFM based on polyarylethersulfone (PAES) from Gambro [Oo *et al.*, 2013], ethylene vinyl alcohol (EVAL) from Kasei Kuraray Medical [Saito *et al.*, 2012; Takahashi *et al.*, 2013] and polyethersulfone (PES) from 3M-Membrana [Chevtchik *et al.*, 2016]. Since the commercial membranes were available in various materials, several groups even compared them in terms of their ability to support cell adhesion. For example, Saito and coworkers reported a comparison between polyimide, PSU and EVAL [Saito, 2006], and their results supported the use of EVAL membranes. In addition for better cell adhesion, EVAL presented a high mechanical strength and therefore HFM had thin walls (25 μm). Table 5.3 summarizes the major HFM materials reported in literature as components of BAK in combination with cells from human origin.

5.4.2 *Membrane permeability and selectivity*

As mentioned earlier, mostly commercially available HD membranes were used for BAK. They usually present high permeability, in the ultrafiltration range. This property is important in allowing the transport of nutrients to the cells during the proliferation and maturation phases. During the function of the BAK, the high permeability should also allow

(1) easy access of the toxins from the blood to the cells,
(2) the excreted toxins to move from the cells to the waste and
(3) the re-absorbed metabolites to move from the cells to the waste/blood.

The high fluxes are achieved thanks to the relatively thin HFM wall and high porosity. The wall thickness reported in the literature varies between 25 and 145 μm. This parameter is strongly dependent on the material used, since the HFM needs to have a sufficient mechanical strength to allow handling. Most of the HD membranes applied are "asymmetric", porous and open on the one side (dialysate) and have a "skin layer" with reduced pore size in contact with the blood. This skin layer really determines the membrane selectivity or MWCO. The HD membranes presents MWCO in the range 40–65 kDa, in order to prevent albumin leakage of the patients. Interestingly, the ideal MWCO for the BAK application is not very well defined in literature. According to most authors, the HFM should prevent albumin leakage. However, if the HFM is covered by a tight monolayer of ciPTEC, the cells should be able to act as a barrier against albumin loss. Moreover, in order to optimize the removal of protein-bound toxins, albumin, the carrier, should be brought in close proximity to the cells. The MWCO of membranes used for BAK are presented in Table 5.3.

5.4.3 *HFM Diameter Size and Curvature*

It has been shown that the increase in substrate curvature could up-regulate the PTEC functions without altering the confluent cell morphology [Chong Shen & Guoliang Zhang, 2013]. Researchers cultured either canine MDCK cells or human HK-2 on HFM from PSf and PSf-PEG, with inner diameters of 0.4, 0.8 and 1.2 mm. Although the cell monolayer morphology was always good, the activity of the brush border enzyme, of the glucose transporter (GLUT) and of the multi-drug resistance-associated protein 2 (MRP2) was higher on HFM with a smaller inner diameter. In the literature, the range of internal diameters of the HFM is rather broad. In reality, since most researchers used commercially available membranes, inner diameters in the range 175–250 μm are used. Larger-diameter membranes (490 μm) were reported too [Oo *et al.*, 2011]. Finally, it is interesting to consider the natural size of the proximal tubule. The diameters for human proximal tubule are ranging from 30 to 60 μm [Qian Li *et al.*, 2009]. Therefore, one could expect that a further decrease in the diameter of the HFM would be beneficial to the BAK function.

5.4.4 *Membranes Surface Modifications for Cell Adhesion*

All HFMs for dialysis therapies are developed to have a low cell adhesion and fouling during blood filtration. The chemical groups present at the membrane surface may explain its ability to support or not cell adhesion. The presence of apolar groups, such as methyl, has been shown to inhibit cellular attachment, whereas polar or charged functional groups, such as amino or carboxylic groups, have been identified as promoting cell attachment [Kirchhof & Groth, 2008]. Therefore, the cytocompatibility of the materials can be tailored by the incorporation of the desired groups to their surface, by synthesis of the copolymers or by surface modification. Most of the time, the easier and more commonly reported solution remains an HFM surface modification.

5.4.4.1 *Chemical Surface Modifications*

Ni *et al.* [2011] reported an extensive list of surface modifications applied to HFM membranes, among others, poly(maleic anhydride-alt-1-octadecene), oxygen plasma treatment and hydrogen peroxide. These techniques mostly aimed at increasing the presence of carboxylic acid groups on the surface of the membranes. The best cell attachment was achieved with a coating of l-3,4-dihydroxyphenylalanine (L-Dopa) (Fig. 5.5). The same coating is used for many materials [Lee *et al.*, 2007; Xi *et al.*, 2009] and various cell lines (human pluripotent stem cells, e.g. HK-2, HPTC and ciPTEC [Kandasamy *et al.*, 2014]). This favorable cell attachment to L-Dopa-coated substrates may be explained by the presence of additional groups such as amines. Ni *et al.* [2011] also reported greater cell attachment while using a natural ECM coating, applied in addition to a surface treatment. These coatings will be described in the next section.

Recent research makes use of the charge properties of the materials. The adhesion of the negatively charged cells is promoted to slightly positive surfaces. The group of Thomas Groth reported the use of poly(ethylene imine) and/or poly(ether imide) as having good hemocompatibility and as promoting cell attachment, proliferation and/or differentiation [Liu *et al.*,

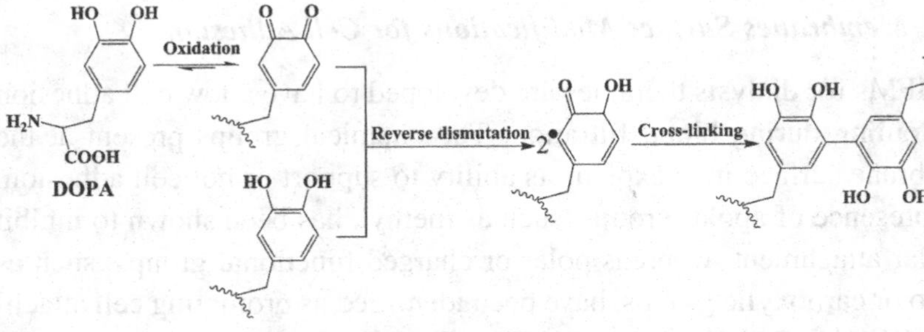

Figure 5.5. Scheme of cross-linking of L-Dopa during coating. Reprinted from Xi *et al.* [2009] with the permission of Elsevier.

2010; Trimpert *et al.*, 2006; Tzoneva *et al.*, 2008]. In the case of membranes for BAK, the patent from Gambro reports coatings of poly(ethylene imine) to improve cell adhesion, too [Luttropp *et al.*, 2009].

5.4.4.2 *Biologically Derived Extracellular Matrices*

It has been shown that cell adhesion is linked to the presence and conformation of specific attachment proteins on material surfaces. The ECM, which surrounds cells in tissues (Fig. 5.6), is composed of structural proteins, like collagens, adhesive proteins and glycosaminoglycans

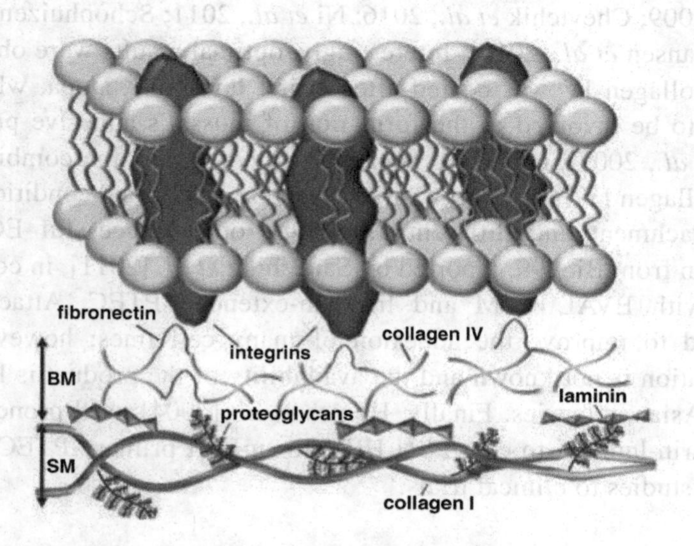

Figure 5.6. Essential extracellular matrix components. The native ECM is a key factor in inter- and intracellular signaling, regeneration and support and is a depot for growth factors, indicating its high relevance in cell maintenance. The cell–ECM adhesion and signaling is mediated by integrins, which are transmembrane receptors located in the PTEC plasma membrane. The ECM composition can be divided into two major components: the basement membrane (BM) and the stromal matrix (SM). The BM is a sheet-like scaffold mainly characterized by fibronectin, proteoglycans, laminin and collagen IV. The SM is made up of larger, fibrous structures, which provide the major structural support of the ECM, mainly Collagen I, proteoglycans and GAGs. Reprinted from Jansen *et al.* [2014a] with the permission of Elsevier.

[Groth & Liu, 2008]. The understanding of the composition of the ECM can help designing the membrane surface properties.

In the last few years, researchers tested various ECM compounds as coatings for adhesion of cell lines (HK-2) or HPTC. ECM coating was applied to the membranes for several hours [Zhang *et al.*, 2009; Chevtchik *et al.*, 2016] and at a fixed concentration, prior to seeding the renal epithelial cells (RECs). The ECM coating stimulates cell adhesion and differentiation; successful cell differentiation causes ECM production by the epithelium [Jansen *et al.*, 2014a, 2014b].

Collagen IV from human sources appears to be one of the best ECM coatings in both PES/PVP and PET membranes to support the adhesion and function of human PTEC (HK-2, HPTC, ciPTEC) [Zhang *et al.*, 2009; Chevtchik *et al.*, 2016; Ni *et al.*, 2011; Schophuizen *et al.*, 2015; Jansen *et al.*, 2015]. Interestingly, optimal results were obtained when collagen IV was coated after a first layer of L-Dopa, which is shown to be involved in the formation of mussel's adhesive proteins [Lee *et al.*, 2007]. L-Dopa is negatively charged, and the combination with collagen IV (positively charged) can create optimal conditions for cell attachment and differentiation. One other successful ECM is Attachin from Bio999, reported by Sanechika *et al.* [2011], in combination with EVAL HFM and lifespan-extended PTEC. Attachin is reported to improve the adhesion of many cell lines; however, its formulation is not known and the availability of the product is limited to the Asian countries. Finally, Humes *et al.* [2004] used pronectin-L and murin laminin to coat PSU HFM to support primary PTEC, from *in vivo* studies to clinical trials.

5.4.5 *HFM Challenges and Perspectives*

The combination of parameters such as surface chemistry and topography can have a significant impact on the cell attachment. Hulshof *et al.* [2017] reported a striking difference between the response of ciPTEC on PS and PES membranes (coated with L-Dopa). While for PS the large topographic features did not adversely affect ciPTEC cell numbers and monolayer formation, the same features fabricated on PES disrupted the cell monolayer.

As discussed earlier, many HFM characteristics have been shown to play a crucial role in cell attachment, growth, morphology and function, such as material, selectivity and curvature. The research to study the impact of those parameters was often performed by modifying one parameter at a time, while keeping the other parameters constant. A more systematic research, including design of experiments or "high-throughput screening" [Hulsman *et al.*, 2015; Hulshof *et al.*, 2017] could allow a better understanding of the impact of several parameters and their combination on the cell attachment and function. In-depth knowledge of the effects of the above-cited parameters could avoid the use of additional surface modification or ECM coatings to favor cell attachment. Finally, the surface properties can be optimized for a given cell line, but be detrimental for another one [Tasnim *et al.*, 2010].

5.5 An Improved Replacement of the Renal Function — The BAK — History and Perspectives

Table 5.3 highlights the major BAK prototypes, using human PTEC, and their characteristics.

The first BAK, composed of PTECs grown inside ultrafiltration HFM, was proposed by Aebisher *et al.* [1987]. They achieved a continuous ultrafiltration for relatively long periods of time when using non-human-derived (canine or porcine) cells. Since then, the group of David Humes developed a RAD system based on PSU HFM seeded first with porcine renal proximal tubule cells (LLC-PK1) and then with human PTEC. They first treated uremic animals [Humes *et al.*, 1999, 2002], showing active vectorial transport of sodium, bicarbonate, glucose and organic anions, enabling functional maintenance. Moreover, endocrine activity with conversion of 25-hydroxy(OH)-vitaminD3 to 1,25-(OH)2 vitD3 was demonstrated in the RAD. Subsequently, the system passed the Phase IIa clinical trials successfully in 2005 for the treatment of patients with AKI and CRF [Tumlin *et al.*, 2008]. The Phase IIb clinical trials, however, were suspended for safety reasons: platelet count levels reached a lower limit of 35,000 per mm^3 [Humes *et al.*, 2004]. Moreover, practical drawbacks such as cell expansion, differentiation, storage and transport issues were reported.

Table 5.3: BAK systems using human kidney cell sources, main characteristics.

System — *Name* — *Cell type* — *Cell seeding/culturing*	Membrane characteristics — *Material/provenance* — *Coating* — *MWCO*	Testing and key output parameters	References
RAD Primary — isolated renal Tubule progenitor cells Internal seeding Culture under perfusion	PSU coated with murine laminin or bovine collagen IV 45 kDa/50 kDa	1. *In vitro* and pre-clinical: increased excretion of ammonia, glutathione metabolism, and production of 1,25-dihydroxyvitamin D3 2. Clinical — phase I and phase IIa: more rapid recovery of kidney function, RAD well-tolerated	1. Humes *et al.* [2002] 2. Tumlin *et al.* [2008]
RAD HK-2 cell-line transfected with pcDNA3.1-hEpo, Internal seeding Static culture	PSF coated with Laminin 50 kDa	*In vitro*: gene expression and secretion of erythropoietin (Epo)	Sun *et al.* [2011]
BAK Primary HPTC Internal seeding Culture under perfusion	PES/PVP/ NMP coated with L-Dopa and human collagen IV <65 kDa	*In vitro*: immunostainings and qPCR gene expression	Oo *et al.* [2011]

BAK Primary: HPTC External seeding Culture under perfusion	PAES (Gambro) No coating PSU (Fresenius) No coating PES/PVP — self-made, coated with L-Dopa and human collagen IV <65 kDa	*In vitro:* OAT transport (Lucifer yellow) and uptake of urea and creatinine, high levels of IL-6 and IL-8	Oo *et al.* [2013], Zink & Zay [2013]
BTD Primary RPTEC with siRNA-mediated lifespan extension Internal seeding culture under perfusion	EVAL — (Asahi Kasei Kuraray Medical) Attachin <65 kDa	1. *In vitro*: re-absorption of water, sodium and glucose, metabolization of β2-microglobulin and pentosidine 2. *In vivo*: (AKI goats) expended lifespan; clearance of small solutes; decreased inflammatory cytokines 3. *In vivo*: (AKI goats) culture in serum-free media with a similar performance	1. Sanechika *et al.* [2011] 2. Saito *et al.* [2012] 3. Takahashi *et al.* [2013]
BAK ciPTEC cell line External seeding Static culture	PES — MicroPES (3M — Membrana) L-Dopa and human collagen IV 150 kDa	*In vitro*: immunostainings and active uptake of organic cations	Chevtchik *et al.* [2016]

To overcome the previous issues, the Humes group recently developed a bioartificial renal epithelial cell system (BRECS) [Buffington *et al.*, 2012] composed of porous, niobium-coated carbon disks, retaining a dense population of allogenic RECs. After the cells reach an optimal density, the BRECS can be cryopreserved at −80 or −140°C, transported and stored. This unique design allows for long-term storage and should permit on-demand use for acute clinical applications. It could also be incorporated to a PD circuit and provide an improved PD wearable dialysis. This device has been recently tested *in vivo* on nephretectomized sheep for 24 h and was demonstrated a stable uraemic state and endocrine support in the form of 1,25 vitamin D3.

Ni *et al.* used PES/PVP, PSU/PVP and PSU HFM in combination with a double coating and human PTEC [Ni *et al.*, 2011; Oo *et al.*, 2013]. The first trials were, however, performed with MDCK cells, which adhered perfectly without coating on PES/PVP HFM [Tasnim *et al.*, 2010]. The human PTEC reacted differently and required an additional coating or a different membrane material.

The same group presented a new model of BAK with PTEC seeded on the extraluminal side of the HFM in 2013 [Oo *et al.*, 2013] and showed improved PTEC performance without using coatings. This BAK configuration was patented in 2013 [Zink & Zay, 2013].

The group of Akira Saito first worked with LLC-PK1 cells (porcine kidney) and MDCK cells (canine kidney) seeded inside coated PSU or cellulose acetate HFM. Later, they switched to human cells and had to re-adapt materials and coatings previously optimized for animal cells. They further developed a RAD using lifespan-extended human PTEC cultured in a newly developed serum-free medium. They compared its performance with BAK prepared with PTEC cultured in serum-containing conventional medium in AKI goats with positive results [Sanechika *et al.*, 2011; Takahashi *et al.*, 2013]. Moreover, the group also considered developing a bioartificial glomerulus using CD133+ progenitor cells to replace the conventional hemofilter which precedes the BAK [Saito, 2009]. Gambro [Luttropp *et al.*, 2009; Krause *et al.*, 2011] proposed combination of a distal tubule part with a proximal tubule part. Their patent is based on internal, confidential reports, and no published research articles are available. As a comparison, the group of Zink patented their BAK system [Zink & Zay, 2013] based on their publication [Oo *et al.*, 2013].

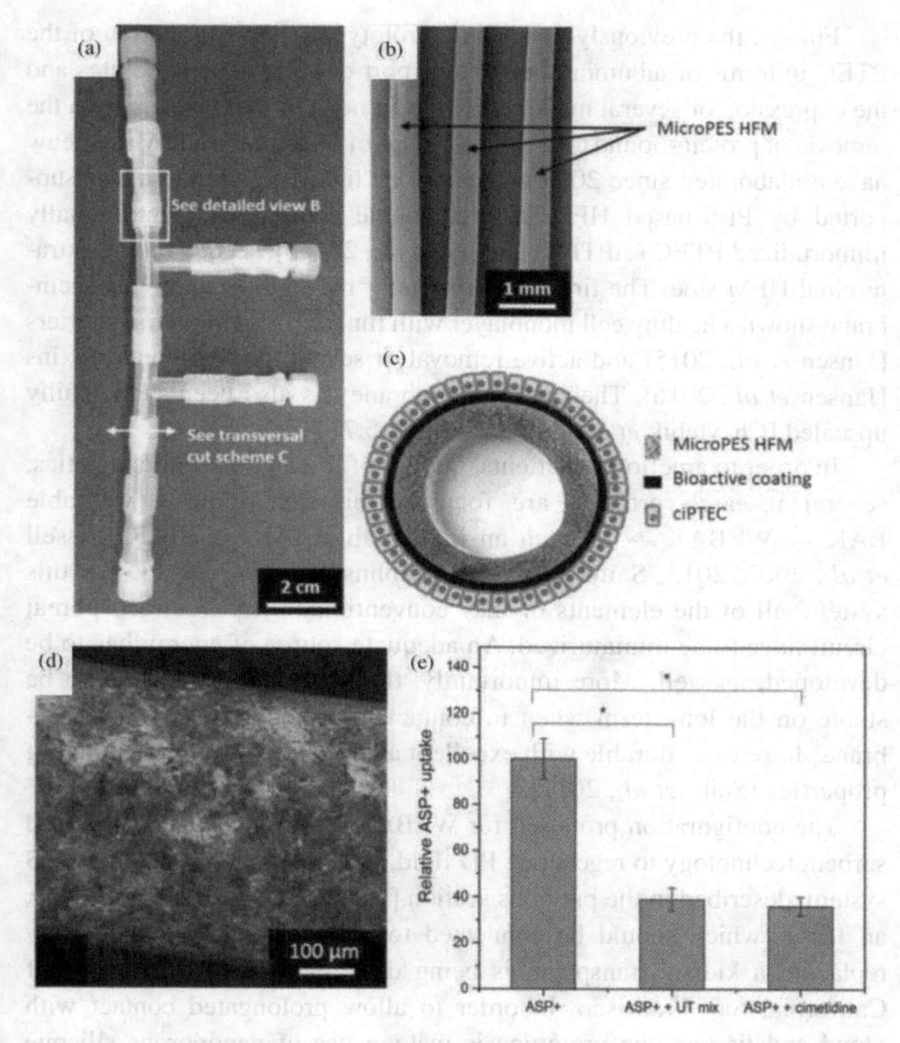

Figure 5.7. Functional upscaled "living membrane". (a) Picture of one module used for upscaled "living membrane" model. Three MicroPES hollow fiber membranes (HFMs) within a housing composed of PE, PP and silicone parts, LuerLock fittings and caps. (b) SEM image of three MicroPES HFMs. (c) Scheme of a transversal cut of one "living membrane". Not at proportional scale. (d) Representative confocal microscopy images of ciPTEC cultured on HFM with DAPI staining of nuclei and immunostaining for ZO-1. (e) Quantification of ASP+ uptake (10 mM) in the absence or presence of specific inhibitors (cationic uremic toxin mix (UTmix), cimetidine (cim,100 mM)) in matured ciPTEC cultured on upscaled HFM. Reprinted from Chevtchik *et al.* [2016] with the permission of Elsevier.

Finally, the previously cited BAK prototypes showed function of the PTEC in terms of albumin uptake, transport of various ionic solutes and the expression of several markers. However, none of them have shown the removal of protein-bound toxins. The groups of Stamatialis and Masereeuw have collaborated since 2009 to propose a "living membrane". It is supported by PES-based HFM with a double coating and conditionally immortalized PTEC (ciPTEC) [Jansen *et al.*, 2014b], seeded on the extraluminal HFM side. The first *in vitro* tests of the small-scale living membrane shown a healthy cell monolayer with function of several transporters [Jansen *et al.*, 2015] and active removal of several protein-bound toxins [Jansen *et al.*, 2016]. Their living membrane has also been successfully upscaled [Chevtchik *et al.*, 2016] (see Fig. 5.7).

In order to ameliorate patients' quality of life and facilitate logistics, several research projects are focussed on developing a wearable BAK — WEBAK — or even an implantable BAK — IBAK [Fissell *et al.*, 2007, 2013; Saito *et al.*, 2011; Johnston *et al.*, 2016]. For this system, all of the elements of the "conventional" BAK extracorporeal circuit have to be miniaturized. An adequate source of energy has to be developed, as well. More importantly, the filtration system has to be stable on the long term when in contact with body fluids. The membranes have to be durable with excellent antifouling and anticoagulating properties [Saito *et al.*, 2011].

The configuration proposed for WEBAK so far made use of PD and sorbent technology to regenerate PD fluid, in combination with a BRECS system, described in the previous section [Humes *et al.*, 2014]. Currently, an IBAK which should be connected to the blood and bladder, fully replacing a kidney transplant, is being developed in the University of California, San Fransisco. In order to allow prolongated contact with blood and tissues, the prototype is making use of nanoporous silicone membranes for the blood filtration step [Fissell *et al.*, 2007, 2009, 2013; Nissenson *et al.*, 2005].

5.6 Conclusion, Challenges and Perspectives

Since the first BAK has been presented 30 years ago [Aebischer *et al.*, 1987], much progress happened in the field. The results clearly indicated the need of a reliable and consistent cell line as well as device-related logistics such as cost-effective manufacturing, storage and distribution process.

New renal cells, from human origin, have been developed and fully characterized. Still many challenges exist, including the generation of cells with defined PTEC activity. Currently available cell lines yield promising results; nonetheless, they are mostly highly valuable research tools. Such cell types face several questions when it comes to its use in an actual biomedical device, namely the immunological considerations. Since these cells are genetically modified, viruses were used to promote transfection of the vectors that enable immortalization and stability, which might provoke safety issues and require systematic testing as set by regulation authorities.

For any cell type, it is important to design the BAK with the right fluidics to maintain cell viability and functionality. Indeed, high sheer stress may damage the cell monolayer. The study of the maximal toxin concentrations to which the device can be exposed is also of crucial importance, as high toxin concentrations are leading to high cell mortality [Perazella, 2009].

The BAK comes with many questions concerning logistics and costs. It should be first produced in a GMP environment, stored, transported and used by qualified personal. Precise estimates for the number of expected AKI patients per day per participating medical center would be required to adjust the production rate and limit the storage time. The BRECS could be a solution to overcome the storage problems of the HFM-based BAK since there it is possibility to store the system using commercially available and FDA-approved cryopreservation media [Buffington *et al.*, 2012]. The BRECS is also tested to be part of a WEBAK. This device is now on the fast track process of FDA registration, showing the importance of a treatment for kidney injury.

Acknowledgments

This work was funded by the EU Marie Curie ITN Project BIOART (grant no. 316690; EU-FP7-PEOPLE-ITN-2012) and Nephrotools (grant no. 289754; EU-FP7-PEOPLE-ITN-2011).

Dimitrios Stmatialis and Rosalinde Masereeuw would like to gratefully thank the EUTox Working Group of the European Renal Association and of European Society for Artificial Organs, for its financial contribution.

List of Abbreviations

AKI	acute kidney injury
ARF	acute renal failure
BAK	bioartificial kidney device
BRECS	bioartificial renal epithelial cell system
BTD	bioartificial renal tubule device
CKD	chronic kidney disease
CRF	chronic renal failure
ESRD	end-stage kidney disease
GFR	glomerular filtration rate
HD	hemodialysis
HF	hollow fiber
HFM	hollow fiber membrane
IBAK	implantable bioartificial kidney
iPS	induced pluripotent stem cells
L-Dopa	3,4-dihydroxy-l-phenylalanine
LCC-PK1	pig kidney epithelial cells
MDCK	Madin–Darby canine kidney cells
MHC	major histocompatibility complex
MWCO	mass weight cutoff
OAT	organic anion transporter
OCT	organic cation transporter
PD	peritoneal dialysis
PSU	polysulfone
PTEC	proximal tubule epithelial cell

RAD	renal assist device
RPTEC	renal PTEC
RRF	residual renal function
RRT	renal replacement therapy
SLC	solute carrier family
WEBAK	wearable bioartificial kidney

References

Aebischer P, Ip TK, Panol G and Galletti PM (1987). The bioartificial kidney: progress towards an ultrafiltration device with renal epithelial cells processing. *Life Support Syst*, 5, pp. 159–168.

Barreto FC, Barreto DV, Liabeuf S, Meert N, Glorieux G, Temmar M, Choukroun G, Vanholder R, Massy ZA and European Uremic Toxin Work G (2009). Serum indoxyl sulfate is associated with vascular disease and mortality in chronic kidney disease patients. *Clin J Am Soc Nephrol*, 4, pp. 1551–1558.

Brunelli SM, Chertow GM, Ankers ED, Lowrie EG and Thadhani R (2010). Shorter dialysis times are associated with higher mortality among incident hemodialysis patients. *Kidney Int*, 77, pp. 630–636.

Buffington DA, Pino CJ, Chen L, Westover AJ, Hageman G and Humes HD (2012). Bioartificial renal epithelial cell system (BRECS): a compact, cryopreservable extracorporeal renal replacement device. *Cell Med*, 4, pp. 33–43.

Chaudhary K (2011). Peritoneal dialysis drop-out: causes and prevention strategies. *Int J Nephrol*, 2011, pp. 434–608.

Chevtchik NV, Fedecostante M, Jansen J, Mihajlovic M, Wilmer M, Rüth M, Masereeuw R and Stamatialis D (2016). Upscaling of a living membrane for bioartificial kidney device. *Eur J Pharmacol*, 790, pp. 28–35

Chong Shen QM and Guoliang Zhang L (2013). Increased curvature of hollow fiber membranes could up-regulate differential functions of renal tubular cell layers. *Biotechnol Bioeng*, 110, pp. 2173–2183.

DesRochers TM, Suter L, Roth A and Kaplan DL (2013). Bioengineered 3D human kidney tissue, a platform for the determination of nephrotoxicity. *PLoS One*, 8, p. e59219.

Dukes JD, Whitley P and Chalmers AD (2011). The MDCK variety pack: choosing the right strain. *BMC Cell Biol*, 12, p. 43.

Edmondson R, Broglie JJ, Adcock AF and Yang L (2014). Three-dimensional cell culture systems and their applications in drug discovery and cell-based biosensors. *Assay Drug Dev Technol*, 12, pp. 207–218.

El-Sheikh AA, Greupink R, Wortelboer HM, van den Heuvel JJ, Schreurs M, Koenderink JB, Masereeuw R and Russel FG (2013). Interaction of immunosuppressive drugs with human organic anion transporter (OAT) 1 and OAT3, and multidrug resistance-associated protein (MRP) 2 and MRP4. *Transl Res*, 162, pp. 398–409.

Eloot S, Ledebo I and Ward RA (2014). Extracorporeal removal of uremic toxins: can we still do better? *Semin Nephrol*, 34, pp. 209–227.

El-Sheikh AA, Koenderink JB, Wouterse AC, van den Broek PH, Verweij VG, Masereeuw R and Russel FG (2014). Renal glucuronidation and multidrug resistance protein 2-/multidrug resistance protein 4-mediated efflux of mycophenolic acid: interaction with cyclosporine and tacrolimus. *Transl Res*, 164, pp. 46–56.

Eurotransplant. Active waiting list (at year-end) in All ET, by year, by organ. http://statistics.eurotransplant.org/: © Eurotransplant International Foundation; 2016, Statistics Report Library.

Fissell WH, Dubnisheva A, Eldridge AN, Fleischman AJ, Zydney AL and Roy S (2009). High-performance silicon nanopore hemofiltration membranes. *J Memb Sci*, 326, pp. 58–63.

Fissell WH, Fleischman AJ, Humes HD and Roy S (2007). Development of continuous implantable renal replacement: past and future. *Transl Res*, 150, pp. 327–336.

Fissell WH, Roy S and Davenport A (2013). Achieving more frequent and longer dialysis for the majority: wearable dialysis and implantable artificial kidney devices. *Kidney Int*, 84, pp. 256–264.

Flythe JE, Curhan GC and Brunelli SM (2013). Shorter length dialysis sessions are associated with increased mortality, independent of body weight. *Kidney Int*, 83, pp. 104–113.

Freedman BS and Steinman TI (2015). iPS cell technology: future impact on renal care. *Nephrol News Issues*, 29(18), pp. 20–11.

Fresenius MC (2013). ESRD patients in 2013. A global perspective. In: Fresenius Medical Care, (Ed.) https://www.freseniusmedicalcare.com/fileadmin/data/de/pdf/investors/News___Publications/Annual_Reports/2013/FMC_Annual_Report_2013_en.pdf.

Gaganis P, Miners JO, Brennan JS, Thomas A and Knights KM (2007). Human renal cortical and medullary UDP-glucuronosyltransferases (UGTs): immunohistochemical localization of UGT2B7 and UGT1A enzymes and kinetic characterization of *S*-naproxen glucuronidation. *J Pharmacol Exp Ther*, 323, pp. 422–430.

GODT (2014). *Organ Donation and Transplantation Activities* (World Health Organization).

Griffith LG and Swartz MA (2006). Capturing complex 3D tissue physiology *in vitro*. *Nat Rev Mol Cell Biol*, 7, pp. 211–224.

Groth T and Liu Z-M (2008). Application of membranes in tissue engineering and biohybrid organ technology. In Peinemann, Ed, *Membranes for the life Sciences*. Federal Republic of Germany: WILEY-VCH.

Hagos Y and Wolff NA (2010) Assessment of the role of renal organic anion transporters in drug-induced nephrotoxicity. *Toxins (Basel)*, 2, pp. 2055–2082.

Hedgeman E, Lipworth L, Lowe K, Saran R, Do T and Fryzek J (2015). International burden of chronic kidney disease and secondary hyperparathyroidism: a systematic review of the literature and available data. *Int J Nephrol*, 2015, p. 184321.

Hill NR, Fatoba ST, Oke JL, Hirst JA, O'Callaghan CA, Lasserson DS and Hobbs FD (2016). Global prevalence of chronic kidney disease — a systematic review and meta-analysis. *PLoS One*, 11, p. e0158765.

Hoenig MP and Zeidel ML (2014). Homeostasis, the milieu interieur, and the wisdom of the nephron. *Clin J Am Soc Nephrol*, 9, pp. 1272–1281.

Hoste EA, Bagshaw SM, Bellomo R, Cely CM, Colman R, Cruz DN, Edipidis K, Forni LG, Gomersall CD, Govil D, Honore PM, Joannes-Boyau O, Joannidis M, Korhonen AM, Lavrentieva A, Mehta RL, Palevsky P, Roessler E, Ronco C, Uchino S, Vazquez JA, Vidal Andrade E, Webb S and Kellum JA (2015). Epidemiology of acute kidney injury in critically ill patients: the multinational AKI-EPI study. *Intensive Care Med*, 41, pp. 1411–1423.

Huang C and Miller RT (2007). Regulation of renal ion transport by the calcium-sensing receptor: an update. *Curr Opin Nephrol Hypertens*, 16, pp. 437–443.

Huls M, Brown CD, Windass AS, Sayer R, van den Heuvel JJ, Heemskerk S, Russel F. G. and Masereeuw R (2008). The breast cancer resistance protein transporter ABCG2 is expressed in the human kidney proximal tubule apical membrane. *Kidney Int*, 73, pp. 220–225.

Hulshof F, Schophuizen C, Mihajlovic M, van Blitterswijk C, Masereeuw R, de Boer J and Stamatialis D (2017). New insights into the effects of biomaterial chemistry and topography on the morphology of kidney epithelial cells. *J Tissue Eng Regen Med*.

Hulsman M, Hulshof F, Unadkat H, Papenburg BJ, Stamatialis DF, Truckenmuller R, van Blitterswijk C, de Boer J and Reinders MJ (2015). Analysis of high-throughput screening reveals the effect of surface topographies on cellular morphology. *Acta Biomater*, 15, pp. 29–38.

Humes HD, Buffington DA, MacKay SM, Funke AJ and Weitzel WF (1999). Replacement of renal function in uremic animals with a tissue-engineered kidney. *Nat Biotech*, 17, pp. 451–455.

Humes HD, Buffington D, Westover AJ, Roy S and Fissell WH (2014). The bioartificial kidney: current status and future promise. *Pediatr Nephrol*, 29, pp. 343–351.

Humes HD, Fissell WH, Weitzel WF, Buffington DA, Westover AJ, MacKay SM and Gutierrez JM (2002). Metabolic replacement of kidney function in uremic animals with a bioartificial kidney containing human cells. *Am J Kidney Dis*, 39, pp. 1078–1087.

Humes HD, Weitzel WF, Bartlett RH, Swaniker FC, Paganini EP, Luderer JR and Sobota J (2004). Initial clinical results of the bioartificial kidney containing human cells in ICU patients with acute renal failure. *Kidney Int*, 66, pp. 1578–1588.

International Transporter C, Giacomini KM, Huang SM, Tweedie DJ, Benet LZ, Brouwer KL, Chu X, Dahlin A, Evers R, Fischer V, Hillgren KM, Hoffmaster KA, Ishikawa T, Keppler D, Kim RB, Lee CA, Niemi M, Polli JW, Sugiyama Y, Swaan PW, Ware JA, Wright SH, Yee SW, Zamek-Gliszczynski MJ and Zhang L (2010). Membrane transporters in drug development. *Nat Rev Drug Discov*, 9, pp. 215–236.

Ip TK, Aebischer P and Galletti PM (1988). Cellular control of membrane permeability. Implications for a bioartificial renal tubule. *ASAIO Trans*, 34, pp. 351–355.

Jansen J (2016). *Innovative Strategies to Improve or Replace Renal Proximal Convoluted Tubule Function* (RU Radboud Universiteit).

Jansen J, De Napoli IE, Fedecostante M, Schophuizen CM, Chevtchik NV, Wilmer MJ, van Asbeck AH, Croes HJ, Pertijs JC, Wetzels JF, Hilbrands LB, van den Heuvel LP, Hoenderop JG, Stamatialis D and Masereeuw R (2015). Human proximal tubule epithelial cells cultured on hollow fibers: living membranes that actively transport organic cations. *Sci Rep*, 5, p. 16702. doi: 10.1038/srep16702.

Jansen J, Fedecostante M, Wilmer MJ, Peters JG, Kreuser UM, van den Broek PH, Mensink RA, Boltje TJ, Stamatialis D, Wetzels JF, van den Heuvel LP, Hoenderop JG and Masereeuw R (2016). Bioengineered kidney tubules efficiently excrete uremic toxins. *Sci Rep*, 6, p. 26715.

Jansen J, Fedecostante M, Wilmer MJ, van den Heuvel LP, Hoenderop JG and Masereeuw R (2014a). Biotechnological challenges of bioartificial kidney engineering. *Biotechnol Adv*, 32, pp. 1317–1327.

Jansen J, Schophuizen CM, Wilmer MJ, Lahham SH, Mutsaers HA, Wetzels JF, Bank RA, van den Heuvel LP, Hoenderop JG and Masereeuw R

(2014b). A morphological and functional comparison of proximal tubule cell lines established from human urine and kidney tissue. *Exp Cell Res*, 323, pp. 87–99.

Jenkinson SE, Chung GW, van Loon E, Bakar NS, Dalzell AM and Brown CD (2012). The limitations of renal epithelial cell line HK-2 as a model of drug transporter expression and function in the proximal tubule. *Pflugers Arch*, 464, pp. 601–611.

Johnston KA, Westover AJ, Rojas-Pena A, Buffington DA, Pino CJ, Smith PL and Humes HD (2016). Development of a wearable bioartificial kidney using the Bioartificial Renal Epithelial Cell System (BRECS). *J Tissue Eng Regen Med*. 10.1002/term.2206.

Kandasamy K, Narayanan K, Ni M, Du C, Wan AC and Zink D (2014). Polysulfone membranes coated with polymerized 3,4-dihydroxy-l-phenylalanine are a versatile and cost-effective synthetic substrate for defined long-term cultures of human pluripotent stem cells. *Biomacromolecules*, 15, pp. 2067–2078.

Karkar A, Hegbrant J and Strippoli GF (2015). Benefits and implementation of home hemodialysis: a narrative review. *Saudi J Kidney Dis Transpl*, 26, pp. 1095–1107.

KDIGO (2012). KDIGO clinical practice guideline for acute kidney injury. *Kidney Int Suppl*, 2. pp. 1–138.

KDIGO (2013a). Chapter 1: Definition and classification of CKD. *Kidney Int Suppl* (2011), 3, pp. 19–62.

KDIGO (2013b). Clinical practice guideline for the evaluation and management of chronic kidney disease. *Kidney Int Suppl*, 3. 99, pp. 1–150.

Kirchhof K and Groth T (2008). Surface modification of biomaterials to control adhesion of cells. *Clin Hemorheol Microcirc*, 39, pp. 247–251.

Klingemann H, Matzilevich D and Marchand J (2008). Mesenchymal stem cells — sources and clinical applications. *Transfus Med Hemother*, 35, pp. 272–277.

Konig J, Muller F and Fromm MF (2013). Transporters and drug–drug interactions: important determinants of drug disposition and effects. *Pharmacol Rev*, 65, pp. 944–966.

Krause B, Neubauer MS, Luttropp AD and Deppisch R (2011). Hybrid bioartificial kidney. In: European Patent Office, 2011.

Lacson E, Jr and Brunelli SM (2011). Hemodialysis treatment time: a fresh perspective. *Clin J Am Soc Nephrol*, 6, pp. 2522–2530.

Lee H, Dellatore SM, Miller WM and Messersmith PB (2007). Mussel-inspired surface chemistry for multifunctional coatings. *Science*, 318, pp. 426–430.

Li Z and Cui Z (2014). Three-dimensional perfused cell culture. *Biotechnol Adv*, 32, pp. 243–254.

Liu ZM, Lee SY, Sarun S, Moeller S, Schnabelrauch M and Groth T (2010). Biocompatibility of poly(l-lactide) films modified with poly(ethylene imine) and polyelectrolyte multilayers. *J Biomater Sci Polym Ed*, 21, pp. 893–912.

Lohr JW, Willsky GR and Acara MA (1998). Renal drug metabolism. *Pharmacol Rev*, 50, pp. 107–141.

Luttropp D, Krause B, Neubauer M, Deppisch R, Deppisch D and Schnell A (2009). Hybrid bioartificial kidney. U.S. Patent.

Masereeuw R, Mutsaers HAM, Toyohara T, Abe T, Jhawar S, Sweet DH and Lowenstein J (2014). The kidney and uremic toxin removal: glomerulus or tubule? *Sem Nephrol*, 34, pp. 191–208.

Medvedev SP, Shevchenko AI and Zakian SM (2010). Induced pluripotent stem cells: problems and advantages when applying them in regenerative medicine. *Acta Nat*, 2, pp. 18–28.

Mehta RL, Cerdá J, Burdmann EA, Tonelli M, García-García G, Jha V, Susantitaphong P, Rocco M, Vanholder R, Sever MS, Cruz D, Jaber B, Lameire NH, Lombardi R, Lewington A, Feehally J, Finkelstein F, Levin N, Pannu N, Thomas B, Aronoff-Spencer E and Remuzzi G (2015). International Society of Nephrology's 0by25 initiative for acute kidney injury (zero preventable deaths by 2025): a human rights case for nephrology. *Lancet*, 385, pp. 2616–2643.

Meijers BK, Claes K, Bammens B, de Loor H, Viaene L, Verbeke K, Kuypers D, Vanrenterghem Y and Evenepoel P (2010). p-Cresol and cardiovascular risk in mild-to-moderate kidney disease. *Clin J Am Soc Nephrol*, 5, pp. 1182–1189.

Motohashi H and Inui K (2013). Organic cation transporter OCTs (SLC22) and MATEs (SLC47) in the human kidney. *AAPS J*, 15, pp. 581–588.

Mutsaers HA, Caetano-Pinto P, Seegers AE, Dankers AC, van den Broek PH, Wetzels JF, van den Brand JA, van den Heuvel LP, Hoenderop JG, Wilmer MJ and Masereeuw R (2015). Proximal tubular efflux transporters involved in renal excretion of p-cresyl sulfate and p-cresyl glucuronide: implications for chronic kidney disease pathophysiology. *Toxicol In Vitro*, 29, pp. 1868–1877.

Mutsaers HA, Wilmer MJ, Reijnders D, Jansen J, van den Broek PH, Forkink M, Schepers E, Glorieux G, Vanholder R, van den Heuvel LP, Hoenderop JG and Masereeuw R (2013). Uremic toxins inhibit renal metabolic capacity through interference with glucuronidation and mitochondrial respiration. *Biochim Biophys Acta*, 1832, pp. 142–150.

National Kidney Foundation (2016a). *Organ donation and transplantation statistics*.

National Kidney Foundation (2016b). *When a transplant fails*.

Ni M, Teo JC, Ibrahim MS, Zhang K, Tasnim F, Chow PY, Zink D and Ying JY (2011). Characterization of membrane materials and membrane coatings for bioreactor units of bioartificial kidneys. *Biomaterials*, 32, pp. 1465–1476.

Nielsen R, Birn H, Moestrup S, Nielsen M, Verroust P and Christensen EI (1998). Characterization of a kidney proximal tubule cell line, LLC-PK1, expressing endocytotic active megalin. *J Am Soc Nephrol*, 9, pp. 1767–1776.

Nielsen R, Christensen EI and Birn H (2016). Megalin and cubilin in proximal tubule protein reabsorption: from experimental models to human disease. *Kidney Int*, 89, pp. 58–67.

Nigam SK, Wu W, Bush KT, Hoenig MP, Blantz RC and Bhatnagar V (2015). Handling of drugs, metabolites, and uremic toxins by kidney proximal tubule drug transporters. *Clin J Am Soc Nephrol*, 10, pp. 2039–2049.

Nissenson AR, Ronco C, Pergamit G, Edelstein M and Watts W (2005). Continuously functioning artificial nephron system: the promise of nanotechnology. *Hemodial Int*, 9, pp. 210–217.

Oo ZY, Deng R, Hu M, Ni M, Kandasamy K, bin Ibrahim MS, Ying JY and Zink D (2011). The performance of primary human renal cells in hollow fiber bioreactors for bioartificial kidneys. *Biomaterials*, 32, pp. 8806–8815.

Oo ZY, Kandasamy K, Tasnim F and Zink D (2013). A novel design of bioartificial kidneys with improved cell performance and haemocompatibility. *J Cell Mol Med*, 17, pp. 497–507.

Palmer LG and Sackin H (1988). Regulation of renal ion channels. *FASEB J*, 2, pp. 3061–3065.

Pavlenko D, van Geffen E, van Steenbergen MJ, Glorieux G, Vanholder R, Gerritsen KG and Stamatialis D (2016). New low-flux mixed matrix membranes that offer superior removal of protein-bound toxins from human plasma. *Sci Rep*, 6, p. 34429.

Perazella MA (2009). Renal vulnerability to drug toxicity. *Clin J Am Soc Nephrol*, 4, pp. 1275–1283.

Pleniceanu O, Harari-Steinberg O, and Dekel B (2010). Concise review: kidney stem/progenitor cells: differentiate, sort out, or reprogram? *Stem Cells*, 28, pp. 1649–1660.

Presnell SC, Bruce AT, Wallace SM, Choudhury S, Genheimer CW, Cox B, Guthrie K, Werdin ES, Tatsumi-Ficht P, Ilagan RM, Kelley RW, Rivera EA, Ludlow JW, Wagner BJ, Jayo MJ and Bertram TA (2011). Isolation, characterization, and expansion methods for defined primary renal cell populations from rodent, canine, and human normal and diseased kidneys. *Tissue Eng Part C Methods*, 17, pp. 261–273.

Qian Li MLO, Andrews PM, Chen C-W, Paek A, Naphas R, Yuan S, Jiang J, Cable A and Chen Y (2009). Automated quantification of microstructural dimensions of the human kidney using optical coherence tomography (OCT). *Optics Express*, 17, pp. 16000–16016.

Rahmoune H, Thompson PW, Ward JM, Smith CD, Hong G and Brown J (2005). Glucose transporters in human renal proximal tubular cells isolated from the urine of patients with non-insulin-dependent diabetes. *Diabetes*, 54, pp. 3427–3434.

Roberts I, Baila S, Rice RB, Janssens ME, Nguyen K, Moens N, Ruban L, Hernandez D, Coffey P and Mason C (2012). Scale-up of human embryonic stem cell culture using a hollow fibre bioreactor. *Biotechnol Lett*, 34, pp. 2307–2315.

Russel FG, Koenderink JB and Masereeuw R (2008). Multidrug resistance protein 4 (MRP4/ABCC4): a versatile efflux transporter for drugs and signalling molecules. *Trends Pharmacol Sci*, 29, pp. 200–207.

Ryan MJ, Johnson G, Kirk J, Fuerstenberg SM, Zager RA and Torok-Storb B (1994). HK-2: an immortalized proximal tubule epithelial cell line from normal adult human kidney. *Kidney Int*, 45, pp. 48–57.

Saito A (2006). Present status and perspectives of bioartificial kidneys. *J Artif Organs*, 9, pp. 130–135.

Saito A (2009). CD133þ endothelial progenitor cells as a potential cell source for a bioartificial glomerulus. *Tissue Eng Part A*, 15, pp. 3173–3182.

Saito A, Sawada K and Fujimura S (2011). Present status and future perspectives on the development of bioartificial kidneys for the treatment of acute and chronic renal failure patients. *Hemodial Int*, 15, pp. 183–192.

Saito A, Sawada K, Fujimura S, Suzuki H, Hirukawa T, Tatsumi R, Kanai G, Takahashi H, Miyakogawa T, Sanechika N, Fukagawa M and Kakuta T (2012). Evaluation of bioartificial renal tubule device prepared with lifespan-extended human renal proximal tubular epithelial cells. *Nephrol Dial Transplant*, 27, pp. 3091–3099.

Sanchez-Romero N, Schophuizen CM, Gimenez I and Masereeuw R (2016). *In vitro* systems to study nephropharmacology: 2D versus 3D models. *Eur J Pharmacol*, 790, pp. 36–45.

Sanechika N, Sawada K, Usui Y, Hanai K, Kakuta T, Suzuki H, Kanai G, Fujimura S, Yokoyama TA, Fukagawa M, Terachi T and Saito A (2011). Development of bioartificial renal tubule devices with lifespan-extended human renal proximal tubular epithelial cells. *Nephrol Dial Transplant*, 26, pp. 2761–2769.

Schophuizen CM, De Napoli IE, Jansen J, Teixeira S, Wilmer MJ, Hoenderop JG, Van den Heuvel LP, Masereeuw R and Stamatialis D (2015). Development of a living membrane comprising a functional human renal proximal tubule cell monolayer on polyethersulfone polymeric membrane. *Acta Biomater*, 14, pp. 22–32.

Schophuizen CM, Wilmer MJ, Jansen J, Gustavsson L, Hilgendorf C, Hoenderop JG, van den Heuvel LP and Masereeuw R (2013). Cationic uremic toxins affect human renal proximal tubule cell functioning through interaction with the organic cation transporter. *Pflugers Arch*, 465, pp. 1701–1714.

Sciancalepore AG, Sallustio F, Girardo S, Passione LG, Camposeo A, Mele E, Di Lorenzo M, Costantino V, Schena FP and Pisignano D (2015). Correction: a bioartificial renal tubule device embedding human renal stem/progenitor cells. *PLoS ONE*, 10, p. e0128261.

Simon-Friedt BR, Wilson MJ, Blake DA, Yu H, Eriksson Y and Wickliffe JK (2015). The RPTEC/TERT1 cell line as an improved tool for *in vitro* nephrotoxicity assessments. *Biol Trace Elem Res*, 166, pp. 66–71.

Song JH and Humes HD (2009). The bioartificial kidney in the treatment of acute kidney injury. *Curr Drug Targets*, 10, pp. 1227–1234.

Stepanenko AA and Dmitrenko VV (2015). HEK293 in cell biology and cancer research: phenotype, karyotype, tumorigenicity, and stress-induced genome-phenotype evolution. *Gene*, 569, pp. 182–190.

Sun J, Wang C, Zhu B, Larsen S, Wu J and Zhao W (2011). Construction of an erythropoietin-expressing bioartificial renal tubule assist device. *Ren Fail*, 33, pp. 54–60.

Takahashi H, Sawada K, Kakuta T, Suga T, Hanai K, Kanai G, Fujimura S, Sanechika N, Terachi T, Fukagawa M and Saito A (2013). Evaluation of bioartificial renal tubule device prepared with human renal proximal tubular epithelial cells cultured in serum-free medium. *J Artif Organs*, 16, pp. 368–375.

Takasato M, Er PX, Chiu HS, Maier B, Baillie GJ, Ferguson C, Parton RG, Wolvetang EJ, Roost MS, Chuva de Sousa Lopes SM and Little MH (2015). Kidney organoids from human iPS cells contain multiple lineages and model human nephrogenesis. *Nature*, 526, pp. 564–568.

Tasnim F, Deng R, Hu M, Liour S, Li Y, Ni M, Ying JY and Zink D (2010). Achievements and challenges in bioartificial kidney development. *Fibrogenesis Tissue Repair*, 3, pp. 3–14.

Tijink MS, Kooman J, Wester M, Sun J, Saiful S, Joles JA, Borneman Z, Wessling M and Stamatialis DF (2014). Mixed matrix membranes: a new asset for blood purification therapies. *Blood Purif*, 37, pp. 1–3.

Tijink MS, Wester M, Glorieux G, Gerritsen KG, Sun J, Swart PC, Borneman Z, Wessling M, Vanholder R, Joles JA and Stamatialis D (2013). Mixed matrix hollow fiber membranes for removal of protein-bound toxins from human plasma. *Biomaterials*, 34, pp. 7819–7828.

Tijink MS, Wester M, Sun J, Saris A, Bolhuis-Versteeg LA, Saiful S, Joles JA, Borneman Z, Wessling M and Stamatialis DF (2012). A novel approach for blood purification: mixed-matrix membranes combining diffusion and adsorption in one step. *Acta Biomater*, 8, pp. 2279–2287.

Trimpert C, Boese G, Albrecht W, Richau K, Weigel T, Lendlein A and Groth T (2006). Poly(ether imide) membranes modified with poly(ethylene imine) as potential carriers for epidermal substitutes. *Macromol Biosci*, 6, pp. 274–284.

Tumlin J, Wali R, Williams W, Murray P, Tolwani AJ, Vinnikova AK, Szerlip HM, Ye J, Paganini EP, Dworkin L, Finkel KW, Kraus MA and Humes HD (2008). Efficacy and safety of renal tubule cell therapy for acute renal failure. *J Am Soc Nephrol*, 19, pp. 1034–1040.

Tzoneva R, Seifert B, Albrecht W, Richau K, Groth T and Lendlein A (2008). Hemocompatibility of poly(ether imide) membranes functionalized with carboxylic groups. *J Mater Sci Mater Med*, 19, pp. 3203–3210.

Vanholder R, De Smet R, Glorieux G, Argiles A, Baurmeister U, Brunet P, Clark W, Cohen G, De Deyn PP, Deppisch R, Descamps-Latscha B, Henle T, Jorres A, Lemke HD, Massy ZA, Passlick-Deetjen J, Rodriguez M, Stegmayr B, Stenvinkel P, Tetta C, Wanner C, Zidek W and European Uremic Toxin Work G (2003a). Review on uremic toxins: classification, concentration, and interindividual variability. *Kidney Int*, 63, pp. 1934–1943.

Vanholder R, De Smet R, Glorieux G and Dhondt A (2003b). Survival of hemodialysis patients and uremic toxin removal. *Artif Organs*, 27, pp. 218–223.

Vanholder RC, Eloot S and Glorieux GL (2015). Future avenues to decrease uremic toxin concentration. *Am J Kidney Dis*, 67, pp. 664–676.

Vanholder R, Schepers E, Pletinck A, Nagler EV and Glorieux G (2014). The uremic toxicity of indoxyl sulfate and p-cresyl sulfate: a systematic review. *J Am Soc Nephrol*, 25, pp. 1–11.

Vasiliou V, Vasiliou K and Nebert DW (2009). Human ATP-binding cassette (ABC) transporter family. *Hum Genomics*, 3, pp. 281–290.

Vats A, Tolley NS, Polak JM and Buttery LD (2002). Stem cells: sources and applications. *Clin Otolaryngol Allied Sci*, 27, pp. 227–232.

Wilmer MJ, Ng CP, Lanz HL, Vulto P, Suter-Dick L and Masereeuw R (2016). Kidney-on-a-chip technology for drug-induced nephrotoxicity screening. *Trends Biotechnol*, 34, pp. 156–170.

Wilmer MJ, Saleem MA, Masereeuw R, Ni L, van der Velden TJ, Russel FG, Mathieson PW, Monnens LA, van den Heuvel LP and Levtchenko EN (2010a). Novel conditionally immortalized human proximal tubule cell line expressing functional influx and efflux transporters. *Cell Tissue Res*, 339, pp. 449–457.

Wilmer MJ, Saleem MA, Masereeuw R, Ni L, van der Velden TJ, Russel FG, Mathieson PW, Monnens LA, van den Heuvel LP and Levtchenko EN (2010b). Novel conditionally immortalized human proximal tubule cell line expressing functional influx and efflux transporters. *Cell Tissue Res*, 339, pp. 449–457.

Wilmes A, Bielow C, Ranninger C, Bellwon P, Aschauer L, Limonciel A, Chassaigne H, Kristl T, Aiche S, Huber CG, Guillou C, Hewitt P, Leonard MO, Dekant W, Bois F and Jennings P (2015). Mechanism of cisplatin proximal tubule toxicity revealed by integrating transcriptomics, proteomics, metabolomics and biokinetics. *Toxicol In Vitro*, 30, pp. 117–127.

Xi Z-Y, Xu .-Y, Zhu L-P, Wang Y and Zhu B-K (2009). A facile method of surface modification for hydrophobic polymer membranes based on the adhesive behavior of poly(DOPA) and poly(dopamine). *J Membrane Sci*, 327, pp. 244–253.

Xing L, Wen JG, Frokiaer J, Djurhuus JC and Norregaard R (2014). Ontogeny of the mammalian kidney: expression of aquaporins 1, 2, 3, and 4. *World J Pediatr*, 10, pp. 306–312.

Yamanaka S and Yokoo T (2015). Current bioengineering methods for whole kidney regeneration. *Stem Cells Int*, 2015, p. 724047.

Zhang H, Tasnim F, Ying JY and Zink D (2009). The impact of extracellular matrix coatings on the performance of human renal cells applied in bioartificial kidneys. *Biomaterials*, 30, pp. 2899–2911.

Zink D and Zay YO (2013). Bioreactor unit for use in bioartificial kidney device. Google Patents.

Zuk A and Bonventre JV (2016). Acute kidney injury. *Annu Rev Med*, 67, pp. 293–307.

Chapter 6
Membrane-Based Bioartificial Liver Devices

S. Khakpour*, †, ‡, H. M. M. Ahmed*, †, ‡ and L. De Bartolo*, §

**Institute on Membrane Technology, National Research Council of Italy, Rende, Italy*

†Department of Chemical Engineering and Materials (DIATIC), University of Calabria, Rende, Italy

‡Authors contributed equally

§l.debartolo@itm.cnr.it

6.1 Introduction

Liver disease, and the subsequent loss of liver function, is an enormous clinical challenge and is currently the 12th most frequent cause of death in the United States and the fourth most frequent for middle-aged adults [Mann *et al.*, 2003]. Emergence of new liver diseases such as steatohepatitis, absence of a hepatitis C vaccine and increasing number of hepatocellular carcinoma patients further worsen the situation [Bosch *et al.*, 2004; Jemal *et al.*, 2010]. Liver transplantation is the only established successful treatment for end-stage liver disease, and currently there are over 117,064 people on the waiting list for a donor organ, and of those, there are around 14,250 candidates awaiting a liver transplant (based on

United Network for Organ Sharing Organ Procurement and Transplantation Network, UNOS OPTN, July 2017). In 2015, there were 5950 liver transplants performed in the United States.

Various surgical options have been pursued, including living-donor partial transplantation and split liver transplants, in order to expand the supply of livers available for transplantation [Clavien *et al.*, 2007]. Despite these surgical advances, organ shortage remains a major hurdle, and thus it is unlikely that liver transplantation procedures alone will ever meet the increasing demand. For these reasons, many researchers have developed various extracorporeal biohybrid artificial liver (BAL) systems. Generally, a BAL system consists of functional liver cells supported by an artificial cell culture material. In particular, it incorporates hepatocytes into a bioreactor in which the cells are immobilized, cultured and induced to perform the hepatic functions by processing the blood or plasma of liver-failure patients. BAL devices act as a bridge for the patients until a donor organ is available for transplantation or until liver regeneration [Strain & Neuberger, 2002].

6.2 Liver in Health and Disease

The human liver is the largest solid organ in the body accounting for 2–5% of body weight and performs a complex array of functions, among which are embryonic hemopoiesis, protein synthesis (albumin, fibrinogen), nutrient storage, glycogen storage as well as metabolic homeostasis by regulating carbohydrate, lipid and amino acid levels. The liver also metabolizes endogenous (e.g. bilirubin, ammonia) and exogenous (drugs and environmental compounds) substances, xenobiotics and endogenous hormones. It also produces bile to aid digestion and as a route of excretion of liver waste [Underhill *et al.*, 2007].

Liver disease usually leads to a variety of life-threatening metabolic and physiologic abnormalities. For example, the absence of these functions leads to bleeding abnormalities, accumulation of neurotoxins causing hepatic encephalopathy, accumulation of serum ammonia and jaundice from elevation of serum bilirubin. It is possible to medically support liver disease patients through therapies targeted at features such as portal hypertension and coagulopathy. However, there are no therapeutic strategies effectively replacing the range of affected functions. Thus, an organ transplant has been the only permanently successful therapy to date. This is different compared to other organs, such as the heart and kidneys, in which patients with failing tissues can be supported by pharmaceuticals and machines, without the need for immediate transplantation.

Consequently, efforts have been focused toward the development of liver support systems that could provide temporary support for patients with liver failure. These measures include extracorporeal support devices analogous to kidney dialysis systems, processing the blood or plasma of liver failure patients [Carpentier *et al.*, 2009; Rademacher *et al.*, 2011]. They range from non-biological-based systems to cell-based therapies, such as BALs.

In vivo, the liver exhibits a unique capacity for regeneration, with the potential for full restoration of liver mass and function even after massive damage [Taub, 2004]. However, a major hurdle to the advancement of cell-based therapeutic strategies is the loss of the proliferative capacity and of the liver-specific functions exhibited by hepatocytes once isolated from the *in vivo* microenvironment. Another obstacle in the progress of cell-based approaches is the limited availability of human hepatocytes. Only a limited supply of primary human hepatocytes is currently available from organs deemed inappropriate for transplantation. Thus, significant research efforts are focused on the potential of alternative cell sources, most notably those based on stem cell differentiation and reprogramming.

6.3 Artificial Liver Support Devices

Over the last three decades, liver support systems have been developed to replace orthotopic liver transplantation, to complement patient care by promoting liver tissue regeneration or to provide a bridge to liver transplantation. A successful liver support system should provide sufficient detoxification, synthesis, biotransformation and excretion functionality as performed by the liver. They are commonly divided into two main categories: biological and non-biological systems.

Accumulation of endogenous hepatotoxic substances is conjectured to induce loss of liver function, which in turn gives rise to accumulation of toxins, production of cytokines and further damage of the liver [Carpentier *et al.*, 2009]. Artificial liver (AL) devices are typically designed to emulate detoxification functions of the liver through filtration and adsorption mechanisms, only, without employing living components. These devices are briefly discussed here, since they are described in detail in Chapter 3.

Molecular Adsorbent Recirculating System (MARS®; Gambro, Stockholm, Sweden) is a prominent, extensively evaluated AL, based on dialysis, adsorption and filtration processes. It removes both water-soluble and albumin-bound toxins using a high-flux polysulfone hemodialyzer hollow fiber (HF) module. Recirculating albumin-enriched dialysate is regenerated through consecutive dialysis, ion exchange and charcoal adsorption units.

Hepa Wash® procedure (Hepa Wash GmbH, Munich, Germany) uses a similar principle as MARS®, except that the albumin dialysate is regenerated through pH and temperature changes. In single-pass albumin dialysis, on the other hand, the albumin solution is discarded instead of being regenerated.

In fractionated plasma separation and adsorption (Prometheus®, Fresenius Medical Care, Bad Homburg, Germany), endogenous albumin is purified by passing through an albumin-permeable polysulfone filter, neutral resin, ion exchanger and high-flux hemodialyzer.

In selective plasma-exchange therapy (SEPET™, Arbios Systems, Allendale, NJ, USA), a size-selective membrane removes smaller molecules (MW < 100 kDa). The albumin fraction associated with toxins is then replaced by electrolytes, albumin and fresh-frozen plasma.

ALs are merely based on physicochemical mechanisms and thus lack synthetic and biochemical functions of the liver. Additionally, hepatic detoxification inside the body is not limited to elimination of albumin-bound toxins. Moreover, the probable adverse effects of unselective adsorption and removal of molecules are yet to be evaluated. Moreover, regulatory functions of the liver are broader than acid–base status and electrolyte levels [Struecker *et al.*, 2014].

Considering the range and complexity of functions performed by the liver, non-biological-based systems merely detoxifying the blood are insufficient to support liver failure patients and thus show limited clinical success [Rademacher *et al.*, 2011]. To provide a larger complement of important liver functions, including synthetic and metabolic processes, biohybrid support devices incorporating living hepatic cells have been developed [Phua & Lee, 2008].

6.4 Bioartificial Liver Systems

In order to address the shortcomings of the ALs and to provide a more comprehensive range of hepatic functions, extensive research has been dedicated to explore and develop cell-based therapies. Such therapeutic interventions include hepatocyte (primary or stem-cell-derived) transplantation by infusion of isolated cells through the portal vein in the liver, extracorporeal bioartificial liver (BAL) devices incorporating hepatic cell culture in a bioreactor and implantation of tissue-engineered grafts. More recent, cutting-edge technologies include repopulation of decellularized liver, tissue/organ biofabrication through 3D printing techniques and induced organogenesis [Bhatia *et al.*, 2014; Lee *et al.*, 2015; Struecker *et al.*, 2014].

Preserving prolonged and stable functionality of hepatocytes *in vitro* is indeed a major issue. Microenvironmental signals, namely soluble mediators, cell–extracellular matrix (ECM) interactions and cell–cell interactions are reported to regulate hepatic functionality. Consequently, a diverse range of *in vitro* hepatic culture models have been developed to fully understand the regulating mechanisms of hepatocytes, some of which include perfused whole organs and wedge biopsies, precision-cut liver slices, isolated primary hepatocytes, immortalized liver cell lines and isolated organelles [Underhill *et al.*, 2007].

BALs provide a promising means toward developing a temporary support, a platform for drug testing and for *in vitro* study of hepatic cultures. Thanks to incorporation of functional hepatocytes, BALs can potentially perform a wide range of vital hepatic functions, namely detoxification, metabolism and synthesis.

In vitro cell cultures are expected to actualize a microenvironment in which *in vivo*-like phenotypic functions of cells are maintained. Viability and functionality of isolated hepatocytes *in vitro* highly depends on external cues, introduced in their microenvironment with respect to both time and space [Khetani *et al.*, 2015]. Consequently, hepatic cultures have been investigated in various configurations, in 2D and 3D, with or without perfusion and in different scales.

Numerous BAL designs have been suggested and explored, which fall into four main categories: flat plate systems, hollow fiber membrane bioreactors (HFMBRs), perfused packed bed/scaffold systems and suspension-/encapsulation-based reactors. Additionally, microfluidic systems and microfabricated reactor systems have been studied recently [Ebrahimkhani *et al.*, 2014]. In the following sections, different bioreactor configurations for membrane-based BAL systems are introduced.

6.4.1 *Flat Plate Membrane Bioreactors*

The primitive Petri dish-based static monolayer (2D) cultures demonstrate several disadvantages, namely: (i) continuous temporal change in cellular microenvironment due to consumption of nutrients and accumulation of cellular metabolic products, (ii) limited oxygen supply due to its low solubility and diffusion length, (iii) poor cell–cell and cell–ECM interactions, (iv) smooth, 2D substrate incomparable to *in vivo* situation and (v) unidirectional mass exchange due to impermeable substrate.

Different strategies have been investigated in bioreactors to address the aforementioned shortcomings. The advantages of perfusion, i.e. medium flow over or through the cellular layer, in the bioreactor have been recognized for a long time. Gebhardt and Mecke [1979], for example, reported improved viability and functionality (in terms of urea synthesis) of primary rat hepatocytes over 6 days under perfusion compared to static culture.

The perfusion significantly improves mass transfer. However, the shear stress exerted on the cells becomes a new limiting factor and needs to be maintained within a safe range well tolerated by hepatocytes.

Incorporation of membranes in flat plate bioreactors introduces many valuable features to the dynamic culture system. Membranes compartmentalize the system, allowing nutrients and oxygen to pass through the cellular compartment while protecting the cells from the fluid shear. They may support one or both surfaces of the cellular layer, allowing for mass transfer to/from cells in all directions. Additionally, oxygen-permeable membranes can also be employed, so that oxygen gradient is applied separately from the fluid flow. Moreover, porous membranes can offer a more *in vivo*-like three-dimensional substrate compared to smooth solid plastic, while facilitating cellular interaction studies [Sheridan *et al.*, 2008].

Other enhancements have also been explored for monolayer-based systems, which can be applied to flat membrane bioreactors as well, including co-cultures [Salerno *et al.*, 2011] and sandwich cultures [Dunn *et al.*, 1992] for improving cell–cell and cell–ECM interactions, micro-grooved substrate [Park *et al.*, 2005] for protection against shear stress and substrate micropatterning [Thery, 2010] for cell morphogenesis studies.

6.4.2 *Hollow Fiber Membrane Bioreactors*

HFMBRs are commonly used in tissue engineering applications for cell-based therapies [Diban & Stamatialis, 2014] including BAL devices [Yu *et al.*, 2012] and large-scale cell cultures [Knazek *et al.*, 1972].

HFMBRs consist of a bundle of semipermeable HFs placed in an outer housing, similar to ultrafiltration or dialysis applications. Depending on the application and the cell types used, different configurations can serve different functions. The cells are more commonly attached to the outer wall of the HFs with the medium flowing in the lumen of the fibers exchanging nutrients and other components similar to blood capillary network. Alternatively, the cells may be seeded in the lumen of the HF, and the module can be operated under different flow patterns [Wung *et al.*, 2014]. More complex configurations have also been suggested, such as multi-bore system [De Bartolo *et al.*, 2007], alginate immobilization [Hoesli *et al.*, 2009] and three-compartment multi-coaxial system [Hilal-Alnaqbi *et al.*, 2013].

HFMBRs can potentially improve mass-transfer rates — for both nutrient provision and waste removal — with respect to limitations imposed by the diffusion length. Thanks to this compartmentalization, the cells are separated from direct fluid flow and are thus protected from shear and air–liquid interfacial stresses. Additionally, HFMBRs provide a large surface area to volume ratio, which allows to culture the same amount of cells in 0.58 L, compared to 1 m^3 in case of using standard flask culture techniques [Shipley *et al.*, 2011].

6.5 Bioreactor Configurations in Bioartificial Liver Designs

So far, only few BAL systems have reached clinical trials, while various designs are explored *in vitro* as dynamic hepatic culture systems. The majority of BALs in clinical trials (Table 6.1) as well as many *in vitro* systems are based on HF bioreactors, further demonstrating their significance in these applications.

6.5.1 *Bioartificial Liver Systems in Clinical Trial*

One of the most well-known BAL systems that has reached clinical trials is HepatAssist™ Device (Alliqua Inc., Langhorne, PA, USA), developed by Demetriou *et al.* Here, porcine hepatocyte cells are maintained in a modified dialysis cartridge based on HF membranes. Patients' plasma is separated, led through an activated charcoal adsorber followed by an oxygenator and then through the bioreactor [Demetriou *et al.*, 1986, 2004]. A randomized controlled trial of HepatAssist™ in 171 acute liver failure patients showed improved survival at 30 days: 71% for HepatAssist device vs 62% for standard medical therapy. In fact, survival in fulminant or sub-fulminant liver failure patients was much higher in HepatAssist group. Unfortunately, this is the only randomized controlled trial carried out on a bioartificial liver support system. The other BAL systems have been assessed in smaller studies [Carpentier *et al.*, 2009].

One of the first clinical devices using HF membranes was Extracorporeal Liver Assist Device (ELAD®) (Vital Therapies Inc., San Diego, CA, USA) developed by Sussman *et al.* It employs C3A human hepatoblastoma cell lines, while the flow circuit is conceptually similar to HepatAssist [Ellis *et al.*, 1996; Sussman *et al.*, 1994].

Chamuleau's group took a different approach in designing the Academisch Medisch Centrum Bioartificial Liver (AMC-BAL). This device consists of non-woven polyester matrix and HFs encased in a housing. HFs distributed within the matrix are used for oxygen supply and CO_2 removal, while the cells are cultured on the matrix in a 3D architecture. Porcine hepatocytes were initially used, but the device has been modified to use immortalized fetal liver cell lines.

Table 6.1: Membrane-based bioartificial systems currently in clinical trials.

Clinical trial	Phase II/III	Phase I	Phase I	Phase I/II	Phase I
Oxygenation	Before bioreactor	Before bioreactor	Inside bioreactor	Before bioreactor	Inside bioreactor
BR flow rate (ml/min)	400	15–200	150	100–250	100–200
Perfusion medium	Plasma	Blood/plasma ultrafiltrate	Plasma	Blood	Plasma
Cell amount	$5–7 \times 10^9$	200–400 g	1010	70–120 g	≤600 g
Cell source	Cryopreserved	C3A	Freshly isolated	Freshly isolated	Freshly isolated
Cell type	Porcine	Human, tumor cell line	Porcine	Porcine	Porcine/human
MWCO (kDa)	3000	70	Membrane for oxygenation only	100	400
Membrane	Polysulfone	Cellulose acetate	Polypropylene membrane, polyester matrix	Cellulose acetate	Polyethersulfone
BR type	HF	HF	HF + matrix	HF	HF
BAL system	HepatAssis	ELAD	AMC-BAL	BLSS	MELS

The unique aspect in AMC-BAL is that after plasmapheresis, the patient's plasma is in direct contact with the cells, enhancing cell–plasma mass transfer [Flendrig *et al.*, 1997].

Patzer *et al.* [1999] developed the Bioartificial Liver Support System (BLSS) based on a hemofilter containing freshly isolated porcine cells. This system differs from the others in two major aspects: whole blood is perfused rather than plasma, and the cells are in suspension, circulating in the extra-capillary space (ECS) [Mazariegos *et al.*, 2002].

The Modular Extracorporeal Liver Support (MELS) developed by Gerlach *et al.* is one of the most complex, yet appealing, HF bioreactor designs, consisting three separate bundles of HFs interwoven together: two sets of hydrophilic polyethersulfone HFs for plasma perfusion (culture medium flows between the two sets semi-interstitially) and one set of hydrophobic multi-layer HFs for local oxygenation. Plasma is perfused into the bioreactor containing primary porcine or primary human liver cells capable of forming tissue-like structures between HFs [Sauer *et al.*, 2001, 2003a, 2003b].

The aforementioned ALs and BALs, their treatment units and clinical findings have been reviewed more extensively, by others [Carpentier *et al.*, 2009; Podoll *et al.*, 2012; Struecker *et al.*, 2014].

6.5.2 *Bioreactor Designs for In Vitro Hepatic Culture Studies*

Various bioreactor designs have been investigated for dynamic hepatic cultures *in vitro*, as BAL devices or drug-testing platforms in pharmaceutical research. Here, few examples with different configurations are exemplified to provide a better understanding of bioreactor design and various design aspects they address.

An oxygen-permeable, flat-membrane bioreactor was developed by De Bartolo *et al.* [2006] (Fig. 6.1). Human hepatocytes were cultured between two fluorocarbon flat semipermeable membranes. The cells were directly oxygenated by the bottom membrane to which they adhered, while their upper surface was in contact with the culture medium which in turn was oxygenated through the upper membrane. Hepatic functionality was evaluated by synthesis of urea and albumin, and diclofenac biotransformation, which were maintained for 32 days.

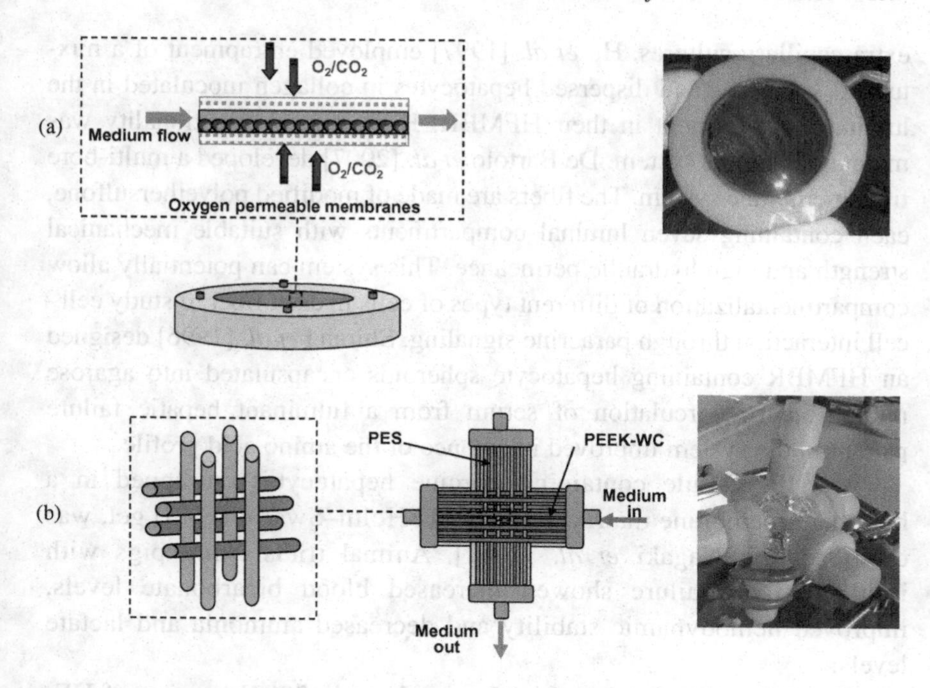

Figure 6.1. Examples of bioreactors used for *in vitro* studies. (a) Oxygen-permeable flat-membrane bioreactor [De Bartolo *et al.*, 2006]. (b) Crossed HFMBR [De Bartolo *et al.*, 2009].

Schmitmeier *et al.* [2006] compared conventional well-plate cultures with a small-scale bioreactor with a gas-permeable membrane at the bottom using a hepatic sandwich culture. Better liver-specific functionality was found for the bioreactor model, without dedifferentiation of cells over 17 days. In another study, formation and cultivation of hepatocyte spheroids in a rotating-wall gas-permeable membrane system (RWMS) was investigated and compared with a rotating-wall gas-impermeable polystyrene system (RWPS). Oxygen, glucose and lactate transfer in both systems were also evaluated by mathematical modeling. Improved viability of cells in RWMS was mathematically predicted and experimentally confirmed [Curcio *et al.*, 2007].

Cultivation of cells in the luminal compartment of HFs is also investigated by researchers, but it is less common compared to extra-capillary cultures. Hu *et al.* [1997] employed entrapment of a mixture of spheroids and dispersed hepatocytes in collagen inoculated in the luminal compartment in their HFMBR. High hepatic functionality was maintained in this system. De Bartolo *et al.* [2007] developed a multi-bore fiber membrane system. The fibers are made of modified polyethersulfone, each containing seven luminal compartments with suitable mechanical strength and high hydraulic permeance. This system can potentially allow compartmentalization of different types of cells in each fiber to study cell–cell interaction through paracrine signaling. Shiraha *et al.* [1996] designed an HFMBR containing hepatocyte spheroids encapsulated into agarose microdroplets. Circulation of serum from a fulminant hepatic failure patient in the system improved imbalance of the amino acid profile.

An HF module containing porcine hepatocytes entrapped in a basement membrane matrix, Engelbreth–Holm–Swarm (EHS) gel, was developed by Nagaki *et al.* [2001]. Animal trials using pigs with ischemic liver failure showed increased blood bicarbonate levels, improved hemodynamic stability and decreased ammonia and lactate levels.

The OXY-HFB developed by Jasmund *et al.* [2002] consists of HFs for oxygenation and for internal heat exchange. Culture medium was circulated in the ECS where primary porcine liver cells were seeded on the HF walls. Hepatic functions of the cells, evaluated in terms of urea, albumin and lactate secretion, glucose consumption, oxygen level and diazepam metabolism, were maintained for 3 weeks.

Another HFMBR developed by De Bartolo *et al.* [2009] consists of two different types of HFs arranged in a crossed configuration, mimicking the blood capillary network. Each type of HF is employed to serve a distinguished function: modified polyetheretherketone (PEEK-WC) for supplying the cells with nutrients and metabolites, and polyethersulfone (PES) for removing the catabolites. Urea, albumin and diazepam transport was mathematically modeled and experimentally evaluated. Primary human hepatocytes maintained their functionality (urea and albumin synthesis, diazepam biotransformation) for 18 days.

Application of adhesive substrates in bioreactors to enhance cellular attachment and functionality has also been studied. Lu *et al.* [2005] reported enhanced albumin synthesis in rat hepatocytes cultured in a galactosylated polyvinylidene difluoride HF bioreactor. In another study, sustained human hepatocyte functionality was found in a galactosylated polyethersulfone flat membrane bioreactor [Memoli *et al.*, 2007].

A closer look at the bioreactor configurations introduced above reveals three main challenges in the development of BAL devices: (i) membranes as artificial support, (ii) cell sources and (iii) mass-transfer considerations. These issues are discussed in the following sections.

6.6 Membranes in Bioartificial Liver Systems

The choice of the membrane material is crucially important in bioartificial systems. The material in direct contact with the cells ideally should be non-toxic and biocompatible, promote favorable cellular interactions and functions, support secretion of ECM components required for tissue regeneration and possess necessary mechanical and physical properties. Depending on the application, e.g. for certain implantable scaffolds, the material should be biodegradable and bioresorbable to avoid inflammation [Kim *et al.*, 2000].

Development of membranes for tissue engineering applications has evolved significantly over the past three decades, from merely inert biomaterials to bioactive, biodegradable/bioresorbable materials. More recently, biomaterials are designed to stimulate specific cellular response. In other words, resorbable polymers can be modified at molecular level to provoke specific interactions with cell integrins — transmembrane glycoproteins that attach cells to ECM proteins — bridging cell–cell and cell–ECM interactions.

Advances in the development of polymeric membranes have made a remarkable contribution to the field of tissue engineering and regenerative medicine. Selectivity, stability and biocompatibility of polymeric membranes make them an appealing choice in biohybrid systems for cell culture. Semipermeable membranes provide a suitable support for attachment of anchorage-dependent cells like hepatocytes, allowing selective provision of metabolites and nutrients to cells and selective removal of catabolites and products [De Bartolo *et al.*, 2000; Unger *et al.*, 2005].

Adhesion, proliferation, viability and functionality of cells are strongly regulated by surface properties of the membranes, namely chemical composition, hydrophilicity/hydrophobicity, charge, free energy and roughness. Cell–biomaterial interactions can be promoted through surface modification, e.g. grafting of functional groups and immobilization of functional molecules [Morelli *et al.*, 2010]. Synthesized components of ECM, including collagen, laminin, elastin and fibronectin, are also used as matrices for tissue engineering applications.

The aforementioned properties are generally expected from biomaterials to be used for *in vitro* culture studies. However, each cell type has its own characteristics, which in turn may call for customized biomaterials that are not always commercially available. Development of cell-specific membranes is in fact a vital and challenging step in realization of bioartificial organs.

Unfortunately, most of the commercial membranes employed for hepatic cultures were initially developed for hemodialysis, thus requiring minimal interactions with proteins and cells in the blood. Consequently, development of membranes promoting adhesion and functionality of hepatocytes is a primary and crucial step in liver tissue engineering in general. Cytocompatibility of membranes can be improved by surface modification strategies such as grafting of functional groups (e.g. COOH, NH_2) or immobilization of biomolecules (e.g. RGD peptide or galactose interacting with cell receptors).

In addition to biocompatibility, a BAL device must also be able to provide and promote: (i) adhesion of cells and secretion of ECM, (ii) immunoprotection of cells and (iii) efficient mass transport between culture medium or blood/plasma compartment and the cellular compartment.

Transport properties of the membranes are determined by pore size and molecular weight cutoff (MWCO), i.e. molecular weight of species retained by 90% within the membrane. Membranes with MWCO between 70 and 100 kDa act as an immunoselective barrier, preventing immunoglobulins from passing while allowing the transport of serum albumin. Mass-transfer considerations are discussed in detail in the following sections.

Morphological properties (e.g. pore size, pore size distribution, roughness) and physicochemical properties (e.g. surface charge, wettability, surface free energy) reportedly influence the adhesion and metabolic function of the hepatocytes [De Bartolo *et al.*, 2002].

6.7 Cell Source

Primary human hepatocytes are ultimately the preferred cell type for cell-based therapies, and the development of primary hepatocyte-based approaches is the focus of substantial ongoing research. Yet, progress has been hindered by the limited supply of these cells and their loss of differentiation *in vitro*.

Immortalized hepatocyte cell lines, such as HepG2 (human hepatoblastoma) [Kelly & Darlington, 1989], the HepG2-derived line C3A [Ellis *et al.*, 1996], HepLiu (SV40 immortalized) [Liu *et al.*, 1998], immortalized fetal human hepatocytes [Yoon *et al.*, 1999] and HepaRG (human hepatoma) [Gripon *et al.*, 2002], have been utilized as readily available alternative to primary hepatocytes. The advantages of using established cell lines include the ability to culture large quantities of cells for an extended period of time and the ability to control the degree of hepatocyte function that is displayed [Allen & Bhatia, 2002]. However, due to the lack of the full functional capacity of primary adult hepatocytes, and the risk of transmittance of oncogenic factors to the patient, the use of these cell lines in a clinical setup remains a major concern [Allen *et al.*, 2001]. Thus, as a potential precautionary measure, the use of conditionally immortalized lines and the incorporation of inducible suicide genes have been considered [Lanza *et al.*, 2011].

Primary porcine hepatocytes have been widely used as the cell source for hybrid ALs. Porcine hepatocytes exhibit liver-specific functions including biotransformation functions, ammonia detoxification and synthesis of urea and albumin [te Velde *et al.*, 1995]. Although these cells can be readily obtained in large quantities and demonstrate similar functions and therapeutic effects to human hepatocytes, their major drawbacks are the risk of xenogeneic infections such as porcine endogenous retrovirus and the lack of metabolic compatibility [Pascher *et al.*, 2002].

An independent approach to generate hepatocytes for therapeutics is to use stem and/or progenitor cells, which may be sourced from various tissues and have a high proliferative capacity. In principle, such cells could be amplified, differentiated into various cell types and used in diverse applications [Bhatia *et al.*, 2014]. Although progress has been made in genetically or immunologically identifying tissue-resident stem cell-like populations that reside in human liver [Lee *et al.*, 2014; Schmelzer *et al.*, 2007], further investigation into the role of these cells in normal liver physiology and repair is needed to determine whether these cell populations represent a clinically relevant source of hepatocytes. Pluripotent stem cells, including human ESC (hESC) and induced pluripotent stem cell (iPSC) lines, represent an interesting source for generating hepatocytes.

Various directed differentiation strategies have been applied to hESC and iPSC cultures and have yielded populations that exhibit some functional and phenotypic characteristics of mature hepatocytes, thus termed "hepatocyte-like cells" [Asplund *et al.*, 2016; Hay *et al.*, 2008; Si-Tayeb *et al.*, 2010; Touboul *et al.*, 2010]. Yet, hepatocyte-like cells resemble fetal hepatocytes rather than mature adult cells as evident by their characteristics, such as distinctive cytochrome P450 activities as well as expression of α-fetoprotein [Schwartz *et al.*, 2014]. Recently, researchers have been attempting to identify small molecules that can potentially induce the maturation of hepatocyte-like cells to enhance the chance for using these cells in a clinically relevant setup [Shan *et al.*, 2013]. Besides, directed differentiation of fibroblasts into hepatocyte-like cells, which exhibit more adult hepatic traits, might provide an autologous stem cell source that would bypass the need for immune suppression [Huang *et al.*, 2014; Sekiya & Suzuki, 2011]. In light of this progress, the strategy of using stem cells as a source for generating hepatocytes as a cellular component in BAL devices holds great promise.

6.8 Mass and Momentum Transfer Considerations

In vivo, hepatocytes are organized in unicellular plates along the sinusoids, sandwiched between layers of ECM and equipped with different types of junctions and bile canaliculi, thus providing a unique microstructure and efficient species transfer enabling their wide range of functions. Ideally, such a delicate, well-defined microenvironment should be emulated in culture models *in vitro* and assessed in terms of species transport.

Membrane-based BAL systems generally consist of three compartments: culture medium (in *in vitro* studies) or blood/plasma (in clinical

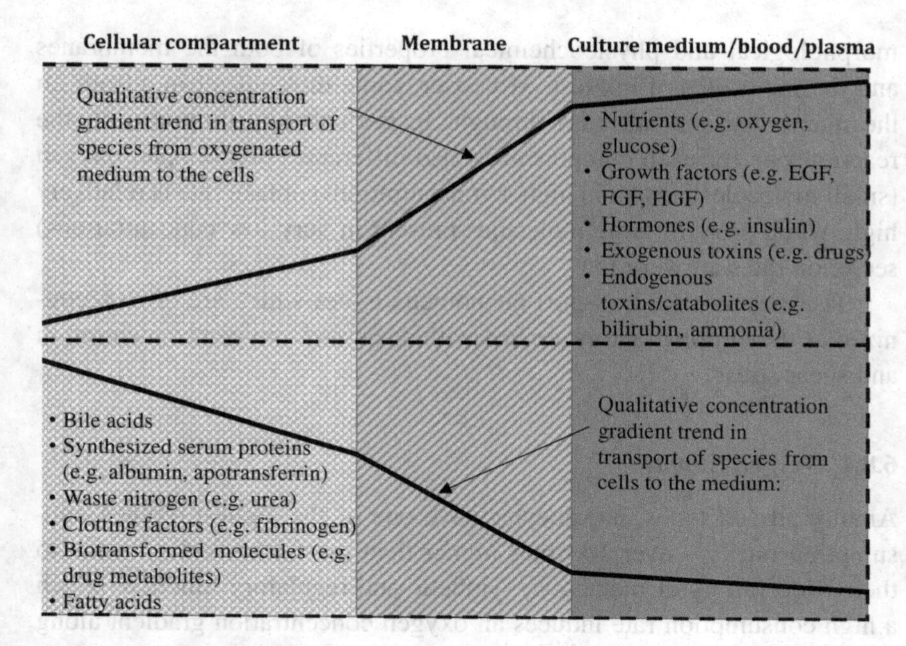

Figure 6.2. Compartmentalization of the membrane-based BALs. Bidirectional mass transfer occurs between the compartments and through the membranes. The concentration gradient trends shown apply to diffusion-controlled mass transfer and are merely qualitative, since the rate and extent of the gradients differ for each component.

studies), membrane and cellular compartment. Oxygen, nutrients, metabolites, growth factors, hormones and other proteins, as well as endogenous catabolites, drugs and toxic compounds (to be metabolized) must be transferred to cells, while catabolites, synthesized proteins and other cellular products need to be efficiently removed from cellular microenvironment (Fig. 6.2).

As one can immediately infer, complex exchange of numerous molecules with a wide range of sizes and physicochemical properties occurs between the compartments. Each component has a different diffusion rate in the liquid solution. Additionally, the three compartments are all coupled together. Therefore, the transport through the porous media (membranes, cells) as well as the consumption or production rates in the cells affects the overall mass transfer. As previously described, the transport rate through the membrane depends on the MWCO, as well as the morphological and physicochemical properties of both the membranes and the molecules of interest. Moreover, some molecules can adsorb on the membrane and not pass through. In the cellular compartment, the reaction rate for each component is also different. For example, oxygen (small molecules present in higher concentrations) uptake rate is relatively high, while protein (large molecules present in very low concentrations) secretion rates are very low.

The most critical transport phenomena issues which are often recognized as the limiting factors are herewith discussed: oxygen concentration and shear stress.

6.8.1 *Oxygen Supply*

Among all cell types, hepatocytes have one of the highest oxygen consumption rates — over 10 times higher than most other cells — due to their wide variety of metabolic, synthetic and regulatory functions. Such a high consumption rate induces an oxygen concentration gradient along the sinusoids. This concentration distribution for oxygen, as well as hormones, nutrients and ECM molecules, is reportedly responsible for the distribution of metabolic functions along the sinusoids [Underhill *et al.*, 2007]. In fact, three metabolic zonations along hepatic sinusoids in the lobule are conventionally recognized: zone 1 around portal vein and hepatic arteriole known as the periportal zone, zone 3 around the central vein known as the perivenous, pericentral or centrilobular zone, and the less well-defined transitional zone 2 in between. Partial pressure of oxygen is decreased by around 50% along the sinusoids, dropping from about 60–65 mmHg (84–91 μmol/L) in the periportal zone to about 30–35 mmHg (42–49 μmol/L) in the perivenous zone, which enables distinguished hepatic metabolism in each section [Allen & Bhatia, 2003; Broughan *et al.*, 2008; Jungermann & Kietzmann, 2000].

Mimicking delicate *in vivo* oxygen conditions, and their realization *in vitro* is indeed very challenging. Sufficient oxygen needs to be supplied to hepatic cultures *in vitro* to avoid hypoxic conditions, which is limited by oxygen's low solubility in culture medium and its short diffusive penetration depth in hepatic tissues. Hyperoxic oxygen tensions, on the other hand, can cause oxidative effects on cells, potentially compromising hepatocytes' viability and functionality. Additionally, a concentration gradient in accordance with the physiological range should also be induced within the hepatic mass inside the bioreactor McClelland *et al.* [2003].

Optimal oxygen tension range reported in the literature for *in vitro* applications is also a controversial topic. Wang *et al.* [2010] briefly review some of the rather contradictory findings about oxygen tension as well as the uptake rate in the literature and conclude that the pericellular oxygen tension of the hepatocytes should mimic the *in vivo* conditions rather than intracellular values.

Among the strategies to improve oxygen supply and to avoid hypoxic/hyperoxic conditions, the two most commonly explored are: (i) oxygen-permeable (HF) membranes to provide sufficient oxygen and to induce an oxygen concentration gradient locally, most notably employed in AMC-BAL and MELS devices introduced before, and (ii) enhancing mass transfer by adding advection.

6.8.2 *Convection-Enhanced Systems and Shear Stress Effects*

In diffusion-controlled, membrane-based BAL systems, chemical potential is the driving force for mass transfer, dominated by the concentration gradient across the membrane. Mass-transport mechanism can be enhanced by convection, through applying a pressure gradient across the membrane.

Adding convection can significantly improve mass transfer, especially considering that various molecules are present covering a wide size range, from oxygen (32 g/mol) to albumin (67 kDa) and apo-transferrin (80 kDa). However, great care must be taken in inducing culture medium flow over/through the cellular compartment. Needless to say, the flow must not result in detachment and elimination of cells from the bioreactor. Moreover, favorable compounds like autocrine factors should not be washed away from the cellular microenvironment. Besides, formation of ECM needs to be promoted and not adversely affected by the medium flow.

One of the most influential yet controversial outcomes of direct perfusion (i.e. convection in the cellular compartment) is the unavoidable shear stress exerted on the cells. In fact, hepatocytes are very sensitive to shear forces, and high flow rates could compromise their viability and functionality [Mazzei *et al.*, 2010]. Studies have shown improved functionality as well as higher release of alanine transaminase — a marker of cell damage — in perfused flat plate systems compared to static culture [Kan *et al.*, 1998, 2004].

Acceptable range of shear stress values well withstood by cells or even beneficial due to favorable stimulation of mechanosensors is still a subject of considerable debate. A review of previous studies actually demonstrates that the effects of shear stress may differ with respect to cell type, culture type (homotypic, heterotypic), culture period and hepatic functions under evaluation, as briefly reviewed by Wang *et al.* [2010] and Ebrahimkhani *et al.* [2014].

6.8.3 *Mathematical Modeling Applications in BAL Devices*

Despite its significant impact, measurement of the concentration of oxygen, nutrients and cellular products at micro-scale within the cellular microenvironment is, if possible, very challenging. Furthermore, the experimental protocols for cell cultures are very costly and time-consuming, inhibiting optimization of the culture conditions through experiments only. Such intrinsic limitations accentuate the value of mathematical modeling of the transport phenomena inside the bioreactor as a powerful tool toward a deeper understanding of the underlying phenomena in bioreactor's performance, a close-to-reality prediction of cellular microenvironment and optimization of the operating conditions.

The mathematical model consists of the differential equations of motion coupled with mass balance equations, incorporating proper boundary conditions. Velocity (U), pressure (P) and species concentrations (c) are the dependent variables of the model, obtained for each domain and coupled between domains through interfacial boundary conditions. Conservation of mass for incompressible fluids reveals:

$$\nabla \cdot \bar{U}_i = 0 \tag{6.1}$$

The subscript i refers to the domain: lumen (l), membrane (m), cellular compartment (cc) and ECS (e). The equation of motion in the free flow regions, i.e. the lumina and possibly the ECS, is described by the Navier–Stokes equations:

$$\rho_f(\bar{U}_i \cdot \nabla)\bar{U}_i - \mu_f \nabla^2 \bar{U}_i + \nabla P_i = 0, \tag{6.2}$$

in which ρ_f and μ_f are the fluid density and dynamic viscosity, respectively.

The fluid transport in the porous media, i.e. membranes and cellular compartment, are described by Darcy's law (Eq. (6.2)) or by Brinkman equation (Eq. (6.3)):

$$\bar{U}_i = -\frac{k_{m_i}}{\mu_f} \nabla P_i, \tag{6.3}$$

$$\mu_{e_i} \nabla^2 \bar{U}_i - \nabla P_i - \frac{\mu_f}{k_{m_i}} \bar{U}_i = 0, \tag{6.4}$$

where K_m is the permeability of the porous medium and μ_e the effective viscosity in the porous medium, which is generally either considered equal to μ_f or defined as a function of porosity. Equation of motion in each domain along with the equation of continuity (Eq. (6.1)) are then coupled through continuity of the normal components of stress and velocity applied at interfacial boundaries. Other boundary conditions must be carefully identified and applied according to the system.

Mass balance for each component in the free fluid regions yields

$$\nabla \cdot (C_{j,i}\bar{U}_i) - \nabla \cdot (D_{j,i} \nabla C_{j,i}) = 0, \tag{6.5}$$

in which D is the diffusion coefficient and subscript j refers to the molecule of interest. Mass balance in the porous media is described by

$$\nabla \cdot (C_{j,i}\bar{U}_i) - \nabla \cdot (D_{e_{j,i}} \nabla C_{j,i}) - R_{j,i} = 0, \tag{6.6}$$

where D_e is the effective diffusion coefficient and R is the reaction rate. In the cellular compartment, R is the metabolic rate of consumption or production of the molecule, which depends on the molecule of interest and the cell type. Oxygen uptake is generally modeled by Michaelis–Menten kinetics:

$$R_o = \frac{V_{\max} c_{o,cc}}{c_{o,cc} + K_M}, \tag{6.7}$$

where V_{max} is the maximum consumption rate and K_M is the concentration at which the rate is half of V_{max}. Reaction term is generally considered in the cellular compartment only. However, if adsorption of proteins to the membrane is also under investigation, it may be modeled as a reaction term within the membrane compartment. Concentration of the same species in different domains is then coupled through continuity of concentration and flux applied at interfacial boundaries. Other boundary conditions must be carefully identified and applied accordingly.

The model is then solved by numerical methods using commercially available software such as FLUENT (ANSYS Inc., Canonsburg, PA, USA) and COMSOL MULTIPHYSICS® (COMSOL Inc., Stockholm, Sweden). Obtained results include fluid velocity field, pressure and species concentrations as the dependent variables. Other highly informative data can then be derived and evaluated, including shear stress and normal stress exerted on cells, and dimensionless numbers comparing rates of convective, diffusive and reactive mechanisms such as Péclet number, Damköhler number and Thiele modulus. These dimensionless numbers elucidate what mechanism is dominant and which one is in fact limiting the process.

6.9 Conceptual Limitations and Future Directions in Development of Bioartificial Liver Systems

In comparison with whole-organ transplantation, the results from clinical trials of liver support systems are limited and not as satisfactory. Blood detoxification by ALs cannot solely support liver failure patients since important metabolic, synthetic and regulatory functions are missing.

Struecker *et al.* [2014] discussed that one key limitation in BAL systems is in fact the membranes. Separation of blood from plasma, and plasma from cells by membranes adversely affects mass-transfer rates. In addition, due to flow resistance, the perfusion in BAL systems is by far less than those *in vivo*.

Majority of BAL systems employ HF membrane bioreactors. However, despite their unique advantages mentioned before, there are also disadvantages potentially limiting their application, especially for *in vitro* studies. Some of such limiting factors include difficult setup, adsorption of proteins and certain species to the membrane, and the consequent change in transport properties of the membrane over time, challenging *in situ* imaging of the cells/tissue, and difficult access to cellular compartment [Ebrahimkhani *et al.*, 2014].

Despite the extensive efforts devoted to development of a BAL able to perform the same *in vivo* liver function, to date none of the proposed devices is ready for routinely clinical treatment of patients with hepatic failure. Key challenges that are still encountered include lack of an ideal cell source, oxygen supply limitations and realization of an *in vivo*-like environment for cells. Future research should focus on the production of highly differentiated hepatocytes from progenitor cells or stem cells in order to have a BAL system functionally active. Another important point is to undertake strategies that favor the creation of microvessels and bile canaliculi by using co-culture of hepatocytes with the other liver cell types. Additionally, more efforts should focus on the development of membrane devices able to provide necessary biological, chemical and mechanical demands or stimuli for the maintenance of liver-specific functions.

Acknowledgments

The authors acknowledge the European Commission for granting the BIOART project within the framework of Marie Curie Initial Training Network, Contract No. FP7-PEOPLE-2012-ITN-316690.

List of Abbreviations

AL	artificial liver
BAL	bioartificial liver
ECM	extracellular matrix
ECS	extra-capillary space
ESC	embryonic stem cell
HF	hollow fiber
HFMBR	hollow fiber membrane bioreactor
iPSC	induced pluripotent stem cell
MWCO	molecular weight cutoff

References

Allen JW and Bhatia SN (2002). Engineering liver therapies for the future. *Tissue Eng*, 8, pp. 725–737.

Allen JW and Bhatia SN (2003). Formation of steady-state oxygen gradients *in vitro*: application to liver zonation. *Biotechnol Bioeng*, 82, pp. 253–262.

Allen JW, Hassanein T and Bhatia SN (2001). Advances in bioartificial liver devices. *Hepatology*, 34, pp. 447–455.

Asplund A, Pradip A, van Giezen M, Aspegren A, Choukair H, Rehnström M, *et al.* (2016). One standardized differentiation procedure robustly generates homogenous hepatocyte cultures displaying metabolic diversity from a large panel of human pluripotent stem cells. *Stem Cell Rev*, 12, pp. 90–104.

Bhatia SN, Underhill GH, Zaret KS and Fox IJ (2014). Cell and tissue engineering for liver disease. *Sci Transl Med*, 6, pp. 245sr2–245sr2.

Bosch FX, Ribes J, Díaz M and Cléries R (2004). Primary liver cancer: worldwide incidence and trends. *Gastroenterology*, 127, pp. S5–S16.

Broughan TA, Naukam R, Tan C, Van De Wiele CJ, Refai H and Teague TK (2008). Effects of hepatic zonal oxygen levels on hepatocyte stress responses. *J Surg Res*, 145, pp. 150–160.

Carpentier B, Gautier A and Legallais C (2009). Artificial and bioartificial liver devices: present and future. *Gut*, 58, pp. 1690–1702.

Clavien P-A, Petrowsky H, De Oliveira ML and Graf R (2007). Strategies for safer liver surgery and partial liver transplantation. *N Engl J Med*, 356, pp. 1545–1559.

Curcio E, Salerno S, Barbieri G, De Bartolo L, Drioli E and Bader A (2007). Mass transfer and metabolic reactions in hepatocyte spheroids cultured in rotating wall gas-permeable membrane system. *Biomaterials*, 28, pp. 5487–5497.

De Bartolo L, Jarosch-Von Schweder G, Haverich A and Bader A (2000). A novel full-scale flat membrane bioreactor utilizing porcine hepatocytes: cell viability and tissue-specific functions. *Biotechnol Prog*, 16, pp. 102–108.

De Bartolo L, Morelli S, Bader A and Drioli E (2002). Evaluation of cell behaviour related to physico-chemical properties of polymeric membranes to be used in bioartificial organs. *Biomaterials*, 23, pp. 2485–2497.

De Bartolo L, Morelli S, Rende M, Campana C, Salerno S, Quintiero N and Drioli E (2007). Human hepatocyte morphology and functions in a multibore fiber bioreactor. *Macromol Biosci*, 7, pp. 671–680.

De Bartolo L, Salerno S, Curcio E, Piscioneri A, Rende M, Morelli S, Tasselli F, Bader A and Drioli E (2009). Human hepatocyte functions in a crossed hollow fiber membrane bioreactor. *Biomaterials*, 30, pp. 2531–2543.

De Bartolo L, Salerno S, Morelli S, Giorno L, Rende M, Memoli B, Procino A, *et al.* (2006). Long-term maintenance of human hepatocytes in oxygen-permeable membrane bioreactor. *Biomaterials*, 27, pp. 4794–4803.

Demetriou AA, Brown RS, Busuttil RW, Fair J, McGuire BM, Rosenthal P, *et al.* (2004). Prospective, randomized, multicenter, controlled trial of a bioartificial liver in treating acute liver failure. *Ann Surg*, 239, pp. 660–667.

Demetriou AA, Whiting J, Levenson SM, Chowdhury NR, Schechner R, Michalski S, Feldman D and Chowdhury JR (1986). New method of hepatocyte transplantation and extracorporeal liver support. *Ann Surg*, 204, pp. 259–271.

Diban N and Stamatialis D (2014). Polymeric hollow fiber membranes for bioartificial organs and tissue engineering applications. *J Chem Technol Biotechnol*, 89, pp. 633–643.

Dunn JC, Tompkins RG and Yarmush ML (1992). Hepatocytes in collagen sandwich: evidence for transcriptional and translational regulation. *J Cell Biol*, 116, pp. 1043–1053.

Ebrahimkhani MR, Neimana JAS, Raredona MSB, Hughesd DJ and Griffitha LG (2014). Bioreactor technologies to support liver function *in vitro*. *Adv Drug Deliv Rev*, 69–70, pp. 132–157.

Ellis AJ, Hughes RD, Wendon JA, Dunne J, Langley PG, Kelly JH, Gislason GT, Sussman NL and Williams R (1996). Pilot-controlled trial of the extracor poreal liver assist device in acute liver failure. *Hepatology*, 24, pp. 1446–1451.

Flendrig LM, la Soe JW, Jörning GG, Steenbeek A, Karlsen OT, Bovée WM, Ladiges NC, te Velde AA and Chamuleau RA (1997). *In vitro* evaluation of a novel bioreactor based on an integral oxygenator and a spirally wound nonwoven polyester matrix for hepatocyte culture as small aggregates. *J Hepatol*, 26, pp. 1379–1392.

Gebhardt R and Mecke D (1979). Perifused monolayer cultures of rat hepatocytes as an improved *in vitro* system for studies on ureogenesis. *Exp Cell Res*, 124, pp. 349–359.

Gripon P, Rumin S, Urban S, Le Seyec J, Glaise D, Cannie I, Guyomard C, Lucas J, Trepo C and Guguen-Guillouzo C (2002). Infection of a human hepatoma cell line by hepatitis B virus. *Proc Natl Acad Sci USA*, 99, pp. 15655–15660.

Hay DC, Zhao D, Fletcher J, Hewitt ZA, McLean D, Urruticoechea-Uriguen A, Black, *et al.* (2008). Efficient differentiation of hepatocytes from human embryonic stem cells exhibiting markers recapitulating liver development *in vivo*. *Stem Cells*, 26, pp. 894–902.

Hilal-Alnaqbi A, Mourad AH, Yousef BF and Gaylor JD (2013). Experimental evaluation and theoretical modeling of oxygen transfer rate for the newly developed hollow fiber bioreactor with three compartments. *Biomed Mater Eng*, 23, pp. 387–403.

Hoesli CA, Luu M and Piret JM (2009). A novel alginate hollow fiber bioreactor process for cellular therapy applications. *Biotechnol Prog*, 25, pp. 1740–1751.

Hu WS, Friend JR, Wu FJ, Sielaff T, Peshwa MV, Lazar A, Nyberg SL, Remmel RP and Cerra FB (1997). Development of a bioartificial liver employing xenogeneic hepatocytes. *Cytotechnology*, 23, pp. 29–38.

Huang P, Zhang L, Gao Y, He Z, Yao D, Wu Z, Cen J, *et al.* (2014). Direct reprogramming of human fibroblasts to functional and expandable hepatocytes. *Cell Stem Cell*, 14, pp. 370–384.

Jasmund I, Langsch A, Simmoteit R and Bader A (2002). Cultivation of primary porcine hepatocytes in an OXY-HFB for use as a bioartificial liver device. *Biotechnol Prog*, 18, pp. 839–846.

Jemal A, Center MM, DeSantis C and Ward EM (2010). Global patterns of cancer incidence and mortality rates and trends. *Cancer Epidemiol Biomarkers Prev*, 19, pp. 1893–1907.

Jungermann K and Kietzmann T (2000). Oxygen: modulator of metabolic zonation and disease of the liver. *Hepatology*, 31, pp. 255–260.

Kan P, Miyoshi H and Ohshima N (2004). Perfusion of medium with supplemented growth factors changes metabolic activities and cell morphology of hepatocyte-nonparenchymal cell coculture. *Tissue Eng*, 10, pp. 1297–1307.

Kan P, Miyoshi H, Yanagi K and Ohshima N (1998). Effects of shear stress on metabolic function of the co-culture system of hepatocyte/nonparenchymal cells for a bioartificial liver. *ASAIO J*, 44, pp. M441–M444.

Kelly JH and Darlington GJ (1989). Modulation of the liver specific phenotype in the human hepatoblastoma line HepG2. *In Vitro Cell Dev Biol*, 25, pp. 217–222.

Khetani SR, Berger DR, Ballinger KR, Davidson MD, Lin C and Ware BR (2015). Microengineered liver tissues for drug testing. *J Lab Autom*, 20, pp. 216–250.

Kim BS, Baez CE and Atala A (2000). Biomaterials for tissue engineering. *World J Urol*, 18, pp. 2–9.

Knazek RA, Gullino PM, Kohler PO and Dedrick RL (1972). Cell culture on artificial capillaries: an approach to tissue growth *in vitro*. *Science*, 178, pp. 65–66.

Lanza R, Langer R and Vacanti JP (2011). *Principles of tissue engineering* (Academic Press, Burlington).

Lee SY, Kim HJ and Choi D (2015). Cell sources, liver support systems and liver tissue engineering: alternatives to liver transplantation. *Int J Stem Cells*, 8, pp. 36–47.

Lee J-H, Park HJ, Jang IK, Kim HE, Lee DH, Park JK, Lee SK and Yoon HH (2014). *In vitro* differentiation of human liver-derived stem cells with mesenchymal characteristics into immature hepatocyte-like cells. *Transplant Proc*, 46, pp. 1633–1637.

Liu J, Pan J, Naik S, Santangini H, Trenkler D, Thompson N, Rifai A, Chowdhury JR and Jauregui HO (1998). Characterization and evaluation of detoxification functions of a nontumorigenic immortalized porcine hepatocyte cell line (HepLiu). *Cell Transplant*, 8, pp. 219–232.

Lu HF, Lim WS, Zhang PC, Chia SM, Yu H, Mao HQ and Leong KW (2005). Galactosylated poly(vinylidene difluoride) hollow fiber bioreactor for hepatocyte culture. *Tissue Eng*, 11, pp. 1667–1677.

Mann RE, Smart RG and Govoni R (2003). The epidemiology of alcoholic liver disease. *Alcohol Res Health*, 27, pp. 209–219.

Mazariegos GV, Patzer JF, Lopez RC, Giraldo M, Devera ME, Grogan TA, *et al.* (2002). First clinical use of a novel bioartificial liver support system (BLSS). *Am J Transplant*, 2, pp. 260–266.

Mazzei D, Guzzardi MA, Giusti S and Ahluwalia A (2010). A low shear stress modular bioreactor for connected cell culture under high flow rates. *Biotechnol Bioeng*, 106, pp. 127–137.

McClelland RE, MacDonald JM and Coger RN (2003). Modeling O_2 transport within engineered hepatic devices. *Biotechnol Bioeng*, 82, pp. 12–27.

Memoli B, De Bartolo L, Favia P, Morelli S, Lopez, L.C, Procino, A., Barbieri, G, *et al.* (2007). Fetuin-A gene expression, synthesis and release in primary human hepatocytes cultured in a galactosylated membrane bioreactor, *Biomaterials*, 28, pp. 4836–4844.

Morelli S, Salerno S, Piscioneri A, Rende M, Campana C and De Bartolo L (2010). Membrane approaches for liver and neuronal tissue engineering. In Drioli E and Giorno L, Eds., *Comprehensive membrane science and engineering*, Vol. 3 (Academic Press Elsevier, Oxford), pp. 229–252.

Nagaki M, Miki K, Kim YI, Ishiyama H, Hirahara I, Takahashi H, Sugiyama A, Muto Y and Moriwaki H (2001). Development and characterization of a hybrid bioartificial liver using primary hepatocytes entrapped in a basement membrane matrix. *Dig Dis Sci*, 46, pp. 1046–1056.

Park J, Berthiaume F, Toner M, Yarmush ML and Tilles AW (2005). Microfabricated grooved substrates as platforms for bioartificial liver reactors. *Biotechnol Bioeng*, 90, pp. 632–644.

Pascher A, Sauer IM and Neuhaus P (2002). Analysis of allogeneic versus xenogeneic auxiliary organ perfusion in liver failure reveals superior efficacy of human livers. *Int J Artif Organs*, 25, pp. 1006–1012.

Patzer JF, II, Mazariegos GV, Lopez R, Molmenti E, Gerber D, Riddervold F, Khanna A, Yin WY, *et al.* (1999). Novel bioartificial liver support system: preclinical evaluation. *Ann NY Acad Sci*, 875, pp. 340–352.

Phua J and Lee KH (2008). Liver support devices. *Curr Opin Crit Care*, 14, pp. 208–215.

Podoll AS, DeGolovine A and Finkel KW (2012). Liver support systems — a review. *ASAIO J*, 58, pp. 443–449.

Rademacher S, Oppert M and Jorres A (2011). Artificial extracorporeal liver support therapy in patients with severe liver failure. *Expert Rev Gastroenterol Hepatol*, 5, pp. 591–599.

Salerno S, Campana C, Morelli S, Drioli E and De Bartolo L (2011). Human hepatocytes and endothelial cells in organotypic membrane systems. *Biomaterials*, 32, pp. 8848–8859.

Sauer IM, Kardassis D, Zeillinger K, Pascher A, Gruenwald A, Pless G, Irgang M, Kraemer M, *et al.* (2003a). Clinical extracorporeal hybrid liver support — phase I study with primary porcine liver cells. *Xenotransplantation*, 10, pp. 460–469.

Sauer IM, Obermeyer N, Kardassis D, Theruvath T and Gerlach JC (2001). Development of a hybrid liver support system. *Ann NY Acad Sci*, 944, pp. 308–319.

Sauer IM, Zeilinger K, Pless G, Kardassis D, Theruvath T, Pascher A, Goetz M, Neuhaus P and Gerlach JC (2003b). Extracorporeal liver support based on primary human liver cells and albumin dialysis — treatment of a patient with primary graft non-function. *J Hepatol*, 39, pp. 649–653.

Schmelzer E, Zhang L, Bruce A, Wauthier E, Ludlow J, Yao HL, Moss N, Melhem A, McClelland R, *et al.* (2007). Human hepatic stem cells from fetal and postnatal donors. *J Exp Med*, 204, pp. 1973–1987.

Schmitmeier S, Langsch A, Jasmund I and Bader A (2006). Development and characterization of a small-scale bioreactor based on a bioartificial hepatic culture model for predictive pharmacological *in vitro* screenings. *Biotechnol Bioeng*, 95, pp. 1198–1206.

Schwartz R, Fleming HE, Khetani SR and Bhatia SN (2014). Pluripotent stem cell-derived hepatocyte-like cells. *Biotechnol Adv*, 32, pp. 504–513.

Sekiya S and Suzuki A (2011). Direct conversion of mouse fibroblasts to hepatocyte-like cells by defined factors. *Nature*, 475, pp. 390–393.

Shan J, Schwartz RE, Ross NT, Logan DJ, Thomas D, Duncan SA, North TE, *et al.* (2013). Identification of small molecules for human hepatocyte expansion and iPS differentiation. *Nat Chem Biol*, 9, pp. 514–520.

Sheridan SD, Gil S, Wilgo M and Pitt A (2008). Microporous membrane growth substrates for embryonic stem cell culture and differentiation. *Methods Cell Biol*, 86, pp. 29–57.

Shipley RJ, Davidson AJ, Chan K, Chaudhuri JB, Waters SL and Ellis MJ (2011). A strategy to determine operating parameters in tissue engineering hollow fiber bioreactors. *Biotechnol Bioeng*, 108, pp. 1450–1461.

Shiraha H, Koide N, Hada H, Ujike K, Nakamura M, Shinji T, Gotoh S and Tsuji T (1996). Improvement of serum amino acid profile in hepatic failure with the bioartificial liver using multicellular hepatocyte spheroids. *Biotechnol Bioeng*, 50, pp. 416–421.

Si-Tayeb K, Noto FK, Nagaoka M, Li J, Battle MA, Duris C, North PE, Dalton S and Duncan SA (2010). Highly efficient generation of human hepatocyte-like cells from induced pluripotent stem cells. *Hepatology*, 51, pp. 297–305.

Strain AJ and Neuberger JM (2002). A bioartificial liver — state of the art. *Science*, 295, pp. 1005–1009.

Struecker B, Raschzok N and Sauer IM (2014). Liver support strategies: cutting-edge technologies. *Nat Rev Gastroenterol Hepatol*, 11, pp. 166–176.

Sussman NL, Hughes RD, Wendon JA, Dunne J, Langley PG, Kelly JH, Gislason GT, Sussman NL and Williams R (1994). The Hepatix extracorporeal liver assist device: initial clinical experience. *Artif Organs*, 18, pp. 390–396.

Taub R (2004). Liver regeneration: from myth to mechanism. *Nat Rev Mol Cell Biol*, 5, pp. 836–847.

te Velde AA, Ladiges NC, Flendrig LM, Chamuleau RA (1995). Functional activity of isolated pig hepatocytes attached to different extracellular matrix substrates. Implication for application of pig hepatocytes in a bioartificial liver. *J Hepatol*, 23, pp. 184–192.

Thery M (2010). Micropatterning as a tool to decipher cell morphogenesis and functions. *J Cell Sci*, 123, pp. 4201–4213.

Touboul T, Hannan NR, Corbineau S, Martinez A, Martinet C, Branchereau S, Mainot S, *et al.* (2010). Generation of functional hepatocytes from human embryonic stem cells under chemically defined conditions that recapitulate liver development. *Hepatology*, 51, pp. 1754–1765.

Underhill GH, Khetani SR, Chen AA and Bhatia SN (2007) Chapter 48 — Liver. In Vacanti R, Lanza R and Langer J, Eds., *Principles of tissue engineering*, 3rd ed (Academic Press, Burlington), pp. 707–731.

Unger RE, Huang Q, Peters K, Protzer D, Paul D and Kirkpatrick CJ (2005). Growth of human cells on polyethersulfone (PES) hollow fiber membranes. *Biomaterials*, 26, pp. 1877–1884.

Wang Y, Susando T, Lei X, Anene-Nzelu C, Zhou H, Liang LH and Yu H (2010). Current development of bioreactors for extracorporeal bioartificial liver. *Biointerphases*, 5, pp. FA116–FA131.

Wung N, Acott SM, Tosh D and Ellis MJ (2014). Hollow fibre membrane bioreactors for tissue engineering applications. *Biotechnol Lett*, 36, pp. 2357–2366.

Yoon J, Lee HV, Lee JS, Park JB and Kim CY (1999). Development of a non-transformed human liver cell line with differentiated-hepatocyte and urea-synthetic functions: applicable for bioartificial liver. *Int J Artif Organs*, 22, pp. 769–777.

Yu Y, Fisher JE, Lillegard JB, Rodysill B, Amiot B and Nyberg SL (2012). Cell therapies for liver diseases. *Liver Transpl*, 18, pp. 9–21.

Chapter 7

Are Co-Culture Approaches Able to Improve Biological Functions of Bioartificial Livers?

V. Pandolfi, U. Pereira, M. Dufresne and C. Legallais*

Université de Technologie de Compiègne (UTC),
Sorbonne Universités UMR CNRS 7338,
Biomechanics and Bioengineering Research Center,
Royallieu CS 60319, 60203 Compiègne Cedex, France
*cecile.legallais@utc.fr

7.1 Introduction

Pre-clinical and clinical trials highlighted the promising role of the bioartificial liver (BAL) systems [Carpentier *et al.*, 2009; Struecker *et al.*, 2014] in taking in charge acute/fulminant liver failure patients until a potential organ tranplantation; however, these devices have not been introduced yet in the routine care. Indeed, none of the clinical studies showed a significant effect of the BAL treatment on patient survival, considered as the major endpoint.

One of the key limitations might come from the relative low performance of the biomass present in BAL. Based on safe surgical resections, common opinions converge on a minimum of the 20% of liver mass with optimal functionality (200 g or 20×10^9 hepatocytes) to maintain liver functions [Chamuleau, 2009; van de Kerkhove *et al.*, 2003]. However, primary human hepatocytes (PHH) obtained from non-transplantable livers, or resection often deriving from pathological conditions, do not ensure such optimal functionalities. In addition, hepatocyte function rapidly drops *in vitro*. To overcome these obstacles, a variety of strategies have been proposed and attempted. Two solutions can be broadly distinguished. On one hand, low availability of PHH can be overcome by looking for alternative cell sources [Allen *et al.*, 2001; Lee *et al.*, 2015; Takebe *et al.*, 2015; van de Kerkhove *et al.*, 2003]. On the other hand, functionalities of isolated PHH should be maximized and preserved by adequate culture conditions.

In this chapter, we will focus only on the second solution. Its rationale is to provide the hepatocytes (HEPs) with some cues recreating *in vivo* microenvironment. To this end, several approaches have been proposed, mostly involving the manipulation of media composition and environment, or the promotion of cell–cell interactions [Allen *et al.*, 2001; LeCluyse *et al.*, 2012; Lee *et al.*, 2015]. Although supplementation of the culture media with hormones or other components (for instance, dexamethasone) was demonstrated as contributing to stabilize HEP survival and functionality, this approach cannot be transferred to actual BAL applications. On the contrary, changes in the environment, by providing a three-dimensional configuration to the cells *via* the introduction of extracellular matrix (ECM) components and/or the establishment of self-assembled aggregates (e.g. spheroids), as well as the inclusion of non-parenchymal cells (NPCs) co-culture setting, are applicable to BAL designs.

Here, we evaluate different publications reporting co-culture strategies and summarize the major outcomes to establish the most promising conditions for translational BAL application.

7.2 Co-Culture: Promising Strategy for Hepatocyte Stabilization in Liver Tissue Engineering

The term "co-culture" refers to a culture setting of multiple, distinct cell types cultivated together within the same environment [Lawrence *et al.*, 1978]. In hepatic research, co-culture appears as an option to maintain HEP survival *in vitro*. Early studies involved primary rodent HEPs and, predominantly, fibroblast cell lines in simple co-culture systems [Langenbach *et al.*, 1979; Michalopoulos *et al.*, 1979].

Guguen-Guillouzo *et al.* [1983] first demonstrated the effectiveness of a co-culture system in enhancing hepatic functionality. The authors speculated about the critical role of cell–cell interactions not only in modulating levels of albumin production, but also in synthetizing ECM components (fibronectin and various collagen types) that in turn might contribute in the maintenance of the protein secretion.

The establishment of a co-culture system engages several critical parameters, and only their correct definition can lead cells toward more physiological interplays and responses. From the scrutiny of a myriad of proposed co-culture models, some elements are identifiable as paramount criteria for the formulation of a promising system; these include the choice of cellular populations, the ratio between different cell types and the design of culture environment (Fig. 7.1). The co-ordination of all these factors regulates cellular events promoting soluble signaling and physical cell–cell and cell–matrix interactions.

Although numerous studies have been carried out to understand the mechanisms underlying the regulation of HEP functions in the case of co-cultivation with other cells [Bale *et al.*, 2014; Bhatia *et al.*, 1998a, 1998b; Catalá *et al.*, 2007; Chia *et al.*, 2005; Cho *et al.*, 2010; Fraslin *et al.*, 1985;

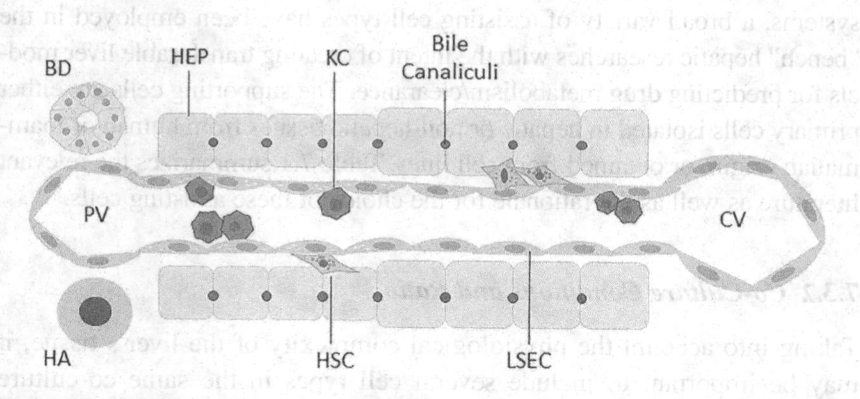

Figure 7.1. Representation of a hepatic sinusoid. It spaces plates of HEPs and runs from the portal triad (including branches of the portal vein (PV), bile ducts (BD) and the hepatic artery (HA)) to the central vein (CV). Liver sinusoidal endothelial cells (LSECs) line the hepatic sinusoids and confer a sieve aspect to these peculiar liver capillaries, thanks to their characteristic fenestrations. Kupffer cells (KCs) and hepatic stellate cells (HSCs) are the other main residents of the sinusoids.

Goers *et al*., 2014; Goulet *et al*., 1988; Milosevic *et al*., 1999; Harimoto *et al*., 2002; Higashiyama *et al*., 2004; Hoebe *et al*., 2001; Jindal *et al*., 2009; Khetani *et al*., 2004; Kim *et al*., 2012; Krause *et al*., 2009; Leite *et al*., 2011; Lu *et al*., 2005; Otsuka *et al*., 2013; Pan *et al*., 2015; Paschos *et al*., 2015; Peterson & Renton, 1986; Seo *et al*., 2006; Underhill *et al*., 2007; YoonáNo, 2013; Zinchenko *et al*., 2006], a clear scheme still remains to be drawn, but this is not the scope of the present chapter.

7.3 Cell Choice and Co-Culture Ratio

The cell types used in co-culture are usually defined *target* and *assisting* (alternatively, supporting or feeder) cells [Goers *et al*., 2014]. In the specific case of the BAL devices, assisting cells co-cultured with target HEPs can ideally allow for the reduction of the high requested hepatic cell mass by enhancing HEP functions, provide an independent therapeutic benefit to disease and improve the preservability of HEP storage before the treatment [Yagi *et al*., 2009].

7.3.1 *Cell Choice*

While few sporadic studies reported the inclusion of supporting cells in BAL systems, a broad variety of assisting cell types have been employed in the "bench" hepatic researches with the intent of creating transferable liver models for predicting drug metabolism/clearance. The supporting cells are either primary cells isolated in hepatic or non-hepatic tissues from human or mammalian origin, or obtained from cell lines. Table 7.1 summarizes the relevant literature as well as the rationale for the choice of these assisting cells.

7.3.2 *Co-Culture Conditions and Ratio*

Taking into account the physiological complexity of the liver's tissue, it may be important to include several cell types in the same co-culture milieu and respect their original relative numbers at seeding time [Kostadinova *et al*., 2013]. A critical aspect in this context is likely represented by the difficulty in sustaining multiple cell types in a unique culture microenvironment. Therefore, most of the defined co-culture systems

Table 7.1: Liver and non-liver derived supporting cells (primary (P), subcultured (SC) or cell lines (CL)) used in co-culture studies with mature HEPs.

Derived Liver Cells		Non-Derived Liver Cells		
Type	Source	Type	Source	Rationale
Hepatic Stellate Cells Higashiyama *et al.* [2004]; Jeong and Lee [2014]; Kasuyact *et al.* [2010]; Krause *et al.* [2009]; Mabuchi *et al.* [2004]; Pan *et al.* [2015]; Riccalton-Banks *et al.* [2003]; Rojkind *et al.* [1995]; Thomas *et al.* [2005]; Wong *et al.* [2011]; YoonáNo [2013]	❖ Human (CL) ❖ Rat (P CL)	*Fibroblasts* Abu-Absi *et al.* [2004a]; Bhandari *et al.* [2001]; Bhatia *et al.* [1997, 1998a]; Chia *et al.* [2005]; Cho *et al.* [2010]; Fukuda *et al.* [2006]; Khetani *et al.* [2004]; Kidambi *et al.* [2007]; Leite *et al.* [2011]; Liu *et al.* [2014]; Nishikawa *et al.* [2008]; Otsuka *et al.* [2013]; Seo *et al.* [2006]; Underhill *et al.* [2007]; Yagi *et al.* [2009]; Yamada *et al.* [2012]; Kim *et al.* [2001]; Takezawa *et al.* [1992]; Utesch *et al.* [1991]	❖ Human derma (P SC) ❖ Mouse embryo (P SC CL)	Production of extracelluler matrix components and in the case of Hepatic Stellate Cell release of growth factors (e.g. hepatocyte growth factor) fundamental for hepatocyte support
Liver sinusoidal endothelial cells Bale *et al.* [2014]; Hwa *et al.* [2007]; Jeong and Lee [2014]; Kaihara *et al.* [2000]; Kang *et al.* [2013]; Kim and Rajagopalan [2010]; Messner *et al.* [2013]	❖ Human (P) ❖ Rat (P)	*Endothelial cells* Harimoto *et al.* [2002]; Jindal *et al.* [2009]; Kang *et al.* [2013]; Kasuya *et al.* [2010]; Kim *et al.* [2012]; Kojima *et al.* [2009]; Lee *et al.* [2004]; Liu *et al.* [2014]; Ota *et al.* [2011]; Otsuka *et al.* [2013]; Prodanov *et al.* [2016]; Salerno *et al.* [2011]; Vozzi *et al.* [2008]	❖ Human umbilical vein and aorta (P SC Cl) ❖ Bovine aorta carotid artery and pulmonary microvessels (P SC CL) ❖ Rat prostate (CL) and heart microvessls (P)	Support of the performance of various metabolism functionalities (such as that of the lipids) as well as the response to inflammatory and toxicant stimuli.

(Continued)

Table 7.1: (*Continued*)

Derived Liver Cells		Non-Derived Liver Cells		
Type	Source	Type	Source	Rationale
Kupffer Cells Catalá *et al.* [2007]; Hoebe *et al.* [2001]; Kaihara *et al.* [2000]; Kowalski-Saunders *et al.* [1992]; Messner *et al.* [2013]; Milosevic [1999]; Peterson and Renton [1986]; Takezawa *et al.* [1992]; Tukov *et al.* [2006]; Wu *et al.* [2006]; Zinchenko and Coger [2005]	❖ Human (P SC) ❖ Rat (P SC) ❖ Porcine (P)	*Monocytes* Prodanov *et al.* [2016]	❖ Human leukemic lymphoma (CL)	Mediation of inflammation toxicity and regulation of hepatic specific functions such as acute-phase response by release of cytokines
Epithelial cells Auth *et al.* [1998]; Begue *et al.* [1984]; Conner *et al.* [1990]; Fraslin *et al.* [1985]; Lerche *et al.* [1997]	❖ Human (P SC) ❖ Rat (P SC)	*Epithelial cells* Donato *et al.* [1991, 1994]	❖ Canine kidney (CL) ❖ Monkey kidney (CL) ❖ Human embryonic lung (CL)	Establishment of hepatime-chanisms dependent on cellular interactions that require peculiar cellular membrane receptors present in biliary epithelial cells

Non-parenchymal cells (*whole fraction*) Bader *et al.* [1996]; Kaihara *et al.* [2000]; Kang *et al.* [2004]; Koike *et al.* [1996]; Kostadinova *et al.* [2013]; Michalopoulos *et al.* [1999]; Mitaka *et al.* [1999]; Shimaoka *et al.* [1987]; Underhill *et al.* [2007]; Yagi *et al.* [1995, 1998]; Yamada *et al.* [2001]	❖ Rat (P)		Closely approaching the *in vivo* complexity of the liver. Support of a combination of hepatic functions
	Mesenchymal stem cells Bao *et al.* [2013]; Gu *et al.* [2009]; Ijima *et al.* [2004]; Yagi *et al.* [2009]	❖ Human/Porcine/Rat Bone Marrow (P) ❖ Human adipose tissue (P)	Production of crucial cytokines and endogenous extra-cellular matrix proteins that sustain the hepatocyte functions

restricted their investigation to only one assisting cell type in addition to the HEPs which were, generally, cultivated in a ratio of 1:1. Few other studies reported more sophisticated co-culture concepts. Beyond the systems including the whole NPC fraction, some groups cultured two or three feeder cell populations with HEPs by controlling their seeding densities. The majority of tri-culture models was established in the 2010s: Kasuya *et al.* [2010] with hepatic stellate cells (HSCs) and (bovine pulmonary microvascular) endothelial cells; Jeong and Lee [2014] with primary subcultured rat HSCs and liver sinusoidal endothelial cells (LSECs); Liu *et al.* [2014] with mouse embryonic NIH3T3 fibroblast cell lines and human umbilical vein endothelial cell lines; and Messner *et al.* [2013] with Kupffer cells (KCs) and LSECs.

Recently, Prodanov *et al.* [2016] presented a co-culture system showing facets of human liver physiology and functions. This system included three different human cell lines in addition to the HEPs as substitutes of the hepatic NPC populations, namely, the human umbilical vein cell line (EA.hy926), the human HSC lines (LX-2) and the human leukemic monocyte lymphoma cell lines (U937), in order to closely approach the actual cellular composition of the organ.

There are disparate viewpoints within the literature regarding the optimum ratio among cell types. Considering similar (spheroidal) co-culture systems, it can be observed that fivefold excess number of sinusoidal endothelial cells [Matsushima *et al.*, 1990] or of (whole fraction) NPCs [Yamada *et al.*, 2001] did not provide the highest level of albumin production which was rather attained with a mixing ratio of 1:1. On the contrary, a surplus (10 times higher) of HEPs over the human adipose mesenchymal stem cell number generated the greatest albumin synthesis [Bao *et al.*, 2013]. In other cases, when murine embryonic fibroblasts outnumbered the HEPs, the level of albumin secretion was augmented [Bhatia *et al.*, 1998a, 1998b; Leite *et al.*, 2011]. Although the several co-culture systems proposed in literature are difficult to compare due to diverse culture conditions (e.g. the medium composition), this analysis indicates that a specific liver function may show a tendency to be stabilized by a precise cellular ratio between HEPs and assisting cells as well as to be dependent on the origin of supporting cells. Finally, these examples also suggest that the ratio of HEPs to a specific NPC type in the natural liver does not exactly coincide with the relative cell proportion that provides the optimal outcomes in *in vitro* co-culture system [Zinchenko *et al.*, 2006].

7.4 Design of an Artificial Co-Culture Microenvironment: Different Techniques

Depending on the research purpose, co-culture systems have been set up on the basis of specific methods. A considerable amount of co-cultures, especially related to initial studies, utilized a "randomly distributed" approach, in which the assisting cell population(s) — generally only one additional type — was simply mixed with the HEPs and cultivated together on coated or bare culture dishes in a two-dimensional manner. Although these investigations primarily aimed to elucidate how the functions of a model tissue were affected by cell–cell interactions [Bhatia *et al.*, 1998a, 1998b], a major limitation was the lack of control of the direct contact between the cells. Here, the cell interactions, as reported by Bhatia *et al.* [1998a, 1998b], are highly variable between each co-culture and depend on the seeding densities, cell aggregation and migration, as well as the cell ratio between the different populations. Such facets lead to disequilibrium in the establishment of the cell interactions, as, for instance, the promotion of homotypic upon heterotypic contacts or vice versa. To overcome this, some other co-culture techniques have been attempted; these will be described in the following sections.

7.4.1 *Microfabrication and Micropatterning*

Various patterning technologies such as soft microlithography [Goubko & Cao, 2009; Xia & Whitesides, 1998] or micropatterning were developed for the purpose of designing more controlled local contacts between neighboring cells [Goubko & Cao, 2009] so that to hold constant the heterotypic interfaces [Bhatia *et al.*, 1998a, 1998b] and, thus, better mimic the *in vivo* milieu [Carter, 1965, 1967; Kleinfeld *et al.*, 1988]. The first study of patterned co-culture was published by Bhatia *et al.* [1997]. There, the authors provided a method for generating two-dimensional, anisotropic surfaces capable of organizing two different cell types (HEPs and

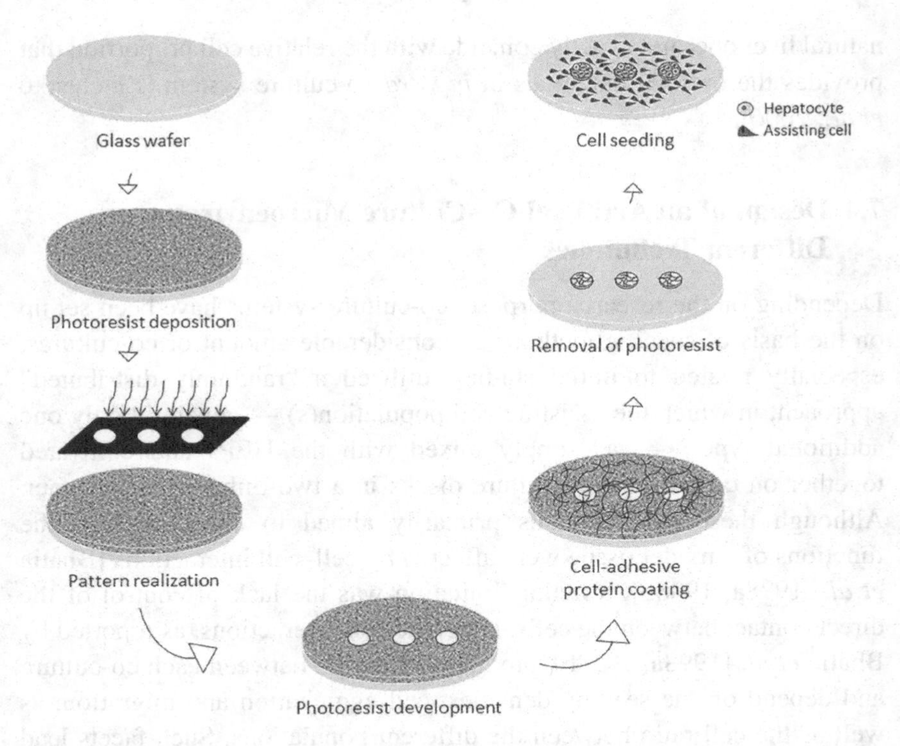

Figure 7.2. Representative scheme of micropatterning method for co-culture of hepatic cells. Adapted from Bhatia *et al.* [1997].

fibroblasts) in discrete spatial locations (Fig. 7.2). Photolithography was used to pattern biomolecules on a glass substrate. Cell-adhesive proteins (collagen) were immobilized on specific micropatterned regions of the substrate, whereas bovine serum albumin (BSA) was bound to the resulting non-adhesive glass background. HEPs were firstly seeded on the substrate in serum-free media, remaining attached only to the collagen-patterned areas. Fibroblasts were then inoculated, as second cell population, in the presence of serum so that they could easily adhere to the BSA non-patterned zones of the substrate.

This process revealed the potentiality in selectively distributing the diverse cell populations on a substrate according to the original pattern and, consequently, to vary initial heterotypic interactions while preserving the ratio of cell populations in culture. Control of the cell–cell interactions appeared markedly enhanced in this micropatterned system compared to that achieved in "randomly distributed" co-cultures. Later, Bhatia *et al.* [1998a, 1998b] also demonstrated the strength of this technology in modulating the HEP functions (albumin and urea production) by playing on the configuration of the micropatterned areas as well as on the seeding number of the fibroblasts. These outcomes mainly resulted from the vicinity of fibroblasts to HEP zones [Bhatia *et al.*, 1998a, 1998b], and thereby from the augmentation of the heterotypic interfaces, which, according to Bhatia *et al.*, may allow the achievement of supraphysiologic hepatocellular functions *in vitro* and the consequential diminution of the cell mass necessary in the BAL devices.

Zinchenko and Coger [2005] established micropatterned co-cultures of HEPs and KCs by taking advantage of the soft lithography technique. HEPs were firstly seeded in circular collagen-coated patterns of the polydimethylsiloxane (PDMS) stencil, whereas KCs were later inoculated and adhered to the remaining BSA-coated regions. In such a configuration, hepatic functions (albumin and urea production) were highly increased compared to random co-cultures, and the HEPs maintained their viability beyond seven culture days, likely thanks to the support given by the KCs. Here, the optimal functional conditions were defined by a dominant presence of HEPs over the KCs. In another study, Cho *et al.* [2010] proved that the hepatic functionalities could be further improved by increasing the heterotypic contact area between both cell types.

Despite the promising features of these reported techniques in controlling cell–cell interactions and modulating the hepatic functions, some shortcomings were identified, such as the difficulty to appropriately seed the second population, to scale-up, or the relative fragility of the systems that make them uneasy to handle [Kidambi *et al.*, 2007; Zinchenko *et al.*, 2006].

7.4.2 *Layer-by-Layer Techniques and Sandwich Approaches*

Decher [1997] developed the layer-by-layer assembly technique that permitted the construction of polymeric thin films, termed "polyelectrolyte multilayers" (PEMs), with nanometer-scale control of ionized species and precise regulation of their complex three-dimensional (3D) topography [Kidambi *et al.*, 2007]. When the deposition of self-assembled monolayers

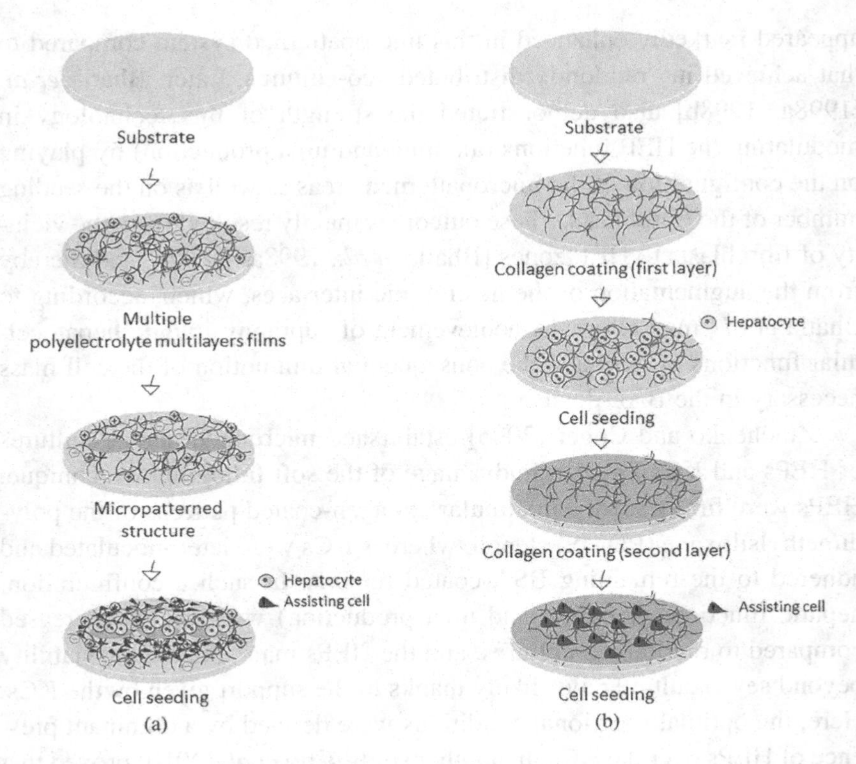

Figure 7.3. Co-culture of hepatic cells by (a) layer-by-layer technique and (b) collagen-sandwich approach.

onto an underlying surface is dictated by a specific micropattern according to a PDMS master, it is common to speak of microcontact printing technique (μCP). Kidambi *et al.* [2007] combined both described methods to generate a composite suitable environment for the co-culture of HEPs and fibroblasts (Fig. 7.3(a)). They utilized two synthetic ionic polymers, the sulfonated polystyrene (SPS) and the poly(diallyldimethylammoniun chloride) (PDAC), to build multiple overlapped PEM films, identified as $(PDAC/SPS)_{10}$, on the top of standard tissue culture polystyrene surfaces. A micropatterned structure of SPS was further added on the topmost of the PEM films by means of the microcontact printing technology in order to avoid previously documented cytophobic effect of the PEM surfaces on HEPs [Yang *et al.*, 2003]. The presence of fibroblast allowed the HEPs to remain attached to the 3D micropatterned PEM framework for up to

3 weeks without the aid of supplemental adhesive proteins. HEP-specific functions (albumin and urea) were also preserved or improved in these conditions.

With this study, the authors aimed to highlight the suitability of both layer-by-layer deposition and μCP techniques in creating templates of patterned co-cultures of HEPs and fibroblasts, permitting the control of cell–surface interactions and the long-term maintenance of the hepatic functions. PEMs can be alternatively constructed with natural polymers. Kim and Rajagopalan [2010] selected chitosan and hyaluronic acid, respectively, as cationic and anionic polyelectrolytes, to assemble PEMs in a 3D manner for the co-culture of HEPs and LSECs and to recapitulate the charged environment of the Space of Disse of the liver. Alternate layers of chitosan and hyaluronic acid were directly assembled on monolayer of HEPs, lying on a collagen-coated substrate. Next, LSECs were added on top of the PEM-coated HEP complex. In this configuration, HEPs and LSECs remained physically separated by the interposed nanoscale PEM (comprising five or fifteen layers with respective heights of 30 and 50 nm); however, intercellular signaling and heterotypic interactions could be potentially promoted, thanks to the high degree of hydration of the PEM. The LSEC–PEM–HEP system, incorporating a minor number of layers, allowed the simultaneous maintenance of phenotype of both cell populations and the maintenance of hepatocellular functions (albumin and urea secretion, as well as CYP450 enzyme activity) over 12 days of culture.

In a similar approach, Bale *et al*. [2014] included both a biomaterial and a 3D configuration for the co-culture of HEPs and LSECs in a sandwich collagen gel model (Fig. 7.3(b)). Because of the common culture parameters, this co-culture model may be compared to that of LSEC–PEM–HEP with the scope to get some insights about the role of the biomaterial and the 3D configuration in favorably contributing to the hepatic functional preservation. Among distinct proposed co-culture configurations, Bale *et al*. seeded the HEPs between two layers of collagen, and then inoculated the LSECs on the topmost layer of collagen which, in turn, were covered with another collagen film. Such 3D cell organization, analogous to that of the LSEC–PEM–HEP system, did not allow direct contacts between HEPs and LSECs. In addition, the collagen, similar to chitosan and hyaluronic acid assembled in PEM in the previous study, was selected as a suitable biomaterial to provide the cells with native cues, since it is one of the major components of the space of Disse. The decision to use a collagen gel sandwich also derived from previous researches demonstrating its beneficial effect in the long-term maintenance of the HEPs. In such co-culture arrangement, the albumin production showed similar level as the control monoculture of only HEPs on day 12. This adverse result was ascribed to the presence of two layers of collagen gel on the top of HEPs which may have negatively affected the metabolic functions of the hepatic cells and the loss of LSEC phenotype. This outcome may induce us to assume that the choice of a biomaterial and its characteristics (as, for instance, the thickness) may principally impact on the hepatic activities and that, accordingly, chitosan-hyaluronic acid in the form of PEM better impacts on the HEPs. However, this is not completely true. In fact, Bale *et al.*, exploring other sandwich-collagen gel co-culture configurations, demonstrated that different cell localization in the system, namely, inverted positioning of HEPs and LSECs, provoked a dramatic increase of albumin secretion after 12 culture days, significantly higher than that measured in the previous co-culture pattern, as well as the preservation of this activity over 30 days. In contrast with other data, this finding proved that the biomaterial was not responsible for the optimal hepatic response. Rather, cellular culture and organization were likely implicated. One major drawback of collagen sandwich culture is its failure in capturing heterotypic interactions [Jindal *et al.*, 2009]. By contrast, layer-by-layer design strategy shows shortcomings due to the solution of the soluble cell-adhesive electrolyte that is directly deposited on the cell monolayer and establishes bonds with the oppositely charged electrolyte on the surface. This solution may be toxic for the cell type, and so care must be taken in this context [Goubko & Cao, 2009].

7.4.3 *Cell Sheet Technology*

A different strategy for constructing 3D patterned co-cultures takes advantage of the properties of thermally responsive polymers, as first introduced by Yamato *et al.* in the early 2000s [Hirose *et al.*, 2000]. Patterned cell sheets are created on thermally responsive polymers, detached by reducing the culture temperature below the lower critical solution temperature of the polymer and transferred onto the monolayer of a second cell population. In this manner, the co-culture setting is constituted. The poly(*N*-isopropylacrylamide) (PIPAAm) is a broadly used thermally responsive polymer. It is usually grafted to the dish and then patterned by using a mask (e.g. glass coverslips in the case of preparation of square cell sheets). HEPs and endothelial cells (ECs) were efficiently co-cultured by using this cell sheet engineering technology, exhibiting an optimal morphological preservation [Harimoto *et al.*, 2002]. Later, Kim *et al.* [2012] revised this technique by offering an approach to create a more precise and uniform stratified dual-layer culture system of HEPs and ECs (Fig. 7.4). In this configuration and in the presence of EC sheet, the HEP-specific functions (albumin and urea production) were improved in comparison with the case of HEP monoculture, thanks to the increased degree of cell interactions as outlined by the stable expression of tight junctions.

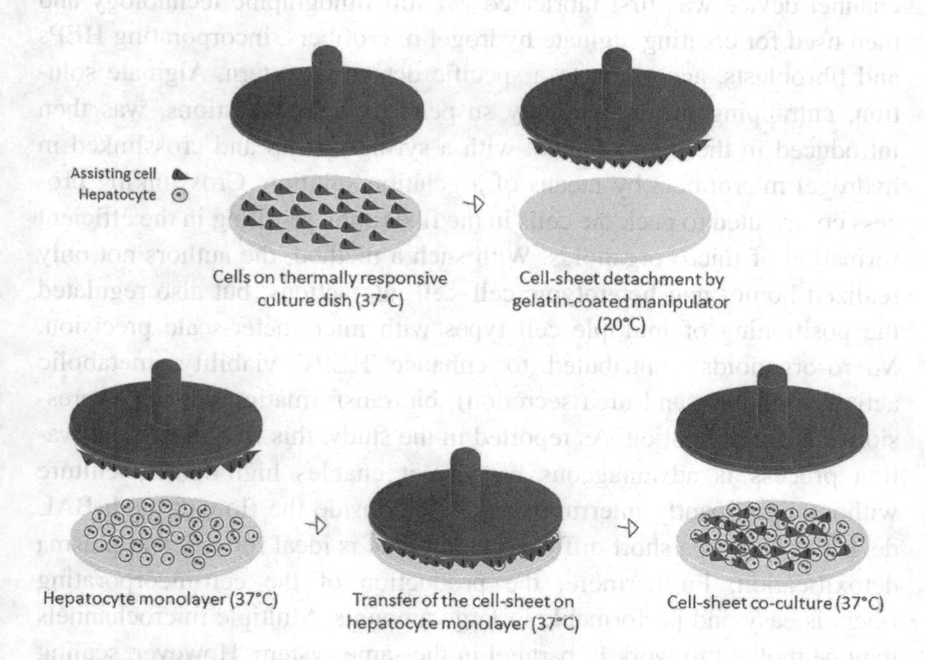

Figure 7.4. Schematic sketch of cell sheet technology for hepatic co-culture. Adapted from Kim *et al.* [2012].

Cheng *et al.* [2004] employed photolithography to generate micro-heater array underneath a PIPAAm surface to control the adhesion of specific cell types in defined patterned areas of the substrate. Subsequent cell types can be aligned to the first one in accordance with the determined patterns permitting a precise special localization of the cell types. However, shortcomings exist linked to temperature gradients around the heaters [Goubko & Cao, 2009].

7.4.4 *Microfluidic Devices*

Other studies intended to maximize the level of preservation of the liver functions by reconstructing the 3D sinusoidal microenvironment [Prodanov *et al.*, 2016; Vozzi *et al.*, 2008; Yamada *et al.*, 2012]. For this goal, microfluidic systems were developed. Interestingly, Yamada *et al.* [2012] proposed an efficient method to produce complex micro-organoids that closely resembled the *in vivo* hepatic cord structure. PDMS micro-channel device was first fabricated *via* soft lithographic technology and then used for creating alginate hydrogel microfibers, incorporating HEPs and fibroblasts, according to a specific designed pattern. Alginate solution, entrapping the individually suspended cell populations, was then introduced in the microchannel with a syringe pump and crosslinked in hydrogel microfibers by means of a gelation solution. Crosslinking process contributed to pack the cells in the fiber core, resulting in the efficient formation of micro-organoids. With such a method, the authors not only realized homo- and heterotypic cell–cell interactions, but also regulated the positioning of multiple cell types with micrometer-scale precision. Micro-organoids contributed to enhance HEPs' viability, metabolic activity (albumin and urea secretion), biotransformation genetic expression and differentiation. As reported in the study, this fiber-based cultivation process is advantageous because it enables high-density culture without significantly interrupting the flow inside the flow-through BAL device as well as a short diffusion length that is ideal for efficient plasma detoxification. Furthermore, the production of the cell-incorporating fibers is easy and performable in large amounts. Multiple microchannels may be thought to work in parallel in the same system. However, scaling up to human size application might be difficult.

7.5 Cellular Self-Assembly Spheroids

In 1989, Koide and coworkers reported the first discovery of the HEP spheroids [Asano *et al.*, 1989]. A spheroid is defined as the final product of the self-aggregation of cells; it mimics natural physiological phenomena and aspects in an *in vitro* context. As stated by Lin and Chang [2008], the formation of a spheroid is a three-step process that involves (i) an initial rapid aggregation of dispersed cells by the establishment of cell–surface integrin binds, (ii) a delay period for cadherin expression and accumulation and (iii) the final cell compaction in the form of the spheroids through homophilic cadherin–cadherin interactions. The spheroid is analogous to avascular tissue with diffusion limitation of about 150–200 μm to many molecules, especially O_2 [Lin & Chang, 2008]. Another study demonstrated that primary porcine HEPs differently expressed more than 65 genes after spheroid formation compared to two-dimensional. This outcome suggested that such transcriptional changes may be the cause of the close similarities of the spheroid features with the liver tissue [Narayanan *et al.*, 2002].

The conjugation of co-culture beneficial conditions and 3D spheroidal configuration thus received interest owing to its ability to better mimic hepatic tissue. Disparate strategies have been developed for the formation of single-cell spheroids (generally called homo-spheroids), which were then adopted for the generation of multiple cell-type spheroids (typically termed hetero-spheroids). These methods share a key aspect that is pivotal for the spheroid production, namely, facilitating the adhesion between cells to the detriment of cell attachment to the culture environment. They can be broadly divided in two categories: chemical-based and physical-based techniques.

7.5.1 *Chemical-based Methods*

The generic approach here is to prevent cells from spreading on a substrate and therefore favor their aggregation. The different materials found in the literature survey are listed in Table 7.2, together with the cell types and specific features for the spheroid formation. In general, hetero-spheroid formation is based first on HEP aggregation that may occur before or concomitantly to support cells addition (Fig. 7.5).

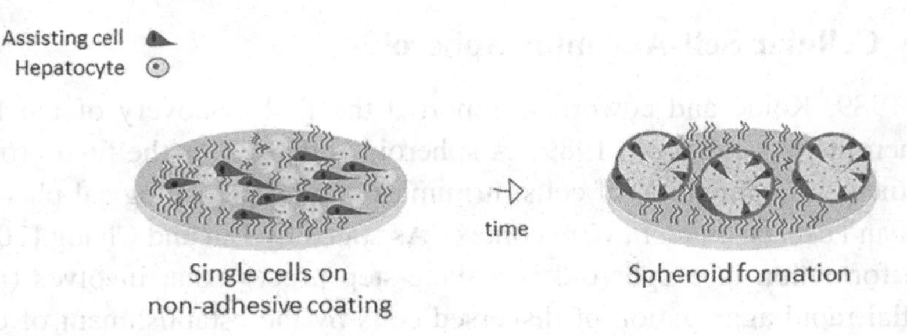

Figure 7.5. Hepatic co-culture on non-adhesive coating for spheroid formation.

In hetero-spheroidal configuration, HEPs generally exhibited higher expression of albumin and CYP450 mRNA, but the enhancement of effective functions (albumin release, urea secretion) is not always as significant, in comparison to the control of HEP homo-spheroids. It is recognized that the establishment of tight homo and hetero interactions may favorably impact HEP functionalities.

Lu *et al*. [2005] demonstrated that galactosylated PVDF membranes can effectively support HEP adhesion and stimulate HEP spheroid formation through the specific interaction between galactose ligands on the substrate and asialoglycoprotein receptors on HEP surface. After HEPs' aggregation in spheroids, fibroblasts were added, preferring to adhere to the HEP spheroids. The hetero-spheroidal configuration provided homo- and heterotypic contacts as well as cell–substrate interactions which may have contributed to the enhancement of the hepatic functionalities.

Another study used Eudragit S100 polymer as a matrix. HEPs and the whole fraction of NPCs, cultured in the presence of this polymer, agglomerated together from the first day of culture. Within four culture days, cells completed the spheroid formation [Yamada *et al*., 2001]. Liver functions (albumin and urea secretion, and ammonia removal) were improved in the hetero-spheroids over the long term (30 days), although the random cell distribution in these 3D constructs was dissimilar from that in the intact liver.

In other studies, spheroid formation between different cell populations was achieved by using several micropatterning techniques so as to

Table 7.2: Some materials employed in chemical-based methods for spheroid production in co-culture conditions. Associated cell type is also listed.

Biomaterial/substrate	Co-cultured cell types	Spheroid formation rationale	Drawbacks	Ref.
<u>*Non- or low adherent*</u>				
• Poly-2-hydroxyethyl methacrylate • Agarose • Commercial low-adhesion plates	HEPs + NPCs (w.f.)	Inability of HEPs to adhere on dish induces their self-assembly Fast spheroid formation	Low production Size heterogeneity Uncontrolled cell composition	[Acikgöz *et al.* 2013]
<u>*Adherent*</u>				
• Falcon Primaria dish • Poly (D,L-lactic acid)-coated Primaria dish • Galactosylated poly(vinylidene difluoride) substrate	HEPs + HSCs HEPs + HSCs HEPs + fibroblasts	Spheroid formation occurs after initial adhesion of HEPs on dish. Self-assembly begins within few days, when HEPs start to detach from dish	Low production Size heterogeneity Uncontrolled cell composition	[Abu-Absi *et al.* 2004] [Riccalton-Banks *et al.* 2003] [Lu *et al.* 2005]
<u>*Other*</u>				
Water-soluble polymer (Eudragit S100)	HEPs + NPCs (w.f.)	Cell aggregation induced by electrostatic and hydrophobic interactions between cell and polymer. Very rapid spheroid formation	Size heterogeneity Uncontrolled cell composition Harvesting difficulty	[Yamada *et al.* 2001]

Note: w.f. = whole fraction.

establish a spatial control on the cells during the process. Fukuda *et al.* [2006] realized a spheroid co-culture system by using soft lithography, specifically employing a micromolding technology. Photo-crosslinkable chitosan polymer was patterned with a PDMS mold and crosslinked with ultraviolet light. The resulting chitosan microwells (200 μm in diameter and 50 μm deep) were used for the spheroid production. HEP cell lines were seeded first, followed by the inoculation of the fibroblasts. Interestingly, cells preferred aggregation between themselves than adhering to chitosan. The authors justified this behavior to be due to the high level of cell–cell adhesion molecules (cadherin and claudin) expressed by the cells and implicated in the spheroid formation. With a similar approach, the group of Lee generated micropatterned hetero-spheroids in PDMS-based concave microwells (300–500 μm in diameter). These latter, fabricated by soft lithography, were coated with BSA in order to impede cell adhesion. In a first study [Wong *et al.*, 2011], HEPs and HSCs were mixed together and simultaneously seeded into the microwells. Later, the investigators extended the complexity of their *in vitro* model by co-culturing HEPs, HSCs and LSECs in accordance with the precedent protocol [Jeong & Lee, 2014]. This technique provided spheroids of highly uniform size, which was dependent on the microwell diameter. Concave microwells crucially controlled the cell aggregation into spheroids. In both studies, the hetero-spheroids generated an improvement of the hepatic functions (albumin production), which was more important when the three types were present. Such a beneficial effect was maintained over 27 culture days. Despite the extreme control of the size and cell composition of the spheroids, a conceivable drawback of this method is the scant number of produced spheroids (one per well) that may be constraining in the case of BAL application. Therefore, this technique might be more suitable for drug screening and predictive toxicology.

7.5.2 *Physical-based Methods*

Concerning the physical-based procedures, the production of spheroids relies on the retained capacity of the cells to re-organize in a tissue structure without the use of scaffold materials. The most common techniques are presented below.

7.5.2.1 *Hanging Drop Technique*

The hanging drop technique takes advantage of gravity to enforce the cells to self-assemble. The method introduced by Kelm *et al.* [2003] uses small aliquots (typically 20 μL) of a cell suspension which are seeded on a tissue culture lid (Fig. 7.6). This latter is subsequently inverted so that the aliquots of cell suspension turn into hanging drops that are kept in place due to surface tension [Breslin & O'Driscoll, 2013]. In this manner, cells, under gravity effect, accumulate at the tip of the drop, at the liquid–air interface, and aggregate together.

Some hanging drop plates have been commercially developed for the purpose of simplifying the cell-seeding step, performed in appropriate wells. Spheroids are harvested thanks to the inclusion of a trap plate under the culture plate. The hanging drop technique is also based on the cells' natural tendency to adhere to each other [Breslin & O'Driscoll, 2013]. Therefore, a single cell population has been generally utilized with this technique in order to avoid the difficulties associated with different adhesion degrees of the several cell types. However, Messner *et al.* [2013] produced well-defined liver microtissues by employing HEPs, LSECs and KCs in a hanging-drop culture platform. The resulting cellular construct resembled liver-like cell composition. HEPs exhibited prolonged lifetime and functionality in comparison with 2D culture, as well as long-term chronic and inflammation-mediated toxicity. The authors proposed to use the model at the early time point in drug development. Similar to the previous methods, the simple and reproducible hanging drop technique, which enables the formation of size-controlled spheroids with a precise cell composition, allows for the production of scant amount of spheroids which may be not scalable for BAL application.

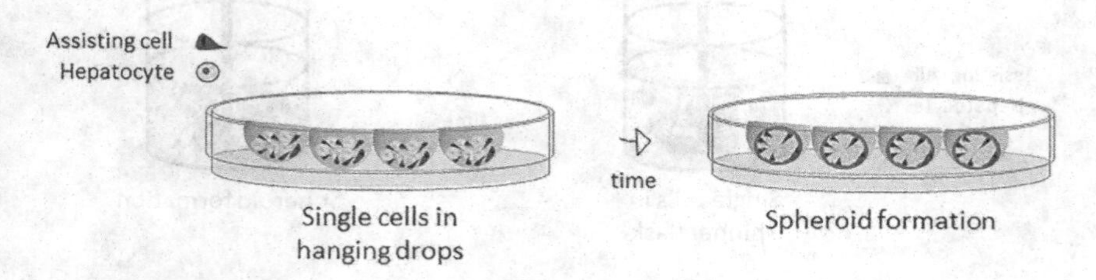

Figure 7.6. Hepatic cells co-cultured in hanging drops and their assembly in spheroids.

7.5.2.2 *Stirring Techniques*

The stirring techniques exploit the motion of suspended cells to obtain massive spheroid production. In principle, a cellular suspension, placed into a container, is kept in movement so that cells do not adhere to the container walls, but instead interact with each other [Breslin & O'Driscoll, 2013]. The motion has been established in different ways, for instance, by the aid of rotating and rocking systems as well as magnetic stirring in a spinner flask (Fig. 7.7).

These systems were broadly used and generally are large, permitting seeding of a large amount of cells enabling large yields of formed spheroids. Moreover, the motion of culture fluids assists the transport of nutrients to, and waste products from, the spheroids [Breslin & O'Driscoll, 2013]. Thomas *et al.* [2005] sustained the production of hetero-spheroids of HEPs and HSCs by rotating motion. The spheroid formation occurred within 2 days following several distinct phases; HSCs first adhered and spread on the culture plate, while the HEPs attached to the former cells, and finally HSCs contracted and pulled the HEPs into focal aggregates which resulted in the formation of spheroids. There, the HSCs, rather than the rotating technique, were crucial for the promotion of spheroid formation. Hepatic functional enhancement was attributed to cell–cell interactions, release of soluble mediators and ECM production. Differently, Bao *et al.* [2013] utilized a rocked mixing

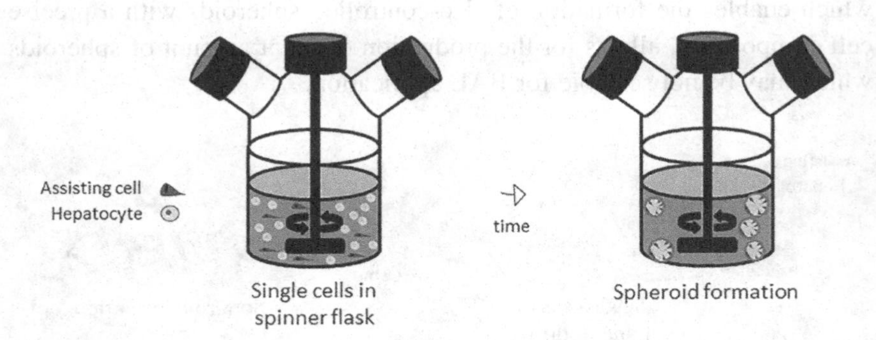

Figure 7.7. Magnetic stirring co-culture of hepatic cells and consequent spheroid formation.

technique to create hetero-spheroids constituted of HEPs and adipose mesenchymal stromal cells. In this co-culture setting, rocking motion maximized the frequency of cell-to-cell contact and rapidly improved the rate and efficiency of spheroid formation. Therefore, spheroids were produced rapidly and exhibited homogenous size as well as composition of the two cell populations. Functional activities (albumin and urea secretion) were highly supported there for 14 days. Besides, the authors stressed the contribution of the mesenchymal stromal cells in forming the spheroids and stabilizing their integrity.

Ota *et al*. [2011] proposed a different technique for rapid formation of size-controlled hetero-spheroids consisting of HEPs and ECs by using microrotation flow. In principle, collagen-coated HEPs and ECs were collected in the center of a chamber by a microrotation flow. Cell aggregation was hydrodynamically controlled, by changing the cell density of the medium, resulting in the regulation of the spheroid size. In addition, the dispersion of ECs in the hetero-spheroids was uniform. Nonetheless, hepatic functions were not evaluated in this study.

Finally, spinner flasks were amply used for the production of homo-spheroids. Lee *et al*. [2004] employed siliconized spinner-flasks in order to prepare large quantities of hetero-spheroids constituted of HEPs and ECs for more specific BAL application. Hetero-spheroids formed 24 h after seeding and exhibited an external layer of ECs covering the HEP spheroid. As stated in this study, such cell disposition may be a restoration of *in vivo* structures. However, ECs tightly adhered to the HEPs, which may be due to their high attachment affinity for the HEPs. ECM production and cell–cell interactions were also observed in these co-culture conditions, both of which may play a role in the preservation of the hepatic functionalities. Similarly, Leite *et al*. [2011] produced hetero-spheroids of HEPs and fibroblasts in spinner vessels. Spheroidal self-assembly of the two cell populations was observed shortly after cell inoculation. In these conditions, drug detoxification (evaluated by phase I and phase II enzyme activities) and synthetic (by measuring albumin secretion) capabilities of the HEPs could be maintained for up to 21 days. A limiting aspect of these latter massive spheroid production methods is the lack of spheroid-size control. This may lead to a dangerous growth of spheroids size that may impede the correct exchange of molecules and determining the appearance of a necrotic core. In addition, depending on the application (e.g. in the drug toxicology field), it might be required to manually select similar sized spheroids in order to set up comparable analysis.

7.6 Conclusion: Which Optimal Parameters Define the Most Promising Co-Culture Setting for an Actual Clinical BAL Application?

It is beyond dispute that co-culture beneficially affects HEPs' viability and functionality *in vitro*. The analysis of the different co-culture approaches proposed here reveals that a large variety of cells can be employed to support HEPs. They can be from liver origin or not. There is no clear consensus about the cell types to be preferentially used.

Hepatocytes receive induction signals from the supporting NPC type in a co-culture system. The propagation of such signals has limited length. Therefore, the distance between different cells should be minimized and cell–cell interactions should be promoted. This is in line with the design criteria of a bioreactor that must be optimized by balancing the highest hepatic functions with the smallest surface area/volume available for cell colonization. As NPCs occupy consistent surface area/volume in a 3D BAL system, the definition of an effective ratio between the target and supporting cells may be necessary, but is not defined yet. Besides, the choice of the methodology for co-culture requires to take into account (i) the large size of co-culture constructs providing the requested biological functions and (ii) the type of BAL to be employed. Compared to other techniques such as micropatterning or sandwich, the production of hetero-spheroids appears easy to scale up, for example, by using spinner vessels. They may represent the optimal choice for use in hollow fibers or in bed bioreactors (after being encapsulated in beads or not), such as those proposed by Erro *et al.* [2013], Figaro *et al.* [2015] and Glorioso *et al.* [2015].

Much remains to be defined in this field to reach real clinical translation of a co-cultured product. However, the available outcomes are very promising, and the above open questions are expected to be solved in the next years.

List of Abbreviations

μCP	microcontact printing technique
2D	two-dimensional
3D	three-dimensional
BAL	bioartificial liver
BSA	bovine serum albumin
CYP450	Cytochrome 450
ECM	extracellular matrix
ECs	endothelial cells
HEPs	hepatocytes
HSCs	hepatic stellate cells
KCs	Kupffer cells
LSECs	liver sinusoidal endothelial cells
mRNA	messenger ribonucleic acid
NPCs	non-parenchymal cells
PDAC	poly(diallyldimethylammoniun chloride)
PDMS	polydimethylsiloxane
PEMs	polyelectrolyte multilayers
PHH	primary human hepatocytes
PIPAAm	poly(*N*-isopropylacrylamide)
SPS	sulfonated polystyrene

References

Abu-Absi SF, Hansen LK and Hu W-S (2004). Three-dimensional co-culture of hepatocytes and stellate cells. *Cytotechnology*, 45(3), pp. 125–140.

Acikgöz A, Giri S, Cho M-G and Bader A (2013). Morphological and functional analysis of hepatocyte spheroids generated on poly-HEMA-treated surfaces under the influence of fetal calf serum and nonparenchymal cells. *Biomolecules*, 3(1), pp. 242–269.

Allen JW, Hassanein T and Bhatia SN (2001). Advances in bioartificial liver devices. *Hepatology*, 34(3), pp. 447–455.

Asano K, Koide N and Tsuji T (1989). Ultrastructure of multicellular spheroids formed in the primary culture of adult rat hepatocytes. *J Clin Electron Microsc*, 22(2), pp. 243–252.

Bale SS, Golberg I, Jindal R, McCarty WJ, Luitje M, Hegde M, Bhushan A, Usta OB and Yarmush ML (2014). Long-term coculture strategies for primary hepatocytes and liver sinusoidal endothelial cells. *Tissue Eng Part C*, 21(4), pp. 413–422.

Bao J, Fisher JE, Lillegard, Wang W, Amiot B, Yu Y, Dietz AB, Nahmias Y and Nyberg SL (2013). Serum-free medium and mesenchymal stromal cells enhance functionality and stabilize integrity of rat hepatocyte spheroids. *Cell Transpl*, 22(2), p. 299.

Bhatia S, Balis U, Yarmush M and Toner M (1998a). Microfabrication of hepatocyte/fibroblast co-cultures: role of homotypic cell interactions. *Biotechnol Progr*, 14(3), pp. 378–387.

Bhatia S, Balis U, Yarmush M and Toner M (1998b). Probing heterotypic cell interactions: hepatocyte function in microfabricated co-cultures. *J Biomater Sci Polym Ed*, 9(11), pp. 1137–1160.

Bhatia SN, Yarmush ML and Toner M (1997). Controlling cell interactions by micropatterning in co-cultures: hepatocytes and 3T3 fibroblasts. *J Biomed Mater Res*, 34(2), pp. 189–199.

Breslin S and O'Driscoll L (2013). Three-dimensional cell culture: the missing link in drug discovery. *Drug Discovery Today*, 18(5), pp. 240–249.

Carpentier B, Gautier A and Legallais C (2009). Artificial and bioartificial liver devices: present and future. *Gut*, 58(12), pp. 1690–1702.

Carter SB (1965). Principles of cell motility: the direction of cell movement and cancer invasion. *Nature*, 208(5016), p. 1183.

Carter SB (1967). Haptotaxis and the mechanism of cell motility. *Nature*, 213, pp. 256–260.

Catalá M, Pagani R and Portolés M (2007). Short term regulation of hepatocyte glutathione content by hepatic sinusoidal cells in co-culture. *Histol Histopathol*, 22(4–6), pp. 399–408.

Chamuleau RA (2009). Future of bioartificial liver support. *World J Gastrointest Surg*, 1(1), p. 21.

Cheng X, Wang Y, Hanein Y, Böhringer KF and Ratner BD (2004). Novel cell patterning using microheater-controlled thermoresponsive plasma films. *J Biomed Mater Res Part A*, 70(2), pp. 159–168.

Chia S-M, Lin P-C and Yu H (2005). TGF-b1 regulation in hepatocyte-NIH3T3 co-culture is important for the enhanced hepatocyte function in 3D microenvironment. *Biotechnol Bioeng*, 89(5), pp. 565–573.

Cho CH, Park J, Tilles AW, Berthiaume F, Toner M and Yarmush ML (2010). Layered patterning of hepatocytes in co-culture systems using microfabricated stencils. *Biotechniques*, 48(1), p. 47.

Decher G (1997). Fuzzy nanoassemblies: toward layered polymeric multicomposites. *Science*, 277(5330), pp. 1232–1237.

Erro E, Bundy J, Massie I, Chalmers SA, Gautier A, Gerontas S, Hoare M, Sharratt P, Choudhury S, Lubowiecki M, Llewellyn I, Legallais C, Fuller B, Hodgson H and Selden C (2013). Bioengineering the liver: scale-up and cool chain delivery of the liver cell biomass for clinical targeting in a bioartificial liver support system. *Biores Open Access*, 2(1), pp. 1–11.

Figaro S, Pereira U, Rada H, Semenzato N, Pouchoulin D and Legallais C (2015). Development and validation of a bioartificial liver device with fluidized bed bioreactors hosting alginate-encapsulated hepatocyte spheroids. *Conf Proc IEEE Eng Med Biol Soc*, 2015, pp. 1335–1338.

Fraslin J, Kneip B, Vaulont S, Glaise D, Munnich A and Guguen-Guillouzo C (1985). Dependence of hepatocyte-specific gene expression on cell–cell interactions in primary culture. *EMBO J* 4(10), p. 2487.

Fukuda J, Khademhosseini A, Yeo Y, Yang X, Yeh J, Eng G, Blumling J, Wang C-F, Kohane DS and Langer R (2006). Micromolding of photocrosslinkable chitosan hydrogel for spheroid microarray and co-cultures. *Biomaterials*, 27(30), pp. 5259–5267.

Glorioso J, Mao S, Rodysill B, Mounajjed T, Kremers W, Elgilani F, Hickey R, Haugaa H, Rose C and Amiot B (2015). Pivotal preclinical trial of the spheroid reservoir bioartificial liver. *J Hepatol.*, 63(2), pp. 388–398.

Goers L, Freemont P and Polizzi KM (2014). Co-culture systems and technologies: taking synthetic biology to the next level. *J Roy Soc Interf*, 11(96), p. 20140065.

Goubko CA and Cao X (2009). Patterning multiple cell types in co-cultures: a review. *Mater Sci Eng C*, 29(6), pp. 1855–1868.

Goulet F, Normand C and Morin O (1988). Cellular interactions promote tissue-specific function, biomatrix deposition and junctional communication of primary cultured hepatocytes. *Hepatology*, 8(5), pp. 1010–1018.

Guguen-Guillouzo C, Clément B, Baffet G, Beaumont C, Morel-Chany E, Glaise D and Guillouzo A (1983). Maintenance and reversibility of active albumin secretion by adult rat hepatocytes co-cultured with another liver epithelial cell type. *Exp Cell Res*, 143(1), pp. 47–54.

Harimoto M, Yamato M, Hirose M, Takahashi C, Isoi Y, Kikuchi A and Okano T (2002). Novel approach for achieving double-layered cell sheets co-culture: overlaying endothelial cell sheets onto monolayer hepatocytes utilizing temperature-responsive culture dishes. *J Biomed Mater Res*, 62(3), pp. 464–470.

Higashiyama S, Noda M, Muraoka S, Uyama N, Kawada N, Ide T, Kawase M and Yagi K (2004). Maintenance of hepatocyte functions in coculture with hepatic stellate cells. *Biochem Eng J*, 20(2), pp. 113–118.

Hirose M, Yamato M, Kwon OH, Harimoto M, Kushida A, Shimizu T, Kikuchi A and Okano T (2000). Temperature-responsive surface for novel co-culture systems of hepatocytes with endothelial cells: 2-D patterned and double layered co-cultures. *Yonsei Med J*, 41(6), pp. 803–813.

Hoebe KH, Witkamp RF, Fink-Gremmels J, Van Miert AS and Monshouwer M (2001). Direct cell-to-cell contact between Kupffer cells and hepatocytes augments endotoxin-induced hepatic injury. *Am J Physiol-Gastrointest Liver Physiol*, 280(4), pp. G720–G728.

Jeong GS and Lee S-H (2014). Immune-protected xenogeneic bioartificial livers with liver-specific microarchitecture and hydrogel-encapsulated cells. *Biomaterials*, 35(32), pp. 8983–8991.

Jindal R, Nahmias Y, Tilles AW, Berthiaume F and Yarmush ML (2009). Amino acid-mediated heterotypic interaction governs performance of a hepatic tissue model. *FASEB J*, 23(7), pp. 2288–2298.

Kasuya J, Sudo R, Mitaka T, Ikeda M and Tanishita K (2010). Hepatic stellate cell-mediated three-dimensional hepatocyte and endothelial cell triculture model. *Tissue Eng Part A*, 17(3–4), pp. 361–370.

Kelm JM, Timmins NE, Brown CJ, Fussenegger M and Nielsen LK (2003). Method for generation of homogeneous multicellular tumor spheroids applicable to a wide variety of cell types. *Biotechnol Bioeng*, 83(2), pp. 173–180.

Khetani SR, Szulgit G, Del Rio JA, Barlow C and Bhatia SN (2004). Exploring interactions between rat hepatocytes and nonparenchymal cells using gene expression profiling. *Hepatology*, 40(3), pp. 545–554.

Kidambi S, Sheng L, Yarmush ML, Toner M, Lee I and Chan C (2007). Patterned co-culture of primary hepatocytes and fibroblasts using polyelectrolyte multilayer templates. *Macromol Biosci*, 7(3), pp. 344–353.

Kim K, Ohashi K, Utoh R, Kano K and Okano T (2012). Preserved liver-specific functions of hepatocytes in 3D co-culture with endothelial cell sheets. *Biomaterials*, 33(5), pp. 1406–1413.

Kim Y and Rajagopalan P (2010). 3D hepatic cultures simultaneously maintain primary hepatocyte and liver sinusoidal endothelial cell phenotypes. *PLoS One*, 5(11), p. e15456.

Kleinfeld D, Kahler K and Hockberger P (1988). Controlled outgrowth of dissociated neurons on patterned substrates. *J Neurosci*, 8(11), pp. 4098–4120.

Kostadinova R, Boess F, Applegate D, Suter L, Weiser T, Singer T, Naughton B and Roth A (2013). A long-term three dimensional liver co-culture system for improved prediction of clinically relevant drug-induced hepatotoxicity. *Toxicol Appl Pharmacol*, 268(1), pp. 1–16.

Krause P, Saghatolislam F, Koenig S, Unthan-Fechner K and Probst I (2009). Maintaining hepatocyte differentiation *in vitro* through co-culture with hepatic stellate cells. *In Vitro Cell Dev Biol-Anim*, 45(5–6), pp. 205–212.

Langenbach R, Malick L, Tompa A, Kuszynski C, Freed H and Huberman E (1979). Maintenance of adult rat hepatocytes on C3H/10T½ cells. *Cancer Res*, 39(9), pp. 3509–3514.

Lawrence TS, Beers WH and Gilula NB (1978). Transmission of hormonal stimulation by cell-to-cell communication. *Nature*, 272(5653), pp. 501–506.

LeCluyse EL, Witek RP, Andersen ME and Powers MJ (2012). Organotypic liver culture models: meeting current challenges in toxicity testing. *Crit Rev Toxicol*, 42(6), pp. 501–548.

Lee S, Kim H and Choi D (2015). Cell sources, liver support systems and liver tissue engineering: alternatives to liver transplantation. *Int J Stem Cells*, 8(1), pp. 36–47.

Lee D-H, Yoon H-H, Lee J-H, Lee K-W, Lee S-K, Kim S-K, Choi J-E, Kim Y-J and Park J-K (2004). Enhanced liver-specific functions of endothelial cell-covered hepatocyte hetero-spheroids. *Biochem Eng J*, 20(2), pp. 181–187.

Leite SB, Teixeira AP, Miranda JP, Tostões RM, Clemente JJ, Sousa MF, Carrondo MJ and Alves PM (2011). Merging bioreactor technology with 3D hepatocyte-fibroblast culturing approaches: improved *in vitro* models for toxicological applications. *Toxicol In Vitro*, 25(4), pp. 825–832.

Lin RZ and Chang HY (2008). Recent advances in three-dimensional multicellular spheroid culture for biomedical research. *Biotechnol J*, 3(9–10), pp. 1172–1184.

Liu Y, Li H, Yan S, Wei J and Li X (2014). Hepatocyte cocultures with endothelial cells and fibroblasts on micropatterned fibrous mats to promote liver-specific functions and capillary formation capabilities. *Biomacromolecules*, 15(3), pp. 1044–1054.

Lu H-F, Chua K-N, Zhang P-C, Lim W-S, Ramakrishna S, Leong KW and Mao H-Q (2005). Three-dimensional co-culture of rat hepatocyte spheroids and NIH/3T3 fibroblasts enhances hepatocyte functional maintenance. *Acta Biomater*, 1(4), pp. 399–410.

Matsushima H, Koide N, Asano K, Sakaguchi K, Kawaguchi M, Takenami T, Takbatake H, Ono R, Tsuji T and Mori M (1990). Possible applicability of mixed cells-spheroid as a bioreactor of a hybrid artificial liver. *Jinko Zoki–J-STAGE Journals*, 19(2), pp. 848–851.

Messner S, Agarkova I, Moritz W and Kelm J (2013). Multi-cell type human liver microtissues for hepatotoxicity testing. *Arch Toxicol*, 87(1), pp. 209–213.

Michalopoulos G, Russell F and Biles C (1979). Primary cultures of hepatocytes on human fibroblasts. *In Vitro*, 15(10), pp. 796–806.

Milosevic N, Schawalder H and Maier P (1999). Kupffer cell-mediated differential down-regulation of cytochrome P450 metabolism in rat hepatocytes. *Eur J Pharmacol*, 368(1), pp. 75–87.

Narayanan R, Rink A, Beattie CW and Hu W-S (2002). Differential gene expression analysis during porcine hepatocyte spheroid formation. *Mammalian Genome*, 13(9), pp. 515–523.

Ota H, Kodama T and Miki N (2011). Rapid formation of size-controlled three dimensional hetero-cell aggregates using microrotation flow for spheroid study. *Biomicrofluidics*, 5(3), p. 034105.

Otsuka H, Sasaki K, Okimura S, Nagamura M and Nakasone Y (2013). Micropatterned co-culture of hepatocyte spheroids layered on non-parenchymal cells to understand heterotypic cellular interactions. *Sci Technol Adv Mater*, 14(6), p. 065003.

Pan X, Wang Y, Yu X, Li J, Zhou N, Du W, Zhang Y, Cao H, Zhu D and Chen Y (2015). Establishment and characterization of an immortalized human hepatic stellate cell line for applications in co-culturing with immortalized human hepatocytes. *Int J Med Sci*, 12(3), p. 248.

Paschos NK, Brown WE, Eswaramoorthy R, Hu JC and Athanasiou KA (2015). Advances in tissue engineering through stem cell-based co-culture. *J Tissue Eng Regener Med*, 9(5), pp. 488–503.

Peterson TC and Renton KW (1986). Kupffer cell factor mediated depression of hepatic parenchymal cell cytochrome P-450. *Biochem Pharmacol*, 35(9), pp. 1491–1497.

Prodanov L, Jindal R, Bale SS, Hegde M, McCarty WJ, Golberg I, Bhushan A, Yarmush ML and Usta OB (2016). Long-term maintenance of a microfluidic 3D human liver sinusoid. *Biotechnol Bioeng*, 113, pp. 241–246.

Riccalton-Banks L, Liew C, Bhandari R, Fry J and Shakesheff K (2003). Long-term culture of functional liver tissue: three-dimensional coculture of primary hepatocytes and stellate cells. *Tissue Eng*, 9(3), pp. 401–410.

Seo S-J, Kim I-Y, Choi Y-J, Akaike T and Cho C-S (2006). Enhanced liver functions of hepatocytes cocultured with NIH 3T3 in the alginate/galactosylated chitosan scaffold. *Biomaterials*, 27(8), pp. 1487–1495.

Struecker B, Raschzok N and Sauer IM (2014). Liver support strategies: cutting-edge technologies. *Nat Rev Gastroenterol Hepatol*, 11(3), pp. 166–176.

Takebe T, Enomura M, Yoshizawa E, Kimura M, Koike H, Ueno Y, Matsuzaki T, Yamazaki T, Toyohara T and Osafune K (2015). Vascularized and complex organ buds from diverse tissues via mesenchymal cell-driven condensation. *Cell Stem Cell*, 16(5), pp. 556–565.

Thomas RJ, Bhandari R, Barrett DA, Bennett AJ, Fry JR, Powe D, Thomson BJ and Shakesheff KM (2005). The effect of three-dimensional co-culture of hepatocytes and hepatic stellate cells on key hepatocyte functions *in vitro*. *Cells Tissues Organs*, 181(2), pp. 67–79.

Underhill GH, Chen AA, Albrecht DR and Bhatia SN (2007). Assessment of hepatocellular function within PEG hydrogels. *Biomaterials*, 28(2), pp. 256–270.

van de Kerkhove MP, Chamuleau R and Van Gulik T (2004). Clinical application of bioartificial liver support systems. *Ann Surg.*, 240(2), pp. 216–230.

Vozzi F, Heinrich J-M, Bader A and Ahluwalia AD (2008). Connected culture of murine hepatocytes and human umbilical vein endothelial cells in a multicompartmental bioreactor. *Tissue Eng Part A*, 15(6), pp. 1291–1299.

Wong SF, Choi YY, Kim DS, Chung BG and Lee S-H (2011). Concave microwell based size-controllable hepatosphere as a three-dimensional liver tissue model. *Biomaterials*, 32(32), pp. 8087–8096.

Xia Y and Whitesides GM (1998). Soft lithography. *Ann Rev Mater Sci*, 28(1), pp. 153–184.

Yagi H, Parekkadan B, Suganuma K, Soto-Gutierrez A, Tompkins RG, Tilles AW and Yarmush ML (2009). Long-term superior performance of a stem cell/hepatocyte device for the treatment of acute liver failure. *Tissue Eng Part A*, 15(11), pp. 3377–3388.

Yamada K, Kamihira M and Iijima S (2001). Self-organization of liver constitutive cells mediated by artificial matrix and improvement of liver functions in long-term culture. *Biochem Eng J*, 8(2), pp. 135–143.

Yamada M, Utoh R, Ohashi K, Tatsumi K, Yamato M, Okano T and Seki M (2012). Controlled formation of heterotypic hepatic micro-organoids in anisotropic hydrogel microfibers for long-term preservation of liver-specific functions. *Biomaterials*, 33(33), pp. 8304–8315.

Yang S, Berg M, Hammond P and Rubner M (2003). Primary hepatocyte and mammalian cell response to polyelectrolyte multilayers containing poly-acrylamide polymers. *Abstracts of Papers of the American Chemical Society* (American Chemical Society, Washington, DC).

YoonáNo D (2013). Spheroid-based three-dimensional liver-on-a-chip to investigate hepatocyte–hepatic stellate cell interactions and flow effects. *Lab on a Chip*, 13(18), pp. 3529–3537.

Zinchenko YS and Coger RN (2005). Engineering micropatterned surfaces for the coculture of hepatocytes and Kupffer cells. *J Biomed Mater Res Part A*, 75(1), pp. 242–248.

Zinchenko YS, Schrum LW, Clemens M and Coger RN (2006). Hepatocyte and Kupffer cells co-cultured on micropatterned surfaces to optimize hepatocyte function. *Tissue Eng*, 12(4), pp. 751–761.

Chapter 8
Membranes for Bioartificial Pancreas: Macroencapsulation Strategies

K. Skrzypek*, M. G. Nibbelink†, M. Karperien†,
A. van Apeldoorn† and D. Stamatialis*,‡

**Faculty of Science and Technology, MIRA Institute,*
Bioartificial Organs Group, Biomaterials Science and Technology Department, University of Twente, The Netherlands

†Developmental BioEngineering,
MIRA Institute of Biomedical Technology, and
Technical Medicine, University of Twente, The Netherlands

‡d.stamatialis@utwente.nl

8.1 Primary Challenge: Diabetes Type 1

Type 1 diabetes mellitus is a chronic disease that mostly manifests in children and young people (usually <30 years) and is caused by destruction of the insulin-producing β-cells due to an autoimmune reaction [Foulis, 1996; Mathis *et al.*, 2001; Hornum & Markholst, 2004; Van Belle *et al.*, 2011]. It is characterized by hyperglycemia as well as relative insulin deficiency. It is known for its severe acute and long-term complications due to micro- and macro-angiopathic lesions and has a significant social and economic impact. Long-term symptoms are retinopathy, neuropathy and nephropathy [Beck *et al.*, 2007; Boron *et al.*, 2005; Kort *et al.*, 2011; Kumar & Clark, 2002; Pirot *et al.*, 2008; Silva & Mateus, 2009; Silva *et al.*, 2006; Steele *et al.*, 2014].

Since blood glucose levels are inadequately maintained due to the lack of insulin, type 1 diabetes mellitus patients need proper diet management in combination with life-long insulin administration, either by multiple daily injections or, more recently, through pump delivery. Glycemic control has also been improved by development of the "artificial pancreas", an integrated closed control system, which combines glucose monitoring with subcutaneous insulin infusion [Klonoff, 2007]. However, this system still shows several limitations mainly related to delayed glucose sensing and insulin absorption into the bloodstream. Moreover, glucose sensors have a relatively short lifetime. In order to enhance the artificial pancreas performance, new glucose-sensing technologies, with higher reliability and longer lifetime, are under development. Additionally, new algorithms, better predicting real-time blood glucose levels and "smart procedures" (miniaturized tools, functionalized materials), are needed to make the implantable artificial pancreas a realistic treatment option for type 1 diabetes patients [Iacovacci *et al.*, 2016; Klonoff, 2007].

Patients with severe glycemic lability, recurrent hypoglycemia, hypoglycemia unawareness or with an insufficient response to the insulin therapy are in need of alternative therapies. One of these is total pancreas transplantation. Despite the increasing rate of successful pancreas transplantations, the intervention involves a complicated abdominal surgery with increased risk of comorbidity [Chhabra & Brayman, 2014]. In addition, the treatment is accompanied with long-term immunosuppressive therapy to avoid rejection of the donor tissue. Due to shortage of donors, a whole pancreas transplantation is restricted to a certain group of patients, often when kidney replacement is necessary, too [Chhabra & Brayman, 2014; Farney *et al.*, 2016]. An alternative for type 1 diabetes treatment is clinical islet transplantation (CIT). Compared to total pancreas transplantation, this treatment is associated with lower surgical risk. Additionally, often when whole pancreas is considered not suitable for transplantation, the islets from donor pancreas still can be utilized and used for CIT [Berney & Johnson, 2010].

8.2 Clinical Islet Transplantation

The CIT consists of the isolation of islets from a donor pancreas and transplantation in the patient *via* infusion in the portal vein (Fig. 8.1). After infusion, the islets will embolize in the microvasculature of the liver and perform their endocrine function.

Over the years, the success rate of CIT has increased from only 24% after 2 years and 15% after 5 years to 50–60% after 2–5 years [Barton *et al.*, 2012; Grundfest-Broniatowski *et al.*, 2009; McCall & James Shapiro, 2012; Shapiro *et al.*, 2006]. However, many islets (60%) are lost in the first days after transplantation [Biarnés *et al.*, 2002; de Vos *et al.*, 2006].

The process of islet loss starts even during isolation, where islets are exposed to a variety of cellular stresses such as mechanical, enzymatic, osmotic and ischemic stresses and disruption of cell matrix and vasculature [Deters *et al.*, 2011]. This has a great impact on islet survival, as islets are particularly well perfused in the pancreas. In fact, although islets consist of only 1% of the entire pancreas, they receive 5–15% of the total blood supply of the pancreas [Ballian & Brunicardi, 2007; Homo-Delarche & Boitard, 1996; Trivedi *et al.*, 2000]. Due to disruption of their

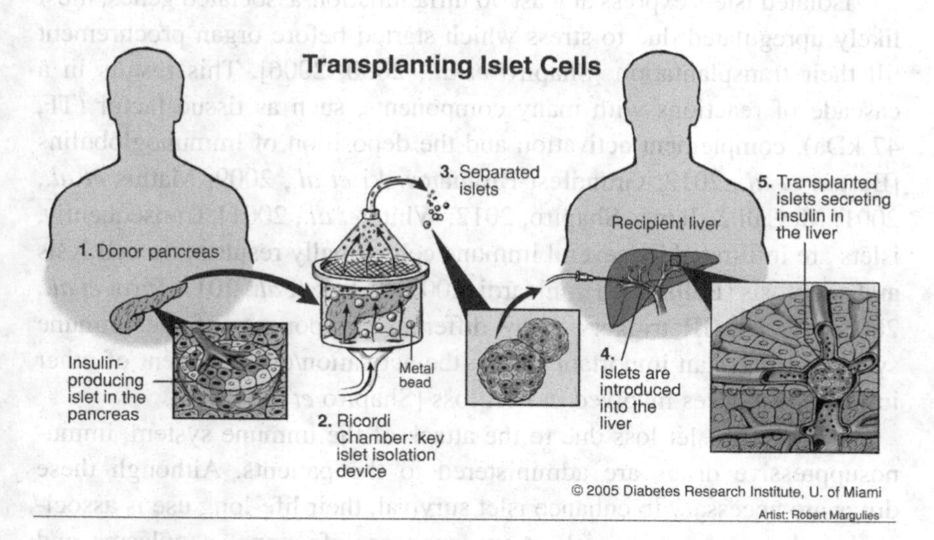

Figure 8.1. Schematic representation of the CIT procedure. Reproduced with permission from Diabetes Research Institute, University of Miami.

vasculature and the exposure to only venous blood in the first weeks after transplantation, the islets are exposed to relative hypoxic conditions. When this situation persists for more than 7 days, hypoxia results, leading to cell death and endocrine dysfunction [Barshes *et al.*, 2005; Beck *et al.*, 2007; Daoud *et al.*, 2010b; Grundfest-Broniatowski *et al.*, 2009; Silva *et al.*, 2006]. Besides, in the liver, islets are immediately exposed to relatively high concentrations of immunosuppressive drugs, glucose and lipids, which can all negatively affect beta cell function and survival [Barshes *et al.*, 2005; Citro *et al.*, 2013; Grundfest-Broniatowski *et al.*, 2009; Harlan *et al.*, 2009; Moberg *et al.*, 2002; Nanji & Shapiro, 2006; Özmen *et al.*, 2002; Kort *et al.*, 2011].

The isolation procedure also brings islets in a pro-inflammatory state as a consequence of cellular stresses [Azzi *et al.*, 2010]. This induces expression of pro-inflammatory cytokines which trigger different immune responses involved in the loss of islets after transplantation. There is in fact one immune response directly related to the transplantation site: Instant Blood Mediated Immune Response (IBMIR), which is triggered by direct contact of islets with ABO blood components in the hepatic portal system [Kort *et al.*, 2011; Pirot *et al.*, 2008].

Isolated islets express at least 50 inflammation-associated genes, most likely upregulated due to stress which started before organ procurement till their transplantation [Shapiro *et al.*, 2000, 2006]. This results in a cascade of reactions with many components, such as tissue factor (TF, 47 kDa), complement activation and the deposition of immunoglobulins [Barton *et al.*, 2012; Grundfest-Broniatowski *et al.*, 2009; Mathis *et al.*, 2001; McCall & James Shapiro, 2012; White *et al.*, 2001]. Consequently, islets are infiltrated by several immune cells, finally resulting in cell lysis and apoptosis [Ballian & Brunicardi, 2007; Deters *et al.*, 2011; Pirot *et al.*, 2008]. As IBMIR triggers many different components of the immune system, it plays an important role in the activation/enhancement of other immune responses involved in islet loss [Shapiro *et al.*, 2006].

To prevent islet loss due to the attack of the immune system, immunosuppressive drugs are administered to the patients. Although these drugs are necessary to enhance islet survival, their life-long use is associated with numerous complications such as infections, neoplasms and failure to control rejection [Mathis *et al.*, 2001]. Additionally, the hepatic location for CIT increases the effect of toxic drugs, as their concentration is high in the liver as the liver metabolizes drugs [Van Belle *et al.*, 2011]. Some drugs have negative effects on islet function by causing metabolic alterations or by direct drug toxicities. For example, calcineurin inhibitors and steroids have shown to interfere with β-cell function [Beck *et al.*, 2007; Foulis, 1996; Hornum & Markholst, 2004; Mathis *et al.*, 2001; Silva & Mateus, 2009; Silva *et al.*, 2006; Steele *et al.*, 2014; Van Belle *et al.*, 2011]. Consequently, multiple donor pancreata are necessary to obtain complete insulin dependency, which is again a problem with limited donor availability [Foulis, 1996; Kumar & Clark, 2002].

Based on the above, it is obvious that methods for islet transplantation which do not require the use of immunosuppressive drugs are highly desirable. To increase CIT efficacy, research has focused on developing devices for either immune protection or improved islet survival. In addition, due to the disadvantages of the portal system as a transplantation site, other transplantation sites are investigated too, such as subcutaneous site, omental pouch, peritoneal cavity, bone marrow or muscle [Iacovacci *et al.*, 2016; Maffi *et al.*, 2013; Yoshimatsu *et al.*, 2015].

8.3 Encapsulation Devices

8.3.1 *Introduction — Requirements*

Combining islet immune protection while maintaining islet viability might be the ultimate solution to overcome issues related to intrahepatic islet transplantation. It is thought that an encapsulation device could both maintain islet viability and act as a barrier for the immune system. Therefore, the encapsulation of islets within a semipermeable membrane, called a bioartificial pancreas (BAP), has been widely investigated for type 1 diabetes treatment (Fig. 8.2) [Iacovacci *et al.*, 2016; Schweicher *et al.*, 2014]. The most essential requirements of this device are [Beck *et al.*, 2007; Colton, 2014; Grundfest-Broniatowski *et al.*, 2009; Lacy *et al.*, 1991a, 1991b; Risbud & Bhonde, 2001; Silva & Mateus, 2009; Silva *et al.*, 2006]:

- Optimal mass-transfer properties, namely, fast nutrient and oxygen transport to the cells and fast and efficient response to high glucose concentration in the blood. In fact, the encapsulated cells should be

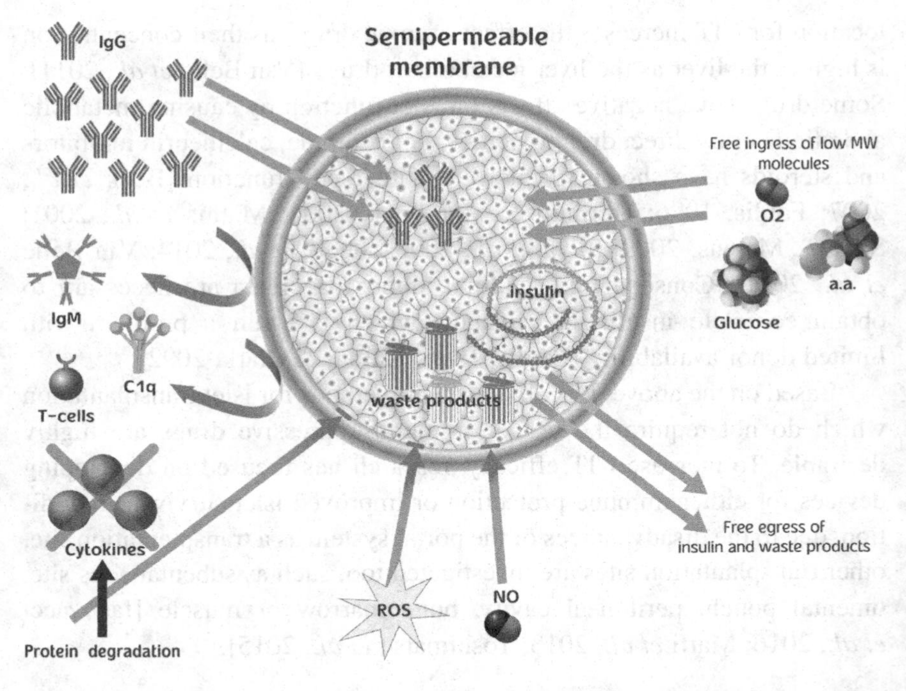

Figure 8.2. Bioartificial pancreas — schematic representation of mechanisms by which semi-permeable membrane protects grafted cells from host immune system. Reproduced with permission from Barkai *et al.* [2016].

able to rapidly detect an increase in blood glucose levels and release insulin to prevent delays in blood glucose regulation.

- Immune protection — islets need to be separated from the bloodstream to avoid contact with immune cells, antibodies, etc., immune protection should not compromise transport of glucose, insulin, oxygen and nutrients as this will lead to islet necrosis and dysfunction of the bioartificial pancreas.
- Biocompatibility — the material used for encapsulation should not activate inflammatory responses and should not stimulate fibrosis.
- The device should be sterilizable and long lasting, preferably non-degradable to sustain its functions over a long period of time.
- Easily implantable — using minimally invasive surgical procedures.
- Retrievable — it should be possible to remove the device in an easy and safe manner in case of failure.

8.3.2 *Encapsulation*

8.3.2.1 *The Need for Immune Protective Device*

When designing an immune-protective device for transplantation of islets, a balance needs to be found between optimal survival of islets and their shielding from the immune system [Tilakaratne *et al.*, 2007]. The challenge then becomes finding the optimal pore size or the molecular weight cut-off (MWCO) for the membrane. MWCO is the molecular weight of the solute that can be retained at least 90% by the membrane.

The overall strategy in the membrane fabrication process is to obtain a highly selective membrane, with high diffusivity of the low-molecular-weight nutrients and low diffusivity of the high-molecular-weight immunoglobulins. Usually membranes used for encapsulation have MWCO of 50–150 kDa [Li, 1998]. The selection of 150 kDa MWCO is often based on the retention of the smallest immunoglobulin — IgG. However, it is important to note that even if the IgG passes through the membrane, it is not an effective cell killer on its own [Barkai *et al.*, 2016]. The immune rejection is mediated by cytotoxic T-cells and therefore the immune-protective encapsulation device needs to prevent cell-to-cell contact. In fact, it has been reported that membranes with 0.4-μm pore size were successful in shielding allogeneic cells from the immune system (e.g. immunoisolation TeraCyte™ device) [Loudovaris *et al.*, 1992, 1999; Nanji & Shapiro, 2006].

Decreasing the membrane pore size would improve retention of potentially harmful molecules (immunoglobulins and some of cytokines); however, it might negatively affect the mass transport properties of the device.

8.3.2.2 *Encapsulation Strategies*

Based on the amount of islet cells encapsulated within the semi-permeable membrane, there are three strategies investigated: nano-, micro- and macro-encapsulation (see Table 8.1).

Nanoencapsulation devices are less than 100-μm in diameter and can envelop single pancreatic β-cells in a semipermeable membrane. The membrane is directly bound to the cell as conformal coating with thickness between nanometers to some micrometers [Iacovacci *et al.*, 2016].

Table 8.1: Overview of encapsulation strategies' advantages and disadvantages.

Encapsulation type	Advantages	Disadvantages
Nanoencapsulation	Very small diffusion distances	Low coating stability Non-retrievable
Microencapsulation	Easy manufacturing procedure	Large diffusion distances No connection to the vasculature Fibrosis Difficult to retrieve
Macroencapsulation (intravascular)	Close proximity to blood Direct access to the nutrients and oxygen Can be reseeded and retrieved Flexible in size	Complex surgical procedure High risk of thrombosis, clot formation Necessity of anticoagulation therapy
Macroencapsulation (extravascular)	Easy to implant retrieve and reload Flexible in size	Large diffusion distances

Several methods of conformal coating have been proposed, including covalent surface attachment of polyethylene glycol (PEG) and layer-by-layer encapsulation [Fotino *et al.*, 2015; Teramura *et al.*, 2013; Zhi *et al.*, 2012]. The advantage of these coatings is that islets are less prone to hypoxia and nutrient deprivation since diffusion distances are reduced to nanometers [Fotino *et al.*, 2015]. The challenge, however, remains to achieve a uniform and stable coating in order to provide sufficient islet immune protection [Fotino *et al.*, 2015; Teramura *et al.*, 2013].

Microencapsulation refers to individual or small clusters of islets enclosed in a polymer gel matrix [Farney *et al.*, 2016]. Most common materials used are hydrogels such as alginate, chitosan, agarose, HEMA-MMA, copolymers of acrylonitrile (AN69) and polyethylene glycol [de Vos *et al.*, 2006]. Alginate has shown advantages over other materials, as it does not interfere with cell function, is mechanically stable and capsules are easily manufactured at physiological conditions [de Vos *et al.*, 2006, 2010; Soon-Shiong *et al.*, 1994]. Additionally, various materials such as PEG and different polycations have been incorporated into alginate to reduce plasma adsorption. Some coatings (e.g. poly-D-lysine (PDL) and poly-L-ornithine (PLO)) may act as pro-inflammatory agents. The poly-L-lysine (PLL) coating was found to be the most optimal since it is the least reactive to the host [Beck *et al.*, 2007; de Vos *et al.*, 2006,

2010; Kendall Jr *et al.*, 2004; Ponce *et al.*, 2006]. As islets are fully embedded in the hydrogel with adequate MWCO, the device can provide sufficient immune protection. Problems there could be large diffusion distances due to thickness of the capsule, fragility, limited islet viability, no connection to the vascular network, fibrosis and lot-to-lot variability of alginates. In addition, microcapsules are difficult to retrieve in case of implant failure [Daoud *et al.*, 2010a; Desai *et al.*, 2000a, 2000b].

Macroencapsulation systems often comprise of the total transplanted cell volume in a single, defined container with centimeter-range dimensions. Macrocapsules can be produced in a relatively simple way and easily implanted with minimally invasive surgical procedure. An even greater advantage is the possibility of their retrieval and/or reload if necessary, but this may come at the expense of mass-transfer limitations [de Vos *et al.*, 2002]. Further, in this chapter, we will focus on the macroencapsulation strategies using polymeric membranes.

8.3.2.3 *Macroencapsulation with Membranes*

Depending on the implantation site, macroencapsulation devices can be distinguished into: extravascular, mostly placed subcutaneously or in the peritoneal cavity; and intravascular devices connected to the patient's cardiovascular system [de Vos *et al.*, 2002].

The intravascular devices contain islets encapsulated within hollow biocompatible tubes or fibers directly attached to the patient's cardiovascular system, allowing for rapid diffusion of the oxygen and nutrients to encapsulated islets [Maki *et al.*, 1993; Sun *et al.*, 1977]. Consequently, the islets are able to react quickly and efficiently to changes in glucose concentration. However, these systems can have several disadvantages including: requiring complex surgical intervention, high risk of thrombosis and clot formation, and life-long, systemic administration of anticoagulation therapy. In the case of material failure, there is a risk of damaging blood vessels, and retrieval of the device is associated with a complex surgical procedure [de Vos *et al.*, 2010; Fotino *et al.*, 2015]. Some of the intravascular devices are listed in Table 8.2.

The first intravascular systems with membranes were made using the copolymer polyacrylonitrile–polivinyl chlorine (PAN-PVC) and were

Table 8.2: Examples of intravascular devices.

Material	Islet source	Animal model	Outcome	Reference
Polyacrylonitrile–polivinyl chlorine (PAN-PVC)	Rat islets Monkey islets	Rat Monkey	Restored normoglycemia	Sun *et al.* [1977]
Polyethylene-vinyl alcohol (EVAL) fibers and poly-amino-urethane-coated, non-woven polytetrafluoroethylene (PTFE) fabric	Porcine isles	Pig	Restored normoglycemia	Ikeda *et al.* [2006]
Polycarbonate membrane	Rat islets	Dog	Restored normoglycemia	Scharp *et al.* [1984]
Nylon microporous membrane	Rabbit fetuses	Human	Restored normoglycemia	Prochorov *et al.* [2008]

reported to reverse diabetes in a rodent model after transplantation [Chick *et al.*, 1975, 1977; Sun *et al.*, 1977; Tze *et al.*, 1976]. Similar results were obtained by Scharp *et al.* [1984] using tubular polycarbonate membrane. While modified versions of intravascular devices have been tested in allogeneic and xenogeneic transplantation models, coagulation and further complications occurred, thus making development of intravascular devices very challenging [Maki *et al.*, 1993, 1996]. In 2008, Prochorov *et al.* [2008] reported the use of a nylon microporous membrane as intravascular macrocapsule transplanted into diabetic human patients. Even though, in this approach, islets from fetal rabbits were used and no immunosuppressive therapy was applied, positive results in several patients were observed even after 2 years of transplantation. The device was immune-protective and thrombosis did not occur. Still, approximately 40% of the islets were lost during the first weeks after transplantation due to poor vascularization of the device. Despite this success, intravascular devices have not been implemented to the clinic so far.

The extravascular devices are mostly placed subcutaneously or in the peritoneal cavity and can be implanted without need of anastomosis, which is advantageous in terms of clinical implementation. Additionally, extravascular devices are relatively easy to implant and retrieve. They can be re-seeded, and they have flexibility in size. However, the design of such devices need to overcome the lack of direct vascular access and the fact that the islets experience diffusional limitations, due to the relatively large size of these devices. Glucose and nutrient transport to the cells can be slower and, as a consequence, the release of insulin is delayed. Additionally, decreased oxygen delivery toward islets may cause necrosis and cell death. Therefore, the membranes used there have to be thin but at the same time mechanically and chemically stable [Schweicher *et al.*, 2014].

Examples of the extravascular devices are listed in Table 8.3. The materials used for extravascular device fabrication can be organic (polymeric) or inorganic. Inorganic materials such as silicon [Desai *et al.*, 1998, 1999, 2000a, 2000b], aluminum/aluminum oxide [La Flamme *et al.*, 2005, 2007] or titanium/titanium oxide [Ainslie *et al.*, 2009; Macak *et al.*, 2007] have been used for the fabrication of nanoporous membranes with controlled pore size and geometry. Their advantages over polymeric membranes are tighter pore distribution and better diffusivity due to reduced

Table 8.3: Examples of extravascular devices.

Material	Transplantation side	Islet source	Model	Configuration	Reference
Modified polyacrylonitrile–polivinyl chlorine (PAN-PVC)	Subcutaneous	Human islets	Patients with diabetes type 1 and 2	Tubular device	Scharp *et al.* [1994]
Cellulose acetate	Intraperitoneally	Human islets	Rat	Tubular device	Altman *et al.* [1984]
Acrylic copolymer (XM-50 Amicon)	Intraperitoneally	Rat	Mice	Tubular device	Lacy *et al.* [1991a, 1991b]
Polysulfone	—	Rat	*In vitro*	Tubular device	Lembert *et al.* [2001]
Nitrocellulose acetate (Millipore)	Intraperitoneally	Mice	Mice	Flat device	Strautz [1970]
2-Hydroxyethyl methacrylate	Sutured to parietal peritoneum	Rat or rabbit pancreatic tissue	Rat	Flat device	Klomp *et al.* [1979]
Acrylonitrile (AN62)	Intraperitoneally	Rat	Rat	Flat device	Kessler *et al.* [1991]
Alginate	Omentum	Dog	Dog	Flat device	Storrs *et al.* [2001]

membrane thickness [Desai *et al.*, 2004]. Since inorganic membrane development is rather new, they have not been extensively tested for cell encapsulation.

8.3.2.4 *Membrane Configuration*

8.3.2.4.1 Hollow Fiber Membranes

Following the development of hollow fiber technology for renal dialysis, hollow fibers have been used for cell encapsulation [Hymer *et al.*, 1981; Monaco *et al.*, 1991; Zekorn *et al.*, 1989]. Hollow fiber extravascular devices were produced from different materials such as modified PAN–PVC [Colton & Avgoustiniatos, 1991; Scharp *et al.*, 1994], regenerated cellulose and polyamide [Zekorn *et al.*, 1989], acrylic copolymer (XM-50 Amicon) [Altman *et al.*, 1984; de Vos *et al.*, 2002; Lacy *et al.*, 1991a, 1991b] and polysulfone [Lembert *et al.*, 2001]. Using these systems, *in vitro* and *in vivo* studies were performed with encapsulated islets. Proper insulin release in response to glucose level changes was obtained and the transplanted islets were viable and functional after several weeks of implantation [Maki *et al.*, 1991, 1995]. However, usually, graft survival was shorter compared to intra-vascular devices, due to limited oxygenation and nutrient transport. In fact, the large volume of islets encapsulated in hollow fiber devices can lead to aggregation and creation of big islet clumps. Consequently, necrosis occurs in the central core of islets resulting in graft failure [Lacy *et al.*, 1991a, 1991b]. This problem can be overcome by using hydrogels (alginate, colla-gen, chitosan) for islet separation [Colton, 1995; Lacy *et al.*, 1991a, 1991b; Metrakos *et al.*, 1993]. Additionally, surface modifications of hollow fiber devices can allow better immunoisolation, biocompatibility and minimal fibrotic response [Lacy *et al.*, 1991a, 1991b; Lanza *et al.*, 1992, 1996].

Hollow fiber devices are adaptable and relatively easy to transplant. However, due to their shape, they tend to bend and break and require a large volume of islets to achieve insulin independence, an important issue in the case of clinical trials [Colton, 1995].

8.3.2.4.2 Flat Devices

Flat devices consist of flat, circular or rectangular membranes encapsu-lating islets. It is believed that this configuration can provide better stability than hollow fiber membranes and can improve oxygen supply to the entire graft. Algire [1943] and Algire and Legallais [1949] used a flat device by gluing two thin microporous membranes made of nitrocellulose acetate and investigated immune rejection mechanisms with non-pancreatic tissue. The Millipore company later adapted the design of Algire and produced an extravascular device with 0.45-μm pore size [Scharp *et al.*, 1984]. Many other researchers used the same device to confirm improved immune protection [Gates *et al.*, 1972; Strautz, 1970]. Besides nitrocellulose, other materials have been applied for development of flat devices such as 2-hydroxyethyl methacrylate [Klomp *et al.*, 1979], acrylonitrile and sodium methalylsulfone [Kessler *et al.*, 1991], poly(vinyl alcohol) hydrogel in combination with a mesh [Aung *et al.*, 1993; Hayashi *et al.*, 1996] and alginate [Lanza *et al.*, 1995; Storrs *et al.*, 2001]. Despite initial successes there, the problem of poor oxygenation and lack of vascularization remained.

Flat devices are mostly implanted subcutaneously or in the peritoneal cavity due to their size and shape. They stay intact and remain in original configuration after transplantation. Nonetheless, if the material is not selected properly, the formation of a thick layer of fibrotic tissue around the device can occur, limiting transport of nutrients and oxygen and contributing to graft failure [Krishnan *et al.*, 2014; Schweicher *et al.*, 2014]. Recently, researchers also focused on the addition of oxygen supply or possibility of device vascularization [Ludwig & Ludwig, 2015]. There are several companies active in this field, developing the products for macroencapsulation. Some of them are described in detail in the next section.

8.3.3 *Upscaling of the Devices*

Encapsulation devices need to fit a certain number of islets to be able to restore normoglycemia. Shapiro *et al.* have shown that about 9,000 islets per kilogram of bodyweight are needed to obtain insulin independency in patients; however, the final number of viable islets is not known [Ryan *et al.*, 2001]. Therefore, optimal macroencapsulation devices, designed for *in vitro* testing, as well as, *in vivo* using smaller animals, should be able to be upscaled in order to be applied to humans. The modeling study of Dulong and Legallais [2007] has shown that, by increasing islet density in the device, the surface of planar devices or the length of tubular devices often needs to be increased in order to encapsulate an optimal number of viable islets, resulting in very large devices not suitable for implantation. Additionally, any compromise of the space required for islet encapsulation may result in mass transport limitation causing cell necrosis and resulting in a less functional device. Decreasing membrane thickness could improve diffusion of nutrients and oxygen; however, it may compromise the membrane mechanical properties. Different approaches can be considered in order to solve these issues. The most obvious is implantation of more than one device in order to obtain the required number of functional islets. In the case of tubular devices, the fibers can be coiled, decreasing the space needed for implantation. To achieve this, the device needs to be mechanically stable to avoid damages and deformations. Besides, for planar devices, multi-layer stacking of the membranes is possible [Papenburg *et al.*, 2009]. Here, optimal transport properties need to be maintained for each layer of encapsulated islets.

8.4 Macroencapsulation Devices under Development

8.4.1 *TheraCyte*™ *System*

In the late 1990s, Baxter Healthcare developed an islet macroencapsulation planar device that is still in use today in several laboratories [Brauker *et al.*, 1995; Loudovaris *et al.*, 1999]. The device is composed of two thin, polytetrafluoroethylene membranes sealed at all sides complemented with a loading port. The device is "teabag"-shaped, 4-cm in length and has at one end a polyethylene port for islet seeding. The outside, 5-μm pore membrane improves strength of the device and allows for infiltration of vasculature, whereas the inner 0.4-μm pore membrane provides immunoisolation. The device is suitable for subcutaneous implantation, but since it is designed to be incorporated into the host vasculature, it is difficult to remove and replace. Animal studies have shown promising results related to biocompatibility and functionality of the device [Brauker *et al.*, 1995, 1996, 1998; Kumagai-Braesch *et al.*, 2013; Rafael *et al.*, 1999; Sweet *et al.*, 2008]. There is also a possibility to improve the system performance by inducing neovascularization before transplantation

[Sorenby *et al.*, 2008], addition of vascular endothelial growth factor [Trivedi *et al.*, 2000] or exploiting encapsulation of human embryonic stem cells (ESCs) derived from islet tissue [Scharp & Marchetti, 2014].

8.4.2 *Cell Pouch System*

Serenova Corporate commercializes a biocompatible macrodevice for subcutaneous implantation that can create a natural environment in the body for long-term survival and function of therapeutic pancreatic cells. The device is made of a non-biodegradable knitted polymer mesh with large pores to allow the development of fibrous tissue rich in vessels. Inside the device, a rod-like polymer plug is positioned to guide the growth of the microvessels and connective tissue in order to create lumen for the future transplantation of islets [Kriz *et al.*, 2012]. When the lumen is created, the rod-like plug is removed and islets can be transplanted. Addition of sertolin, a testicular protein, provides immune protection and reduces the need for immunosuppressive therapy [http://www.sernova.com/technology/].

8.4.3 *Islet Sheet*

Islet sheet is another planar device. Its development began in the late 1990s. First, islets were seeded on a collagen matrix in order to create a cell monolayer that allows for better diffusion of nutrients and oxygen in comparison to islet clusters. This monolayer was then embedded in 3% (w/v) alginate gel creating an islet sheet [Dufrane *et al.*, 2010]. Alginate layers formed a uniform immune-protective barrier for the encapsulated cell and the sheet thickness was maintained as small as possible (~250-μm). The main advantage of this device is the easy implantation (in peritoneal cavity or subcutaneous site) and removal or replacement. Studies in rodent models have demonstrated satisfactory insulin secretion; however, the implantation into larger animals has limited success due to short graft survival [Storrs *et al.*, 2001].

8.4.4 *βAir® Device*

Beta-O_2 Technologies Ltd. has focused on an important problem of extravascular macrodevices: their insufficient oxygen supply after

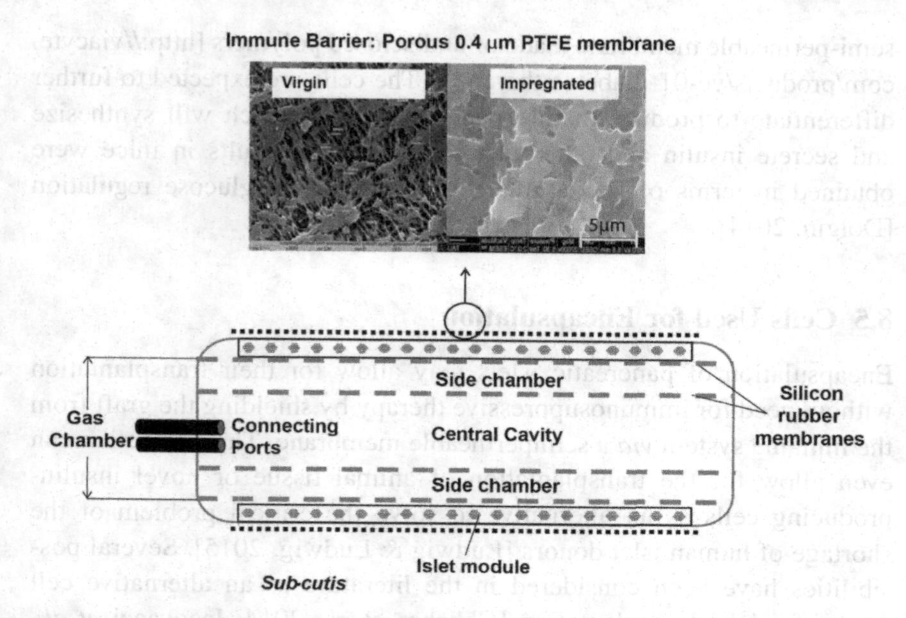

Figure 8.3. Schematic view of the βAir® device. Adapted with permission from Neufeld *et al.* [2013].

implantation resulting in large islet loss at the early stage. Therefore, they developed an oxygen-refueled macrochamber composed of islets immobilized in two flat alginate, immune-protective sheets with an oxygen supply chamber placed between the membranes (Fig. 8.3) [http://beta-o2.com/]. A subcutaneous port connected to the implanted device permits daily replacement of oxygen, which slowly diffuses into the islet compartment. The chamber is housed in a plastic case, providing mechanical protection, and is wrapped in a porous PTFE membrane impregnated with hydrophobically modified alginate to avoid immune responses [Dolgin, 2014; Iacovacci *et al.*, 2016]. Studies in animals and patients with type 1 diabetes have shown proper device functionality and regulated insulin secretion without need for immunosuppressive agents [Ludwig *et al.*, 2013; Neufeld *et al.*, 2013].

8.4.5 *VC-01 System*

ViaCyte developed a subcutaneous macrocapsule based on embryonic stem-cell-derived precursors of insulin-producing β-cells and a semi-permeable membrane made of undisclosed polymers [http://viacyte.com/products/vc-01-diabetes-therapy/]. The cells are expected to further differentiate to produce mature pancreatic cells, which will synthesize and secrete insulin and other factors. Promising results in mice were obtained in terms of neovascularization and blood glucose regulation [Dolgin, 2014].

8.5 Cells Used for Encapsulation

Encapsulation of pancreatic islets may allow for their transplantation without need for immunosuppressive therapy by shielding the graft from the immune system *via* a semipermeable membrane. This protection can even allow for the transplantation of animal tissue or novel insulin-producing cells as an alternative to solve the critical problem of the shortage of human islet donors [Ludwig & Ludwig, 2015]. Several possibilities have been considered in the literature as an alternative cell source for islet transplantation [Chhabra *et al.*, 2014; Iacovacci *et al.*, 2016; Liu *et al.*, 2016; Robles *et al.*, 2014].

8.5.1 *Porcine Islets*

Porcine islets contain physiologically compatible insulin-producing cells [Dufrane & Gianello, 2012]. Pigs are readily available species, and there is close homology between porcine and human insulin. Additionally, porcine islets are morphological similar to human islets; however, they are less sensitive to destruction by autoimmunity in comparison to human islets and there are no ethical issues [Dufrane *et al.*, 2006; Marigliano *et al.*, 2011]. Since porcine islets have less insulin-secreting capacity than humans, new protocols to isolate large quantities of porcine islets have recently been developed [Graham *et al.*, 2011; Qiao *et al.*, 2010]. Furthermore, effective methods have been established for genetic modification of pigs to improve xenotransplantation outcomes [Cooper *et al.*, 2013; Dufrane & Gianello, 2012; Dufrane *et al.*, 2006; Elliott, 2011; Marigliano *et al.*, 2011]. Despite all this, one of the issues in using porcine cells is the risk of retroviral disease transmission, and there is also absolute need for immune-protective encapsulation strategies.

8.5.2. *Exocrine Cells*

Recently, a new approach has been proposed based on reprogramming of exocrine acinar cells to insulin-producing β-cells [Furuya *et al.*, 2013; Lee *et al.*, 2013; Lemper *et al.*, 2015]. Normally, the exocrine pancreatic tissue is discarded after the islet isolation procedure, but it appears to be still useful and valuable. However, in order to guarantee high efficacy and safety, the techniques of reprogramming still need improvement.

8.5.3 *Stem Cells*

Stem cells represent a novel approach for the production of transplantable β-cells, thanks to their regenerative and proliferative abilities [Chhabra & Brayman, 2011, 2013; Chhabra *et al.*, 2009]. Theoretically, they can be used to generate insulin-producing β-cells, multi-cellular islets or even the whole pancreas [Lanzoni *et al.*, 2013; Tan *et al.*, 2014]. Viable insulin-producing β-cells can be derived from various kinds of stem cells, such as human embryonic (hESC) or induced pluripotent stem cells (iPSCs) [Alipio *et al.*, 2010; Chhabra & Brayman, 2013; Chhabra *et al.*, 2009; Kelly *et al.*, 2011; Pagliuca *et al.*, 2014; Schulz *et al.*, 2012]. However, there are still concerns regarding the limited ability to retain insulin independence using β-cells generated from stem cells in pre-clinical models [Iacovacci *et al.*, 2016]. Additionally, the use of immune-protective encapsulation devices is of high importance there since the non-differentiated cells can form tumors [Yang & Yoon, 2015]. Therefore, the risk of cells escaping from the device should be prevented.

8.6 Conclusions and Outlook

CIT, although successful, is associated with several complications hindering the transplantation outcomes. The development of a bioartificial pancreas seems to be a promising strategy to overcome the issues related to intrahepatic transplantation. The use of porous membranes for macroencapsulation devices gives the opportunity to optimize the device properties regarding the transport of nutrients and the exchange of glucose and insulin. Here, the great advantage of macroencapsulation devices is that they can be easily retrieved, replaced or reloaded. The promising results obtained with macroencapsulation devices have led to first clinical studies. However, there is still room for improvement in order to develop a life-long, fully functional islet encapsulation device for type 1 diabetes treatment.

Macroencapsulation systems are advantageous because they contain a high density of islets in a single device. Therefore, cells are in close proximity to each other (similar to healthy pancreas), improving communication and synchronization regarding insulin secretion [Prochorov *et al.*, 2008]. At the same time, a high number of islets placed in one location may lead to their fusion, which negatively affects islet native structure. As a result, large cell aggregates form and islets suffer from limited nutrient diffusion [Lehmann *et al.*, 2007]. In order to avoid islet aggregation, islets can be immobilized using gels [Lacy *et al.*, 1991a, 1991b; Silva & Mateus, 2009]. However, the gel brings an additional barrier for diffusing nutrients and oxygen, impeding proper insulin secretion and device function. In order to improve islet separation without the use of gels, a microwell array has been proposed [Buitinga *et al.*, 2013; Nibbelink, 2016]. Buitinga *et al.* [2013] described an open, microwell scaffold for vessel ingrowth, where individual islets are captured in separate microwell pockets (Fig. 8.4(a)).

The authors of this chapter have also developed a macroencapsulation device where islets are seeded in a microwell membrane and closed with a flat membrane lid (Fig. 8.4(b)) [Skrzypek *et al.*, 2017]. The device can preserve islet morphology and prevent aggregation while maintaining its function *in vitro* (islets respond to glucose concentration changes — Fig. 8.4(c)).

Lower aggregation allows for better transport of nutrients, increasing islet viability and survival. After improving islet performance, and therefore providing more functional islets, one could consider using a lower density of islets without conceding the function of the macroencapsulation device.

Since the islets are highly metabolically active, they require large amounts of oxygen and access to nutrients to function properly within the encapsulation devices. Different strategies to improve islet performance, such as additional supply of oxygen to the construct, the use of growth factors and induction of pre-vascularization, are required. In fact, administration of growth factors has been shown to improve graft functionality by increasing angiogenesis. However, it can also result in

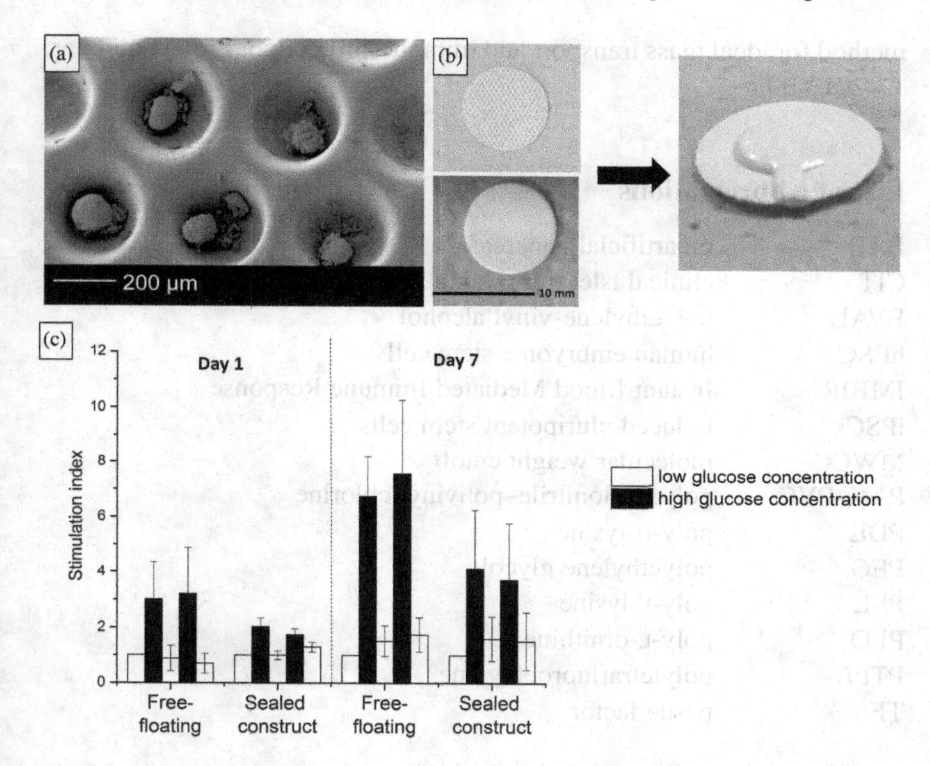

Figure 8.4. Microwell membranes for islet transplantation: (a) Islets seeded in microwell film. Adapted with permission from Buitinga *et al.* [2013]. (b) Macroencapsulation device composed of microwell and flat membrane. (c) Human islet function encapsulated in microwell membrane.

abnormal and unsustainable vasculature formation [Pareta *et al.*, 2012]. Therefore, the addition of a pre-vascularized layer as part of the encapsulation device seems to be a promising strategy, which would overcome the need for an external oxygen supply. The use of pre-vascular networks leads to a long-term solution for vasculature reconnection to the host [Sarker *et al.*, 2015].

Acknowledgments

The authors acknowledge the financial support of Juvenile Diabetes Research Foundation (JDRF). Project title: New islet encapsulation method for ideal mass transport and immune-protection. Project number: 17-2013-303.

List of Abbreviations

BAP	bioartificial pancreas
CIT	clinical islet transplantation
EVAL	polyethylene-vinyl alcohol
hESC	human embryonic stem cells
IMBIR	Instant Blood Mediated Immune Response
iPSCs	induced pluripotent stem cells
MWCO	molecular weight cutoff
PAN–PVC	polyacrylonitrile–polivinyl chlorine
PDL	poly-D-lysine
PEG	polyethylene glycol
PLL	poly-L-lysine
PLO	poly-L-ornithine
PTFE	polytetrafluoroethylene
TF	tissue factor

References

Ainslie KM, Tao SL, Popat KC, Daniels H, Hardev V, Grimes CA and Desai TA (2009). *In vitro* inflammatory response of nanostructured titania, silicon oxide, and polycaprolactone. *J Biomed Mater Res A*, 91(3), pp. 647–655.

Algire GH (1943). An adaptation of the transparent-chamber technique to the mouse. *J Natl Cancer Inst*, 4(1), pp. 1–11.

Algire GH and Legallais FY (1949). Recent developments in the transparent-chamber technique as adapted to the mouse. *J Natl Cancer Inst*, 10(2), pp. 225–253, incl 228 pl.

Alipio Z, Liao W, Roemer EJ, Waner M, Fink LM, Ward DC and Ma Y (2010). Reversal of hyperglycemia in diabetic mouse models using induced-pluripotent stem (iPS)-derived pancreatic beta-like cells. *Proc Natl Acad Sci USA*, 107(30), pp. 13426–13431.

Altman JJ, Houlbert D, Chollier A, Leduc A, McMillan P and Galletti PM (1984). Encapsulated human islet transplantation in diabetic rats. *ASAIO J*, 30(1), pp. 382–386.

Aung T, Kogire M, Inoue K, Fujisato T, Gu Y, Burczak K, Shinohara S, Mitsuo M, Maetani S, Ikada Y, *et al.* (1993). Insulin release from a bioartificial pancreas using a mesh reinforced polyvinyl alcohol hydrogel tube. An *in vitro* study. *ASAIO J*, 39(2), pp. 93–96.

Azzi J, Geara AS, El-Sayegh S and Abdi R (2010). Immunological aspects of pancreatic islet cell transplantation. *Expert Rev Clin Immunol*, 6(1), pp. 111–124.

Ballian N and Brunicardi FC (2007). Islet vasculature as a regulator of endocrine pancreas function. *World J Surg*, 31(4), pp. 705–714.

Barkai U, Rotem A and de Vos P (2016). Survival of encapsulated islets: more than a membrane story. *World J Transp*, 6(1), pp. 69–90.

Barshes NR, Wyllie S and Goss JA (2005). Inflammation-mediated dysfunction and apoptosis in pancreatic islet transplantation: implications for intrahepatic grafts. *J Leukoc Biol*, 77(5), pp. 587–597.

Barton FB, Rickels MR, Alejandro R, Hering BJ, Wease S, Naziruddin B, Oberholzer J, Odorico JS, Garfinkel MR, Levy M, Pattou F, Berney T, Secchi A, Messinger S, Senior PA, Maffi P, Posselt A, Stock PG, Kaufman DB, Luo X, Kandeel F, Cagliero E, Turgeon NA, Witkowski P, Naji A, O'Connell PJ, Greenbaum C, Kudva YC, Brayman KL, Aull MJ, Larsen C, Kay TWH, Fernandez LA, Vantyghem M-C, Bellin M and Shapiro AMJ (2012). Improvement in outcomes of clinical islet transplantation: 1999–2010. *Diabetes Care*, 35(7), pp. 1436–1445.

Beck J, Angus R, Madsen B, Britt D, Vernon B and Nguyen KT (2007). Islet encapsulation: strategies to enhance islet cell functions. *Tissue Eng*, 13(3), pp. 589–599.

Berney T and Johnson PR (2010). Donor pancreata: evolving approaches to organ allocation for whole pancreas versus islet transplantation. *Transplantation*, 90(3), pp. 238–243.

Biarnés M, Montolio M, Nacher V, Raurell M, Soler J and Montanya E (2002). β-Cell death and mass in syngeneically transplanted islets exposed to short- and long-term hyperglycemia. *Diabetes*, 51(1), pp. 66–72.

Boron WF, Boulpaep EL and Barret EJ (2005). *The endocrine pancreas.* (Elsevier Saunders, Philadelphia), pp. 1066–1085.

Brauker J, Frost GH, Dwarki V, Nijjar T, Chin R, Carr-Brendel V, Jasunas C, Hodgett D, Stone W, Cohen LK and Johnson RC (1998). Sustained expression of high levels of human factor IX from human cells implanted within an immunoisolation device into athymic rodents. *Hum Gene Ther*, 9(6), pp. 879–888.

Brauker JH, Carr-Brendel VE, Martinson LA, Crudele J, Johnston WD and Johnson RC (1995). Neovascularization of synthetic membranes directed by membrane microarchitecture. *J Biom Mater Res*, 29(12), pp. 1517–1524.

Brauker J, Martinson LA, Young SK and Johnson RC (1996). Local inflammatory response around diffusion chambers containing xenografts: nonspecific destruction of tissues and decreased local vascularization. *Transplantation*, 61(12), pp. 1671–1677.

Buitinga M, Truckenmüller R, Engelse MA, Moroni L, Ten Hoopen HWM, van Blitterswijk CA, de Koning EJP, van Apeldoorn AA and Karperien M (2013). Microwell scaffolds for the extrahepatic transplantation of islets of Langerhans. *PLoS ONE*, 8(5), p. e64772.

Chhabra P and Brayman KL (2011). Current status of immunomodulatory and cellular therapies in preclinical and clinical islet transplantation. *J Transp*, 2011, Article ID 637692.

Chhabra P and Brayman KL (2013). Stem cell therapy to cure type 1 diabetes: from hype to hope. *Stem Cells Transl Med*, 2(5), pp. 328–336.

Chhabra P and Brayman KL (2014). Overcoming barriers in clinical islet transplantation: current limitations and future prospects. *Curr Prob Surg*, 51(2), pp. 49–86.

Chhabra P, Mirmira RG and Brayman KL (2009). Regenerative medicine and tissue engineering: contribution of stem cells in organ transplantation. *Curr Opin Org Transp*, 14(1), pp. 46–50.

Chhabra P, Sutherland DER and Brayman KL (2014). Overcoming barriers in clinical islet transplantation: current limitations and future prospects. *Curr Prob Surg*, 51(2), pp. 49–86.

Chick WL, Like AA and Lauris V (1975). Beta cell culture on synthetic capillaries: an artificial endocrine pancreas. *Science (New York, N.Y.)*, 187(4179), pp. 847–849.

Chick WL, Perna JJ, Lauris V, Low D, Galletti PM, Panol G, Whittemore AD, Like AA, Colton CK and Lysaght MJ (1977). Artificial pancreas using living beta cells: effects on glucose homeostasis in diabetic rats. *Science (New York, N.Y.)*, 197(4305), pp. 780–782.

Citro A, Cantarelli E and Piemonti L (2013). Anti-inflammatory strategies to enhance islet engraftment and survival. *Curr Diab Rep*, 13(5), pp. 733–744.

Colton CK (1995). Implantable biohybrid artificial organs. *Cell Transplant*, 4(4), pp. 415–436.

Colton CK (2014). Oxygen supply to encapsulated therapeutic cells. *Adv Drug Deliv Rev*, 67–68, pp. 93–110.

Colton CK and Avgoustiniatos ES (1991). Bioengineering in development of the hybrid artificial pancreas. *J Biom Eng*, 113(2), pp. 152–170.

Cooper DK, Hara H, Ezzelarab M, Bottino R, Trucco M, Phelps C, Ayares D and Dai Y (2013). The potential of genetically-engineered pigs in providing an alternative source of organs and cells for transplantation. *J Biomed Res*, 27(4), pp. 249–253.

Daoud J, Petropavlovskaia M, Rosenberg L and Tabrizian M (2010a). The effect of extracellular matrix components on the preservation of human islet function *in vitro*. *Biomaterials*, 31(7), pp. 1676–1682.

Daoud J, Rosenberg L and Tabrizian M (2010b). Pancreatic islet culture and preservation strategies: advances, challenges, and future outlook. *Cell Transplant*, 19(12), pp. 1523–1535.

Desai TA, Chu WH, Tu JK, Beattie GM, Hayek A and Ferrari M (1998). Microfabricated immunoisolating biocapsules. *Biotechnol Bioeng*, 57(1), pp. 118–120.

Desai TA, Hansford DJ and Ferrari M (2000a). Micromachined interfaces: new approaches in cell immunoisolation and biomolecular separation. *Biomol Eng*, 17(1), pp. 23–36.

Desai TA, Hansford DJ, Kulinsky L, Nashat AH, Rasi G, Tu J, Wang Y, Zhang M and Ferrari M (1999). Nanopore technology for biomedical applications. *Biomed Microdev*, 2(1), pp. 11–40.

Desai TA, Hansford DJ, Leoni L, Essenpreis M and Ferrari M (2000b). Nanoporous anti-fouling silicon membranes for biosensor applications. *Biosensors Bioelectron*, 15(9–10), pp. 453–462.

Desai TA, West T, Cohen M, Boiarski T and Rampersaud A (2004). Nanoporous microsystems for islet cell replacement. *Adv Drug Deliv Rev*, 56(11), pp. 1661–1673.

Deters NA, Stokes RA and Gunton JE (2011). Islet transplantation: factors in short-term islet survival. *Arch Immunol Ther Exp*, 59(6), pp. 421–429.

de Vos P, Faas MM, Strand B and Calafiore R (2006). Alginate-based microcapsules for immunoisolation of pancreatic islets. *Biomaterials*, 27(32), pp. 5603–5617.

de Vos P, Hamel AF and Tatarkiewicz K (2002). Considerations for successful transplantation of encapsulated pancreatic islets. *Diabetologia*, 45(2), pp. 159–173.

de Vos P, Spasojevic M and Faas MM (2010). Treatment of diabetes with encapsulated islets. *Adv Exp Med Biol*, 670, pp. 38–53.

Dolgin E (2014). Encapsulate this. *Nat Med*, 20(1), pp. 9–11.

Dufrane D, D'Hoore W, Goebbels RM, Saliez A, Guiot Y and Gianello P (2006). Parameters favouring successful adult pig islet isolations for xenotransplantation in pig-to-primate models. *Xenotransplantation*, 13(3), pp. 204–214.

Dufrane D and Gianello P (2012). Pig islet for xenotransplantation in human: structural and physiological compatibility for human clinical application. *Trans Rev*, 26(3), pp. 183–188.

Dufrane D, Goebbels RM and Gianello P (2010). Alginate macroencapsulation of pig islets allows correction of streptozotocin-induced diabetes in primates up to 6 months without immunosuppression. *Transplantation*, 90(10), pp. 1054–1062.

Dulong JL and Legallais C (2007). A theoretical study of oxygen transfer including cell necrosis for the design of a bioartificial pancreas. *Biotech Bioeng*, 96(5), pp. 990–998.

Elliott RB (2011). Towards xenotransplantation of pig islets in the clinic. *Curr Opin Org Transp*, 16(2), pp. 195–200.

Farney AC, Sutherland DE and Opara EC (2016). Evolution of islet transplantation for the last 30 years. *Pancreas*, 45(1), pp. 8–20.

Fotino N, Fotino C and Pileggi A (2015). Re-engineering islet cell transplantation. *Pharm Res*, 98, pp. 76–85.

Foulis AK (1996). The pathology of the endocrine pancreas in type 1 (insulin-dependent) diabetes mellitus. *APMIS*, 104(3), pp. 161–167.

Furuya F, Shimura H, Asami K, Ichijo S, Takahashi K, Kaneshige M, Oikawa Y, Aida K, Endo T and Kobayashi T (2013). Ligand-bound thyroid hormone receptor contributes to reprogramming of pancreatic acinar cells into insulin-producing cells. *J Biol Chem*, 288(22), pp. 16155–16166.

Gates RJ, Hunt MI, Smith R and Lazarus NR (1972). Return to normal of blood-glucose, plasma-insulin, and weight gain in New Zealand obese mice after implantation of islets of Langerhans. *Lancet (London, England)*, 2(7777), pp. 567–570.

Graham ML, Bellin MD, Papas KK, Hering BJ and Schuurman HJ (2011). Species incompatibilities in the pig-to-macaque islet xenotransplant model affect transplant outcome: a comparison with allotransplantation. *Xenotransplantation*, 18(6), pp. 328–342.

Grundfest-Broniatowski SF, Tellioglu G, Rosenthal KS, Kang J, Erdodi G, Yalcin B, Cakmak M, Drazba J, Bennett A, Lu L and Kennedy JP (2009). A new bioartificial pancreas utilizing amphiphilic membranes for the immunoisolation of porcine islets a pilot study in the canine. *ASAIO J*, 55(4), pp. 400–405.

Harlan DM, Kenyon NS, Korsgren O and Roep BO (2009). Current advances and travails in islet transplantation. *Diabetes*, 58(10), pp. 2175–2184.

Hayashi H, Inoue K, Aung T, Tun T, Wenjing W, Gu YJ, Shinohara S, Echigo Y, Kaji H, Setoyama H, Kawakami Y, Imamura M, Morikawa N, Iwata H, Ikada Y and Miyazaki J (1996). Long survival of xenografted bioartificial pancreas with a mesh-reinforced polyvinyl alcohol hydrogel bag employing a B-cell line (MIN6). *Transp Proc*, 28(3), pp. 1428–1429.

Homo-Delarche F and Boitard C (1996). Autoimmune diabetes: the role of the islets of Langerhans. *Immunol Today*, 17(10), pp. 456–460.

Hornum L and Markholst H (2004). New autoimmune genes and the pathogenesis of type 1 diabetes. *Curr Diab Rep*, 4(2), pp. 135–142.

Hymer WC, Wilbur DL, Page R, Hibbard E, Kelsey RC and Hatfield JM (1981). Pituitary hollow fiber units *in vivo* and *in vitro*. *Neuroendocrinology*, 32(6), pp. 339–349.

Iacovacci V, Ricotti L, Menciassi A and Dario P (2016). The bioartificial pancreas (BAP): biological, chemical and engineering challenges. *Biochem Pharm*, 100, pp. 12–27.

Ikeda H, Kobayashi N, Tanaka Y, Nakaji S, Yong C, Okitsu T, Oshita M, Matsumoto S, Noguchi H, Narushima M, Tanaka K, Miki A, Rivas-Carrillo JD, Soto-Gutierrez A, Navarro-Alvarez N, Tanaka K, Jun HS, Tanaka N and Yoon JW (2006). A newly developed bioartificial pancreas successfully controls blood glucose in totally pancreatectomized diabetic pigs. *Tissue Eng*, 12(7), pp. 1799–1809.

Kelly OG, Chan MY, Martinson LA, Kadoya K, Ostertag TM, Ross KG, Richardson M, Carpenter MK, D'Amour KA, Kroon E, Moorman M, Baetge EE and Bang AG (2011). Cell-surface markers for the isolation of pancreatic cell types derived from human embryonic stem cells. *Nat Biotechnol*, 29(8), pp. 750–756.

Kendall Jr, WF, Darrabie MD, El-Shewy HM and Opara EC (2004). Effect of alginate composition and purity on alginate microspheres. *J Microencap*, 21(8), pp. 821–828.

Kessler L, Pinget M, Aprahamian M, Dejardin P and Damge C (1991). *In vitro* and *in vivo* studies of the properties of an artificial membrane for pancreatic islet encapsulation. *Horm Metab Res*, 23(7), pp. 312–317.

Klomp GF, Ronel SH, Hashiguchi H, D'Andrea M and Dobelle WH (1979). Hydrogels for encapsulation of pancreatic islet cells. *ASAIO J*, 25(1), pp. 74–76.

Klonoff DC (2007). The artificial pancreas: how sweet engineering will solve bitter problems. *J Diab Sci Technnol*, 1(1), pp. 72–81.

Kort HD, Koning EJD, Rabelink TJ, Bruijn JA and Bajema IM (2011). Islet transplantation in type 1 diabetes. BMJ 342(1), pp. d217–d217.

Krishnan R, Alexander M, Robles L, Foster III, CE and Lakey JR (2014). Islet and stem cell encapsulation for clinical transplantation. *RDS*, 11(1), pp. 84–101.

Kriz J, Vilk G, Mazzuca DM, Toleikis PM, Foster PJ and White DJ (2012). A novel technique for the transplantation of pancreatic islets within a vascularized device into the greater omentum to achieve insulin independence. *Am J Surg*, 203(6), pp. 793–797.

Kumagai-Braesch M, Jacobson S, Mori H, Jia X, Takahashi T, Wernerson A, Flodstrom-Tullberg M and Tibell A (2013). The TheraCyte device protects against islet allograft rejection in immunized hosts. *Cell Transpl*, 22(7), pp. 1137–1146.

Kumar P and Clark M (2002). *Diabetes mellitus and other disorders of metabolism* (W. B. Saunders, London), pp. 1069–1121.

La Flamme KE, Mor G, Gong D, La Tempa T, Fusaro VA, Grimes CA and Desai TA (2005). Nanoporous alumina capsules for cellular macroencapsulation: transport and biocompatibility. *Diab Tech Therapeut*, 7(5), pp. 684–694.

La Flamme KE, Popat KC, Leoni L, Markiewicz E, La Tempa TJ, Roman BB, Grimes CA and Desai TA (2007). Biocompatibility of nanoporous alumina membranes for immunoisolation. *Biomaterials*, 28(16), pp. 2638–2645.

Lacy PE, Hegre OD, Gerasimidi-Vazeou A, Gentile FT and Dionne KE (1991b). Maintenance of normoglycemia in diabetic mice by subcutaneous xenografts of encapsulated islets. *Science (N.Y.)*, 254(5039), pp. 1782–1784.

Lacy PE, Hegre OD, Gerasimidi-Vazeou A, Gentile FT, Dionne E, Science S, Series N, Dec N and Dionne KE (1991a). Maintenance of normoglycemia in diabetic mice by subcutaneous xenografts of encapsulated islets maintenance of normoglycemia in diabetic mice by subcutaneous xenografts of encapsulated islets. *Science*, 254(5039), pp. 1782–1784.

Lanza RP, Borland KM, Staruk JE, Appel MC, Solomon BA and Chick WL (1992). Transplantation of encapsulated canine islets into spontaneously diabetic BB/Wor rats without immunosuppression. *Endocrinology*, 131(2), pp. 637–642.

Lanza RP, Ecker D, Kuhtreiber WM, Staruk JE, Marsh J and Chick WL (1995). A simple method for transplanting discordant islets into rats using alginate gel spheres. *Transplantation*, 59(10), pp. 1485–1487.

Lanza RP, Hayes JL and Chick WL (1996). Encapsulated cell technology. *Nat Biotech*, 14(9), pp. 1107–1111.

Lanzoni G, Oikawa T, Wang Y, Cui CB, Carpino G, Cardinale V, Gerber D, Gabriel M, Dominguez-Bendala J, Furth ME, Gaudio E, Alvaro D, Inverardi L and Reid LM (2013). Concise review: clinical programs of stem cell therapies for liver and pancreas. *Stem Cells (Dayton, Ohio)*, 31(10), pp. 2047–2060.

Lee J, Sugiyama T, Liu Y, Wang J, Gu X, Lei J, Markmann JF, Miyazaki S, Miyazaki J-i, Szot GL, Bottino R and Kim SK (2013). Expansion and conversion of human pancreatic ductal cells into insulin-secreting endocrine cells. *eLife*, 2, p. e00940.

Lehmann R, Zuellig RA, Kugelmeier P, Baenninger PB, Moritz W, Perren A, Clavien PA, Weber M and Spinas GA (2007). Superiority of small islets in human islet transplantation. *Diabetes*, 56(3), pp. 594–603.

Lembert N, Petersen P, Wesche J, Zschocke P, Enderle A, Doser M, Planck H, Becker HD and Ammon HP (2001). *In vitro* test of new biomaterials for the development of a bioartificial pancreas. *Ann NY Acad Sci*, 944, pp. 271–276.

Lemper M, Leuckx G, Heremans Y, German MS, Heimberg H, Bouwens L and Baeyens L (2015). Reprogramming of human pancreatic exocrine cells to β-like cells. *Cell Death Differ*, 22(7), pp. 1117–1130.

Li RH (1998). Materials for immunoisolated cell transplantation. *Adv Drug Deliv Rev*, 33(1–2), pp. 87–109.

Liu X, Li X, Zhang N, Zhao Z and Wen X (2016). Bioengineering strategies for the treatment of Type I diabetes. *J Biomed Nanotechnol*, 12(4), pp. 581–601.

Loudovaris T, Charlton B and Mandel T (1992). The role of T cells in the destruction of xenografts within cell-impermeable membranes. *Transpl Proc*, 24(6), p. 2938.

Loudovaris T, Jacobs S, Young S, Maryanov D, Brauker J and Johnson RC (1999). Correction of diabetic nod mice with insulinomas implanted within Baxter immunoisolation devices. *J Mol Med*, 77(1), pp. 219–222.

Ludwig B and Ludwig S (2015). Transplantable bioartificial pancreas devices: current status and future prospects. *Langenbeck's Arch Surg*, 400(5), pp. 531–540.

Ludwig B, Reichel A, Steffen A, Zimerman B, Schally AV, Block NL, Colton CK, Ludwig S, Kersting S, Bonifacio E, Solimena M, Gendler Z, Rotem A, Barkai U and Bornstein SR (2013). Transplantation of human islets without immunosuppression. *PNAS*, 110(47), pp. 19054–19058.

Macak JM, Albu SP and Schmuki P (2007). Towards ideal hexagonal self-ordering of TiO_2 nanotubes. *Rap Res Lett*, 1(5), pp. 181–183.

Maffi P, Balzano G, Ponzoni M, Nano R, Sordi V, Melzi R, Mercalli A, Scavini M, Esposito A, Peccatori J, Cantarelli E, Messina C, Bernardi M, Del Maschio A, Staudacher C, Doglioni C, Ciceri F, Secchi A and Piemonti L (2013). Autologous pancreatic islet transplantation in human bone marrow. *Diabetes*, 62(10), pp. 3523–3531.

Maki T, Lodge JP, Carretta M, Ohzato H, Borland KM, Sullivan SJ, Staruk J, Muller TE, Solomon BA, Chick WL, *et al.* (1993). Treatment of severe diabetes mellitus for more than one year using a vascularized hybrid artificial pancreas. *Transplantation*, 55(4), pp. 713–717; discussion 717–718.

Maki T, Mullon CJ, Solomon BA and Monaco AP (1995). Novel delivery of pancreatic islet cells to treat insulin-dependent diabetes mellitus. *Clin Pharmacokinet*, 28(6), pp. 471–482.

Maki T, Otsu I, O'Neil JJ, Dunleavy K, Mullon CJ, Solomon BA and Monaco AP (1996). Treatment of diabetes by xenogeneic islets without immunosuppression. Use of a vascularized bioartificial pancreas. *Diabetes*, 45(3), pp. 342–347.

Maki T, Ubhi CS, Sanchez-Farpon H, Sullivan SJ, Borland K, Muller TE, Solomon BA, Chick WL and Monaco AP (1991). Successful treatment of diabetes with the biohybrid artificial pancreas in dogs. *Transplantation*, 51(1), pp. 43–51.

Marigliano M, Bertera S, Grupillo M, Trucco M and Bottino R (2011). Pig-to-nonhuman primates pancreatic islet xenotransplantation: an overview. *Curr Diab Rep*, 11(5), p. 402.

Mathis D, Vence L and Benoist C (2001). β-Cell death during progression to diabetes. *Nature*, 414(6865), pp. 792–798.

McCall M and James Shapiro AM (2012). Update on islet transplantation. *Cold Spring Harb Perspect Med*, 2(7), p. a007823.

Metrakos P, Yuan S, Agapitos D and Rosenberg L (1993). Intercellular communication and maintenance of islet cell mass — implications for islet transplantation. *Surgery*, 114(2), pp. 423–427.

Moberg L, Johansson H, Lukinius A, Berne C, Foss A, Källen R, Østraat Ø, Salmela K, Tibell A, Tufveson G, Elgue G, Nilsson Ekdahl K, Korsgren O and Nilsson B (2002). Production of tissue factor by pancreatic islet cells as a trigger of detrimental thrombotic reactions in clinical islet transplantation. *Lancet*, 360(9350), pp. 2039–2045.

Monaco AP, Maki T, Ozato H, Carretta M, Sullivan SJ, Borland KM, Mahoney MD, Chick WL, Muller TE, Wolfrum J, *et al.* (1991). Transplantation of islet allografts and xenografts in totally pancreatectomized diabetic dogs using the hybrid artificial pancreas. *Ann Surg*, 214(3), pp. 339–360; discussion 361–332.

Nanji SA and Shapiro AMJ (2006). Advances in pancreatic islet transplantation in humans. *Diabetes, Obes Metab*, 8(1), pp. 15–25.

Neufeld T, Ludwig B, Barkai U, Weir GC, Colton CK, Evron Y, Balyura M, Yavriyants K, Zimermann B, Azarov D, Maimon S, Shabtay N, Rozenshtein T, Lorber D, Steffen A, Willenz U, Bloch K, Vardi P, Taube R, de Vos P, Lewis EC, Bornstein SR and Rotem A (2013). The efficacy of an immunoisolating membrane system for islet xenotransplantation in minipigs. *PLoS ONE*, 8(8), p. e70150.

Nibbelink, GM. (2016). A route towards immune protection. (Enschede: Universiteit Twente, The Netherlands).

Özmen L, Ekdahl KN, Elgue G, Larsson R, Korsgren O and Nilsson B (2002). Inhibition of thrombin abrogates the instant blood-mediated inflammatory reaction triggered by isolated human islets: possible application of the thrombin inhibitor Melagatran in clinical islet transplantation. *Diabetes*, 51(6), pp. 1779–1784.

Pagliuca FW, Millman JR, Gurtler M, Segel M, Van Dervort A, Ryu JH, Peterson QP, Greiner D and Melton DA (2014). Generation of functional human pancreatic beta cells *in vitro*. *Cell*, 159(2), pp. 428–439.

Papenburg BJ, Liu J, Higuera GA, Barradas AM, de Boer J, van Blitterswijk CA, Wessling M and Stamatialis D (2009). Development and analysis of multi-layer scaffolds for tissue engineering. *Biomaterials*, 30(31), pp. 6228–6239.

Pareta R, Farney AC, Opara EC and McQuilling JP (2012). *Bioartificial pancreas: evaluation of crucial barriers to clinical application* (INTECH Open Access Publisher).

Pirot P, Cardozo AK and Eizirik DL (2008). Mediators and mechanisms of pancreatic beta-cell death in type 1 diabetes. *Arq Bras Endocrinol Metabol*, 52(2), pp. 156–165.

Ponce S, Orive G, Hernández R, Gascón AR, Pedraz JL, de Haan BJ, Faas MM, Mathieu HJ and de Vos P (2006). Chemistry and the biological response against immunoisolating alginate-polycation capsules of different composition. *Biomaterials*, 27(28), pp. 4831–4839.

Prochorov AV, Tretjak SI, Goranov VA, Glinnik AA and Goltsev MV (2008). Treatment of insulin dependent diabetes mellitus with intravascular transplantation of pancreatic islet cells without immunosuppressive therapy. *Adv Med Sci*, 53(2), pp. 240–244.

Qiao AY, Zhang WH, Chen XJ, Zhang J, Xiao GH, Hu YX and Tang DC (2010). Isolation and purification of islet cells from adult pigs. *Transpl Proc*, 42(5), pp. 1830–1834.

Rafael E, Wernerson A, Arner P, Wu GS and Tibell A (1999). *In vivo* evaluation of glucose permeability of an immunoisolation device intended for islet transplantation: a novel application of the microdialysis technique. *Cell Transpl*, 8(3), pp. 317–326.

Risbud MV and Bhonde RR (2001). Islet immunoisolation: experience with biopolymers. *J Biomater Sci, Polym Ed*, 12(11), pp. 1243–1252.

Robles L, Storrs R, Lamb M, Alexander M and Lakey JRT (2014). Current status of islet encapsulation. *Cell Transpl*, 23(11), pp. 1321–1348.

Ryan EA, Lakey JR, Rajotte RV, Korbutt GS, Kin T, Imes S, Rabinovitch A, Elliott JF, Bigam D, Kneteman NM, Warnock GL, Larsen I and Shapiro AM (2001). Clinical outcomes and insulin secretion after islet transplantation with the Edmonton protocol. *Diabetes*, 50(4), pp. 710–719.

Sarker M, Chen XB and Schreyer DJ (2015). Experimental approaches to vascularisation within tissue engineering constructs. *J Biomat Sci, Polym Ed*, 26(12), pp. 683–734.

Scharp DW and Marchetti P (2014). Encapsulated islets for diabetes therapy: history, current progress, and critical issues requiring solution. *Adv Drug Deliv Rev*, 67–68, pp. 35–73.

Scharp DW, Mason NS and Sparks RE (1984). Islet immuno-isolation: the use of hybrid artificial organs to prevent islet tissue rejection. *World J Surg*, 8(2), pp. 221–229.

Scharp DW, Swanson CJ, Olack BJ, Latta PP, Hegre OD, Doherty EJ, Gentile FT, Flavin KS, Ansara MF and Lacy PE (1994). Protection of encapsulated human islets implanted without immunosuppression in patients with type I or type II diabetes and in nondiabetic control subjects. *Diabetes*, 43(9), pp. 1167–1170.

Schulz TC, Young HY, Agulnick AD, Babin MJ, Baetge EE, Bang AG, Bhoumik A, Cepa I, Cesario RM, Haakmeester C, Kadoya K, Kelly JR, Kerr J, Martinson LA, McLean AB, Moorman MA, Payne JK, Richardson M, Ross KG, Sherrer ES, Song X, Wilson A. Z, Brandon EP, Green CE, Kroon EJ, Kelly OG, D'Amour KA and Robins AJ (2012). A Scalable system for production of functional pancreatic progenitors from human embryonic stem cells. *PLoS ONE*, 7(5), p. e37004.

Schweicher J, Nyitray C and Desai TA (2014). Membranes to achieve immunoprotection of transplanted islets. *Front Biosci (Landmark Ed)*, 19, pp. 49–76.

Shapiro AMJ, Ricordi C, Hering BJ, Auchincloss H and Lindblad R (2000). Islet transplantation in seven patiens with type 1 diabetes mellitus using a glucocorticoid-free immunosuppressive regimen. *N Engl J Med*, 343(4), pp. 230–238.

Shapiro AMJ, Ricordi C, Hering BJ, Auchincloss H, Lindblad R, Robertson RP, Secchi A, Brendel MD, Berney T, Brennan DC, Cagliero E, Alejandro R, Ryan EA, DiMercurio B, Morel P, Polonsky KS, Reems J-A, Bretzel RG, Bertuzzi F, Froud T, Kandaswamy R, Sutherland DER, Eisenbarth G, Segal M, Preiksaitis J, Korbutt GS, Barton FB, Viviano L, Seyfert-Margolis V, Bluestone J and Lakey JRT (2006). International trial of the Edmonton protocol for islet transplantation. *N Engl J Med*, 355(13), pp. 1318–1330.

Silva AI, de Matos AN, Brons IG and Mateus M (2006). An overview on the development of a bio-artificial pancreas as a treatment of insulin-dependent diabetes mellitus. *Med Res Rev*, 26(2), pp. 181–222.

Silva AI and Mateus M (2009). Development of a polysulfone hollow fiber vascular bio-artificial pancreas device for *in vitro* studies. *J Biotechnol*, 139(3), pp. 236–249.

Skrzypek, K., M. Groot Nibbelink, J. van Lente, M. Buitinga, M. A. Engelse, E. J. P. de Koning, M. Karperien, A. van Apeldoorn and D. Stamatialis (2017).

Pancreatic islet macroencapsulation using microwell porous membranes. *Sci Rep*, 7(1), p. 9186.

Soon-Shiong P, Heintz RE, Merideth N, Yao QX, Yao Z, Zheng T, Murphy M, Moloney MK, Schmehl M, Harris M, Mendez R and Sandford PA (1994). Insulin independence in a type 1 diabetic patient after encapsulated islet transplantation. *Lancet*, 343(8903), pp. 950–951.

Sorenby AK, Kumagai-Braesch M, Sharma A, Hultenby KR, Wernerson AM and Tibell AB (2008). Preimplantation of an immunoprotective device can lower the curative dose of islets to that of free islet transplantation: studies in a rodent model. *Transplantation*, 86(2), pp. 364–366.

Steele JAM, Hallé JP, Poncelet D and Neufeld RJ (2014). Therapeutic cell encapsulation techniques and applications in diabetes. *Adv Drug Deliv Rev*, 67(0), pp. 74–83.

Storrs R, Dorian R, King SR, Lakey J and Rilo H (2001). Preclinical development of the islet sheet. *Ann NY Acad Sci*, 944(1), pp. 252–266.

Strautz RL (1970). Studies of hereditary-obese mice (obob) after implantation of pancreatic islets in Millipore filter capsules. *Diabetologia*, 6(3), pp. 306–312.

Sun AM, Parisius W, Healy GM, Vacek I and Macmorine HG (1977). The use, in diabetic rats and monkeys, of artificial capillary units containing cultured islets of Langerhans (artificial endocrine pancreas). *Diabetes*, 26(12), pp. 1136–1139.

Sweet IR, Yanay O, Waldron L, Gilbert M, Fuller JM, Tupling T, Lernmark A and Osborne WRA (2008). Treatment of diabetic rats with encapsulated islets. *J Cell Mol Med*, 12(6B), pp. 2644–2650.

Tan G, Elefanty AG and Stanley EG (2014). b-Cell regeneration and differentiation: how close are we to the 'holy grail'? *J Mol Endocrinol* 53(3), pp. R119–R129.

Teramura Y, Oommen OP, Olerud J, Hilborn J and Nilsson B (2013). Microencapsulation of cells, including islets, within stable ultra-thin membranes of maleimide-conjugated PEG-lipid with multifunctional crosslinkers. *Biomaterials*, 34(11), pp. 2683–2693.

Tilakaratne HK, Hunter SK, Andracki ME, Benda JA and Rodgers VGJ (2007). Characterizing short-term release and neovascularization potential of multi-protein growth supplement delivered via alginate hollow fiber devices. *Biomaterials*, 28(1), pp. 89–98.

Trivedi N, Steil GM, Colton CK, Bonner-Weir S and Weir GC (2000). Improved vascularization of planar membrane diffusion devices following continuous infusion of vascular endothelial growth factor. *Cell Transpl*, 9(1), pp. 115–124.

Tze WJ, Wong FC, Chen LM and O'Young S (1976). Implantable artificial endocrine pancreas unit used to restore normoglycaemia in the diabetic rat. *Nature*, 264(5585), pp. 466–467.

Van Belle TL, Coppieters KT and Von Herrath MG (2011). Type 1 diabetes: etiology, immunology, and therapeutic strategies. *Physiol Rev*, 91(1), pp. 79–118.

White SA, James RFL, Swift SM, Kimber RM and Nicholson ML (2001). Human islet cell transplantation — future prospects. *Diab Med*, 18(2), pp. 78–103.

Yang HK and Yoon KH (2015). Current status of encapsulated islet transplantation. *J Diabetes Complications*, 29(5), pp. 737–743.

Yoshimatsu G, Sakata N, Tsuchiya H, Minowa T, Takemura T, Morita H, Hata T, Fukase M, Aoki T, Ishida M, Motoi F, Naitoh T, Katayose Y, Egawa S and Unno M (2015). The co-transplantation of bone marrow derived mesenchymal stem cells reduced inflammation in intramuscular islet transplantation. *PLoS ONE*, 10(2), p. e0117561.

Zekorn T, Siebers U, Filip L, Mauer K, Schmitt U, Bretzel RG and Federlin K (1989). Bioartificial pancreas: the use of different hollow fibers as a diffusion chamber. *Transpl Proc*, 21(1 Pt 3), pp. 2748–2750.

Zhi ZL, Kerby A, King AJF, Jones PM and Pickup JC (2012). Nano-scale encapsulation enhances allograft survival and function of islets transplanted in a mouse model of diabetes. *Diabetologia*, 55(4), pp. 1081–1090.

Chapter 9
Early Health Economic Evaluation of Bioartificial Organs: Involving Users in the Design of the Bioartificial Pancreas for Diabetes

M. J. IJzerman*,‡, T. Wissing*
and E. de Koning†

** University of Twente, Department Health Technology and Services Research, MIRA Institute for Biomedical Technology and Technical Medicine, Enschede, The Netherlands*

†Leiden University Medical Center, Department of Medicine, Leiden, The Netherlands

‡m.j.ijzerman@utwente.nl

9.1 Introduction

With increasing pressure on health systems worldwide, there is a growing interest in health economic evaluation of new medical technologies. Such evaluation may particularly be interesting in the early stages of medical technology development as this would allow for further design improvements and thus better targeting of the specific needs of the patient population.

This chapter first introduces "early health technology assessment" as a new paradigm in health economics to evaluate medical technologies in the early stages of development. The concept of "value" is then discussed in more detail with reference to how different users, such as patients, physicians or the general public, may perceive value of a new technology. The chapter then introduces Multi-Criteria Decision Analysis (MCDA) as one specific approach to support decisions in the development stage of new medical technologies in more detail. MCDA is commonly used to compare the relative value of different therapeutic scenarios, by elicitation and combining criteria weights and expected performance of therapeutic alternatives on these criteria.

In the second section, MCDA is used to elicit the importance of transplantation characteristics and the preference for three potential bioartificial pancreas (BAP) scenarios for type I diabetes mellitus according to both patients and endocrinologists. From the results, it is concluded that therapeutic effectiveness (glycemic control) is most important for patients, whereas impact and safety of the treatment is more important for physicians. Using these results, it is possible to weigh different treatment scenarios against what is preferred by its users in order to maximize treatment value.

9.2 Health Economic Evaluation

9.2.1 *The Need for Health Technology Assessment*

Innovation in medical technologies is critical to improvements in patient care, but it is also costly and uncertain. In Europe, medical technology sales amounted about 1% of the GDP, which was close to €100 billion in 2015 [MedTech Europe, 2015]. On one hand, large amounts of resources are spent on med-tech R&D, and a highly skilled workforce is employed by these companies worldwide. On the other hand, healthcare systems are increasingly concerned with the added costs of new medical technologies. According to the World Health Organization (WHO), health technology assessment (HTA) refers to the systematic evaluation of properties, effects and/or impacts of health technology. It is a multi-disciplinary process to evaluate the social, economic, organizational and ethical issues of a health intervention or health technology. The main purpose of HTA is to inform a policy decision-making, i.e. decisions on market authorization

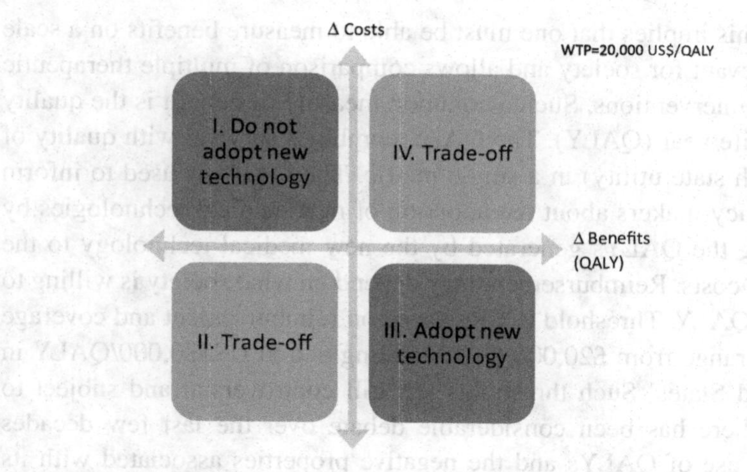

Figure 9.1. Cost-effectiveness plane, illustrating the four outcomes from an economic evaluation. In most cases, new medical technologies will be more beneficial and costlier (quadrant IV). This implies that one has to determine what society is willing to pay for the additional benefits (e.g. US$ 20,000/QALY).

and reimbursement. Following the definition of HTA, health technology includes a wide range of interventions, such as medicines, medical devices, vaccines, procedures and systems developed to solve a health problem and to improve the quality of life.

One of the central elements in HTA is the systematic comparison of the added benefits produced by the new medical technology in relation to the additional costs, also referred to as health economic evaluation. In health economic evaluation, the incremental cost-effectiveness ratio (ICER) is the ratio between the additional costs and the additional benefits of the new intervention compared to current care. The ICER plane typically has four quadrants (Fig. 9.1), i.e. (I) higher cost and less benefits, (II) lower cost and less benefits, (III) lower cost and more benefits and (IV) higher cost and more benefits. The (I) and (III) quadrants are usually referred to as "dominant", implying that either the new or the old intervention dominates. However, in virtually all new medical procedures, the new intervention incurs more costs and thus needs to be compared with the additional benefits produced (quadrant IV).

Health economic evaluation is based on the premise that society aims to allocate scarce resources in a way that it produces most benefits for society. This implies that one must be able to measure benefits on a scale that is relevant for society and allows comparison of multiple therapeutic areas and interventions. Such a common measure of benefit is the quality adjusted life year (QALY). The QALY combines survival with quality of life (health state utility) in a single metric. The QALY is used to inform health policy-makers about the adoption of new medical technologies by comparing the QALYs generated by the new medical technology to the additional costs. Reimbursement may depend on what society is willing to pay for a QALY. Threshold ICERs based on reimbursement and coverage decisions range from £20,000/QALY in England to US$80,000/QALY in the United States. Such thresholds are still controversial and subject to debate. There has been considerable debate over the last few decades about the use of QALYs and the negative properties associated with its measurement, such as the methods to map preference values or utilities to health states [Smith *et al.*, 2009]. Nevertheless, the QALY is still the single most preferred metric in health economic evaluation. While the simplicity and ease of application of the ICER threshold make it very appealing, one cannot escape the deficiencies of the QALY as an outcome measure and the arbitrariness of the threshold [Shiroiwa *et al.*, 2010].

9.2.2 *The Concept of "Value" in Health Economics*

Value has different meanings to different people. In health economics, value is usually referred to as the relative worth or desirability of a service or good. In this interpretation, economists usually refer to the concept of "utility". Accordingly, a health-state utility is a relative desirability for a health state or condition. Health-state utilities are dimensionless numbers on a scale ranging from worst imaginable health state (0) to perfect health (1). One of the most widely used instruments to estimate health-state utilities (and the QALY) is the EQ-5D. In its original form, the EQ-5D included five domains, including mobility, self-care, pain, depression and usual activities [EuroQol Group, 1990]. Each domain has three options (no problems, some problems and extremely problematic), which would then generate 243 different health-state descriptions. Each of the health states is valued by a representative population from society, and thus has a utility tariff associated with it (Fig. 9.2).

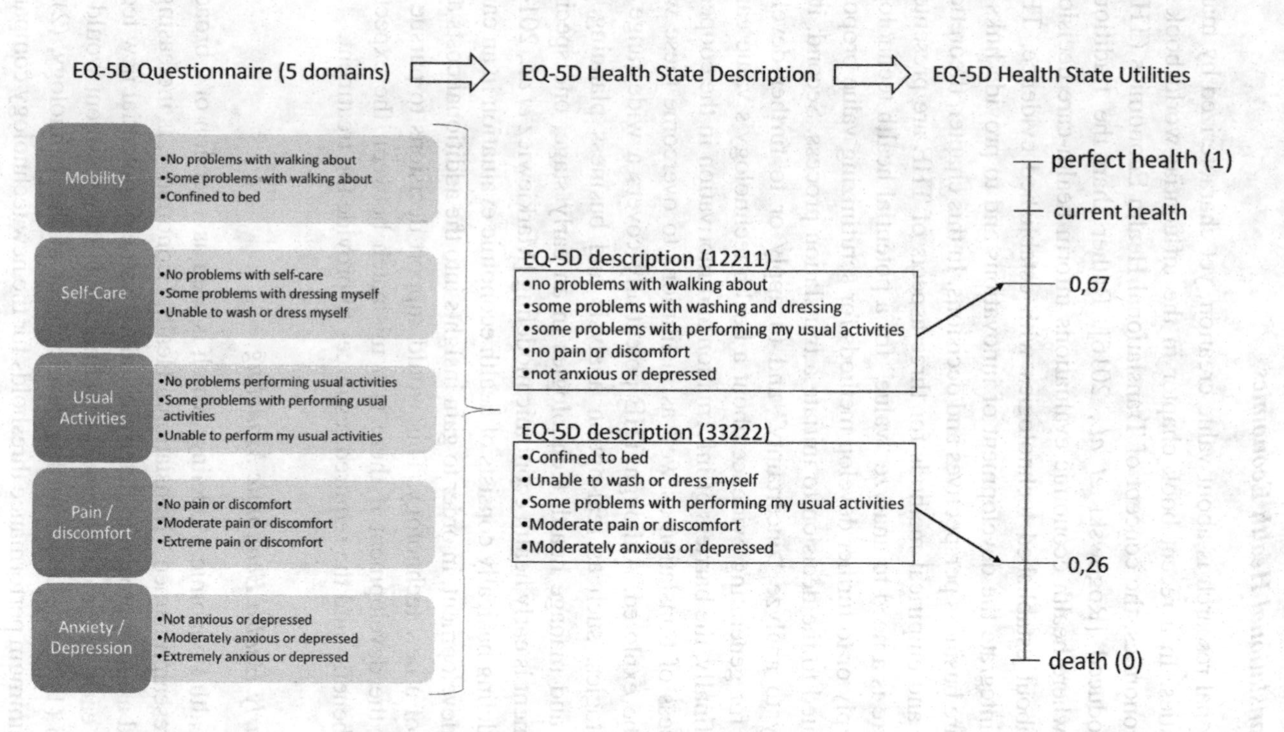

Figure 9.2. Calculation of health-state utilities based on the EQ-5D.questionnaire. See text for further explanation.

9.2.3 *Translational Health Economics*

Translational research is about value creation, yet characterized by many uncertainties. In a recent book chapter in the influential world book of health economics, the concept of Translational Health Economics (THE) was introduced [Rogowski *et al.*, 2016]. Rather than the traditional concept where health economic evaluations inform health-care decision-makers about established technologies with established evidence, THE seeks to integrate the development of innovations and to provide links to health-care business perspectives and decisions. In this chapter, theoretical concepts and empirical methods for three aspects of THE are presented. First, there is a need to analyze "value" for a potential health technology and to apply or to further develop methods for scrutinizing value propositions related to the decision to initiate a translation process. Second, it is necessary to analyze "uncertainty" and to apply or to further develop methods for generating evidence about a health technology's value early on. And finally, the barriers of information and motivation in the cooperative process of translation as well as institutions to overcome these will have to be explored. Although THE potentially covers a wide range of methodologies, such as real-option analysis and business planning, to evaluate and manage health technologies in an early stage, one specific development is early health economic modeling [Markiewicz *et al.*, 2014]. This modeling basically consists of health economic evaluation in an early stage of development, in order to gain insights into the additional costs and benefits of a new technology. This would support decisions to pursue or abandon the development if there is a mismatch between the expected societal benefits and the required resources to provide the treatment.

9.2.4 *Early Health Economic Modeling*

Early Health Economic Modeling, which is seen as a section of a broader field of research named "Translational Health Economics", is increasingly promoted as an approach to determine added value of potential new technologies early in the development pipeline. Such an assessment would be useful to (1) decide about further development of the technology, (2) to define minimum performance thresholds for the new technology compared to currently available technologies and (3) to support pricing and

Table 9.1: Differences between early and mainstream health economics.

	Early health economics	Health economics
Objective	Assess the expected safety, effectiveness and cost-effectiveness of a new medical technology in development	Assess safety, effectiveness and cost-effectiveness of a new medical technology
Decision support	Decision support for manufacturers and investors about design and management of a new technology	Decision support for regulators, patients about market authorization and reimbursement
Evidence	Evidence from early bench, or early clinical trials and registries. Expert elicitation to predict performance range of the new technology	Evidence from clinical trials with the new medical technology
Influence on technology performance	Potentially significant impact on (future) clinical performance of the new technology	Limited or no influence on future clinical performance of the new technology

reimbursement in early stages of development [IJzerman & Steuten, 2011]. The so-called headroom method is the very first and simple start of a health economic analysis in a very early stage [van de Wetering *et al.*, 2012].

Early health economic modeling deviates from mainstream health economic modeling in that it deviates from mainstream health economic modeling in that primarily is used to inform R&D decisions instead of government agencies which are responsible for reimbursement decisions (Table 9.1). This has several important implications. Where HTA is based on a rigorous assessment of clinical evidence obtained from clinical trials or systematic reviews, the evidence base for new technologies in development is much more limited. There are several approaches to deal with such uncertainties, including the use of probability elicitation methods [Kadane & O'Hagan, 2005], setting an arbitrary minimum performance threshold based on competing alternatives and the use of (probabilistic) sensitivity analysis.

Before implementing and conducting early HTA, it is essential to carefully address the type of decision that needs to be informed. Stage-gate decision models assume many different decisions to be made during R&D,

while each decision is affecting a different group of stakeholders and with different strategic and business consequences. Moreover, to estimate the value of new technologies to the health system, it is essential to understand how decisions in different health systems are being made and how society determines value. If an investigator fails to understand these different objectives and requirements, the early assessment will remain a theoretical exercise and will not produce any additional value to inform R&D decisions.

9.2.5 *Multi-criteria Decision Analysis to Value Treatments*

The very first step in THE is the early identification of value of a new technology [Rogowski *et al.*, 2016]. Although different interpretations of value exist, this chapter adopts the health economic view and the QALY, in particular, as a metric of value. One of the current debates in health economics is that the QALY as such is not an appropriate measure of societal value. Because the QALY is a measure that only considers the health outcomes, several economists have argued that the QALY is not able to pick up important treatment features that are related to the process of care [Brennan & Dixon, 2013; Weernink *et al.*, 2016]. On the other hand, it has been stated that the process of care only has value in that it is a commodity which can be exchanged to derive health gains [Donaldson & Shackley, 1997]. In lay terms, this suggests that the burden of life-long use of immunosuppressive drugs by transplanted patients is not considered in our economic value judgment, because it is assumed that this will contribute to an overall net positive benefit which is measured. Thus, it is implicitly assumed the net health benefit accounts for the burden of immunosuppressive drugs. Although this is the classic economic view, there is a growing dissatisfaction with this principle, in particular, in patients with chronic diseases and life-long disease management programs. For instance, Lloyd *et al.* [2010] conclude that the general public and patients with diabetes place a significant value on reducing the need for insulin injection.

For this reason, several people have explored other methods to include process utility, such as conjoint analysis [Ryan *et al.*, 2014]. Conjoint analysis is a methodology that allows to consider multiple attributes simultaneously, such as positive health outcomes, adverse events and process of care. By presenting pairs of hypothetical treatment scenarios where each attribute (e.g. survival) is varied over a range of outcomes (2, 6 or 12 months), it is possible to estimate the importance of the different attributes. Such attribute weights can then be used to estimate the relative value or preference for actual treatments being considered. Conjoint analysis has really taken off in the last few years, and the reader is referred to the literature for more details [Bridges *et al.*, 2011; de Bekker-Grob *et al.*, 2010].

Another emerging methodology to systematically evaluate different components of value is multi-criteria decision analysis (MCDA). MCDA is an umbrella term to describe a collection of formal approaches which seek to take explicit account of multiple criteria in helping individuals or groups explore decisions that matter [Belton & Stewart, 2002]. MCDA has emerged from different disciplines, such as economics, operations research, psychology and engineering [Köksalan *et al.*, 2013]. Its strength is that it allows a systematic and transparent approach to explicitly weigh a set of criteria relevant for comparing treatment alternatives.

It is beyond the scope of this chapter to fully discuss the different approaches for doing MCDA, and the reader is referred to the literature for practical guidance [Marsh *et al.*, 2016; Keeney & Raiffa, 1993; Thokala *et al.*, 2016].

9.3 The Bio-Artificial Pancreas for Diabetes

9.3.1 *Type 1 Diabetes*

Type 1 diabetes mellitus (T1DM) results from an absolute deficiency of insulin secretion by autoimmune destruction of the β-cells of the pancreas [American Diabetes Association, 2010]. Immune-mediated diabetes occurs particularly in childhood and adolescence and accounts for 5–10% of diabetes cases [American Diabetes Association, 2010]. Despite its relatively low prevalence rates compared with type 2 diabetes (T2DM), the economic burden of T1DM is substantial. First, patients with extensive β-cell destruction require exogenous insulin for adequate glycemic control. Moreover, glucose control can be very complicated, in particular, for T1DM patients. The chance of complications depends on the duration of diabetes and the degree of glycemic control. Large changes in blood glucose levels are associated with an increased risk of complications.

Frequent complications include damage to the heart, brain and limbs (macro-vascular) and eyes, kidney and nerves (microvascular). One of these complications is nephropathy, which occurs in 20–30% of patients with T1DM, and develops to end-stage renal disease (ESRD) in 50% of patients within 10 years [Molitch *et al*., 2004].

Pancreas transplantation is recommended in those patients with ESRD who have had or will receive a kidney transplant in order to improve glycemic control and partially reverse long-term complications [Robertson *et al*., 2006]. Islet transplantation is less invasive compared to pancreas transplantation and is also an acceptable method to re-establish and maintain physiological normoglycemia in patients with type 1 diabetes [Lakey *et al*., 2006]. Yet, the islets isolated from only one donor organ are often insufficient to establish normoglycemia because of a considerable amount of islet loss before, during and after islet transplantation [de Kort *et al*., 2011]. Islet loss after transplantation may be attributable to an immediate blood-mediated inflammatory reaction (IBMIR) triggered by the direct contact of islets with blood components, non-native mechanical stress and exposure to toxins, including elevated glucose levels (glucotoxicity), allograft rejection and the recurrence of autoimmunity [Gremizzi *et al*., 2010; Gruessner *et al*., 2010]. Because of these adverse events, there is a strong need to support the development of devices and/or scaffolds to explore alternative transplantation sites and to develop methods to exclude/minimize these inflammatory and immunological responses [Giraldo *et al*., 2010; Silva *et al*., 2006].

9.3.2 *Healthcare Costs in Type 1 Diabetes*

Subgroups of T1DM patients incur high costs, particularly those with a long duration of diabetes and poorly controlled blood glucose levels, which results in a high frequency of complications.

Different figures exist for the average cost of an islet transplantation, dependent on follow-up duration, specific subgroups of patients and country specificity. Roughly, costs vary between €78,000 [Guignard *et al*., 2004] and US$ 139,000 [Moassesfar *et al*., 2016]. The four main cost components were: islet preparation (30% of the total cost), adverse events (24%), drugs (14%) and hospitalization (13%) [Guignard *et al*.,

2004]. A more recent study looked into the cost-effectiveness of islet transplantation and life-long insulin therapy. They conclude that the 20-year cumulative cost of insulin therapy is about US$ 663,000. The 20-year cumulative cost of islets transplantation was estimated at US$ 519,000 [Beckwith *et al.*, 2012]. However, these cost estimates cannot be directly compared as the costs of islet transplantation do not include the effects of secondary complications and re-transplantation procedures.

A comprehensive review about the use of islet transplantation was published by the Institute of Health Economics in Alberta [2013]. They directly compared insulin therapy with islets transplantation and concluded that the incremental cost (i.e. additional cost compared to insulin injections) of islets transplantation is $374,604 if secondary complications are avoided and $506,429 if secondary complications are not prevented [Institute of Health Economics, 2013]. Following their report, they concluded that islet transplantation is associated with clinically significant improvements, but it is not cost-saving. Hence, islet transplantation is not a dominant (better and cheaper) treatment strategy. A more efficient use of islets and a reduction of re-transplantation procedures may potentially lead to a treatment strategy that dominates insulin injections.

9.3.3 *Patient and Physician Values for the BAP*

Over the last 30 years, several initiatives have been taken to combine biomaterials with islets as to ameliorate the survival of transplanted donor islets [Giraldo *et al.*, 2010; Silva *et al.*, 2006]. The developments of these so-called bioartificial organs have the potential to overcome some adverse effects after islet transplantation, by providing an islet-friendly environment that improves viability and physiological insulin secretion. These initiatives all have the potential to improve current type 1 diabetes care, yet little is known about the clinical performance and, hence, the potential success of these new technologies.

For ultimate success of any BAP, it is important to remain focused on the clinical status and the needs of the diabetes patients that have to be met. Regarding the latter, there have been several studies reporting the preference of patients for particular interventions in diabetes management [Joy *et al.*, 2013; Guimarães *et al.*, 2010; Lloyd *et al.*, 2010]. However, no

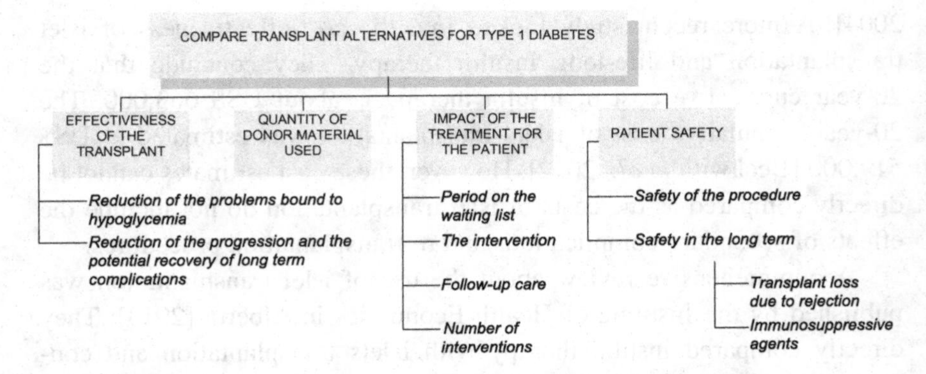

Figure 9.3. The decision tree for evaluating BAP scenarios in T1DM patients. There are four main criteria to be evaluated. Three of these also have subcriteria to further specify the components of value.

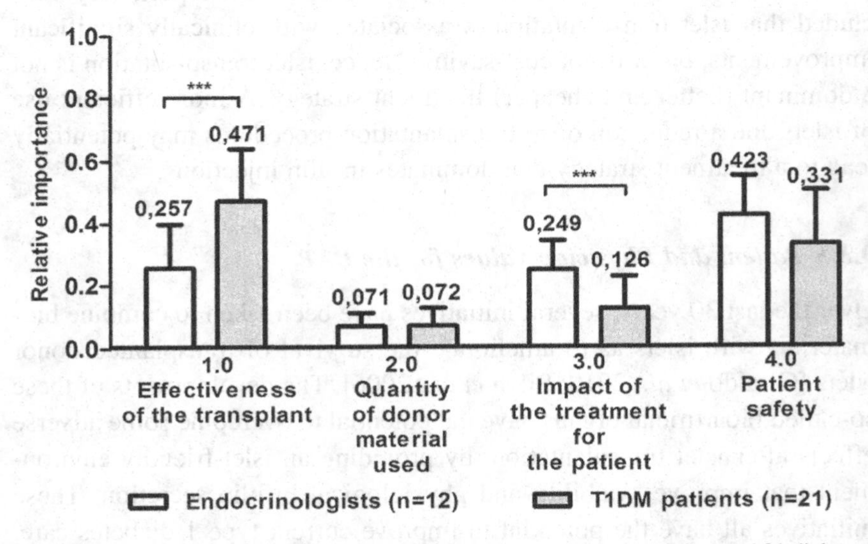

Figure 9.4. Main results from the value judgment by 12 endocrinologists and 21 diabetes patients. The weights of the four main criteria are presented (add up to 1), where *** represents a significant difference [Wissing *et al.*, 2013].

literature is known addressing T1DM patients' and endocrinologists' preferences for transplantation therapy in general nor for the development of the BAP. Because the decision to undergo transplantation surgery is preference-sensitive (i.e. benefits are weighed against the risks of treatment), such systematic evaluation of patient preferences is relevant for future adoption of BAP.

9.3.4 *Weight Elicitation for BAP Treatment Characteristics*

To illustrate the relative value of islets and pancreas transplantation scenarios, the current standard of care and treatment characteristics that determine clinical decisions for a particular transplantation method were analyzed based on a literature search, semi-structured interviews and focus groups with researchers involved in the design, as well as nephrologists, endocrinologists and specialized diabetes nurses. Following the identification of criteria, a decision tree that included the most relevant attributes for transplant decision-making could be constructed (Fig. 9.3).

Two questionnaires were then developed: one for patients and one for endocrinologists. In both questionnaires, the importance of pairs of criteria using an 18-point rating scale needed to be rated, as proposed in the Analytic Hierarchy Process as developed by Saaty [2008]. To ensure all participants made pairwise comparisons from the same point of view, a clinical vignette, i.e. a description of a typical patient, was used to serve as a reference. The T1DM patient was asked to consider a situation in which they would experience the same burden as the hypothetical patient when rating the criteria. The endocrinologist was asked to consider a situation in which they were responsible for the hypothetical patient's treatment. The relative contribution of a decision criterion (transplant attribute) in the overall preference for a transplantation method was then computed according to Saaty [2008].

Figure 9.4 shows some interesting observations. First, it can be concluded that T1DM patients have quite different views than the endocrinologists. On the one hand, patients place a much higher weight on the effectiveness of the transplant, i.e. the ability to restore normoglycemia and the long-term complications. On the other hand, patients consider "impact of the treatment" and "patient safety" to be less important. Endocrinologists, however, have a different and, in fact, opposite view. Although transplant effectiveness is important, patient safety is considered considerably more important. The figure also demonstrates that, although the impact of the treatment (surgery and use of immune-suppressive agents) is important, it is not a major issue for patients compared to the life-long insulin injections which cause a major burden [Guimarães *et al.*, 2010].

9.4 Conclusions and Future Use of the Results

This chapter has introduced some of the basics of health economic evaluation in healthcare and the concept of value of new medical technologies. The chapter then introduced MCDA as an approach to identify and value criteria that are used to determine the acceptability of new BAP designs in T1DM patients with ESRD. Such information may be applied to guide future development of the BAP as well as the acceptance by patients and physicians. Further, the results presented here may support reimbursement decisions if future BAP designs show additive value compared to current standard of care.

Although it is interesting to know what criteria are considered important for the development of future treatment strategies, we also can use the results in a different way. For instance, in consultation with the BAP development team, it is possible to identify potential treatment scenarios based on the criteria. Each of the BAP treatment scenarios likely has a different performance on the different design objectives, e.g. glycemic control, the quantity of donor material needed, transplantation site, surgical procedure and the immunosuppressive agent dose. Such expected performance improvements may then be considered in view of the importance of the attributes according to the users as well as the overall added value to a range of stakeholders including health-care insurance.

List of Abbreviations

BAP	bioartificial pancreas
EQ-5D	EuroQol group, 5 dimensions (questionnaire)
ESRD	end-stage renal disease
IBMIR	immediate blood-mediated inflammatory reaction
ICER	incremental cost-effectiveness ratio

MCDA	multi-criteria decision Analysis
QALY	quality-adjusted life year
T1DM	diabetes mellitus, type 1
THE	translational health economics
WHO	World Health Organization

References

American Diabetes Association (2010). Diagnosis and classification of diabetes mellitus. *Diabetes Care*, 33(Suppl 1), pp. S62–S69.

Beckwith J, *et al.* (2012). A health economic analysis of clinical islet transplantation. *Clin Transpl*, 26(1), pp. 23–33.

Belton V, Stewart TJ. *Multi-criteria decision analysis: an integrated approach.* Springer Science+Business; Dordrecht, 2002.

Brennan VK and Dixon S (2013). Incorporating process utility into quality adjusted life years: a systematic review of empirical studies. *PharmacoEconomics*, 31(8), pp. 677–691.

Bridges JFP, *et al.* (2011). Conjoint analysis applications in health — a checklist: a report of the ISPOR Good Research Practices for Conjoint Analysis Task Force. *Value Health*, 14(4), pp. 403–413.

de Bekker-Grob EW, Ryan M and Gerard K (2010). Discrete choice experiments in health economics: a review of the literature. *Health Econ*, 21(2), pp. 145–172.

de Kort H, *et al.* (2011). Islet transplantation in type 1 diabetes. *BMJ (Clin Res ed.)*, 342, p. d217.

Donaldson C and Shackley P (1997). Does "process utility" exist? A case study of willingness to pay for laparoscopic cholecystectomy. *Soc Sci Med (1982)*, 44(5), pp. 699–707.

EuroQol Group (1990). EuroQol — a new facility for the measurement of health-related quality of life. *Health Policy* (Amsterdam, Netherlands), 16(3), pp. 199–208.

Giraldo JA, Weaver JD and Stabler CL (2010). Tissue engineering approaches to enhancing clinical islet transplantation through tissue engineering strategies. *J Diabetes Sci Technol*, 4(5), pp. 1238–1247.

Gremizzi C, *et al.* (2010). Impact of pancreas transplantation on type 1 diabetes-related complications. *Curr Opin Organ Transpl*, 15(1), pp. 119–123.

Gruessner AC, Sutherland DER and Gruessner RWG (2010). Pancreas transplantation in the United States: a review. *Curr Opin Organ Transpl*, 15(1), pp. 93–101.

Guignard AP, *et al*. (2004). Cost analysis of human islet transplantation for the treatment of type 1 diabetes in the Swiss–French Consortium GRAGIL. *Diabetes Care*, 27(4), pp. 895–900.

Guimarães C, *et al*. (2010). A discrete choice experiment evaluation of patients' preferences for different risk, benefit, and delivery attributes of insulin therapy for diabetes management. *Patient Preference Adherence*, 4, pp. 433–440.

IJzerman MJ and Steuten LMG (2011). Early assessment of medical technologies to inform product development and market access. *Appl Health Econ Health Policy*, 9(5), pp. 331–347.

Institute of Health Economics. (2013). *Islet transplantation for the treatment of type 1 diabetes*. Edmonton AB: Institute of Health Economics.

Joy SM, *et al*. (2013). Patient preferences for the treatment of type 2 diabetes: a scoping review. *PharmacoEconomics*, 31(10), pp. 877–892.

Kadane J and O'Hagan A (2005). Statistical methods for eliciting probability distributions. *J Am Statist …*, 100(470), pp. 680–701.

Keeney RL and Raiffa H. (1993). *Decisions with Multiple Objectives: preferences and value trade-offs*. Cambridge University Press. Cambridge & New York.

Köksalan M, Wallenius J and Zionts S (2013). An early history of multiple criteria decision making. *J Multi-Crit Decis Anal*, 20, pp. 87–94.

Lakey JRT, Mirbolooki M and Shapiro AMJ (2006). Current status of clinical islet cell transplantation. *Methods Mol Biol (Clifton, N.J.)*, 333, pp. 47–104.

Lloyd A, *et al*. (2010). A valuation of infusion therapy to preserve islet function in Type 1 diabetes. *Value Health*, 13(5), pp. 636–642.

Markiewicz K, van Til JA and IJzerman MJ. (2014). Medical devices early assessment methods: systematic literature review. *Int J Technol Assess Health Care*. May 7; 30(2): 137–46.

Marsh K, *et al*. (2016). Multiple criteria decision analysis for health care decision making-emerging good practices: Report 2 of the ISPOR MCDA Emerging Good Practices Task Force. *Value Health*, 19(2), pp. 125–137.

MedTech Europe (2015). *The European Medical Technology industry — in figures*, 2015. Available at: http://www.medtecheurope.org/sites/default/files/resource_items/files/MEDTECH_FactFigures_ONLINE3.pdf.

Moassesfar S, *et al*. (2016). A comparative analysis of the safety, efficacy, and cost of islet versus pancreas transplantation in nonuremic patients with Type 1 diabetes. *Am J Transpl*, 16(2), pp. 518–526.

Molitch ME, *et al.* (2004). Nephropathy in diabetes. *Diabetes Care*, 27(Suppl 1), pp. S79–S83.

Robertson RP, *et al.* (2006). Pancreas and islet transplantation in type 1 diabetes. *Diabetes Care*, 29(4), p. 935.

Rogowski WH, John J and IJzerman MJ. (2016). Translational Health Economics. In: World Scientific Handbook of Global Health Economics and Public Policy. 3rd ed. Page 405–439. World Scientific Publishing Company; Singapore.

Ryan M, *et al.* (2014). Valuing patients' experiences of healthcare processes: towards broader applications of existing methods. *Soc Sci Med (1982)*, 106, pp. 194–203.

Saaty TL. (2008). Decision making with the analytic hierarchy process. *Int J Ser Sci*, 1 (1): 83–98.

Shiroiwa T, *et al.* (2010). International survey on willingness-to-pay (WTP) for one additional QALY gained: what is the threshold of cost effectiveness? *Health Econ*, 19(4), pp. 422–437.

Silva AI, *et al.* (2006). An overview on the development of a bio-artificial pancreas as a treatment of insulin-dependent diabetes mellitus. *Med Res Rev*, 26(2), pp. 181–222.

Smith MD, Drummond M and Brixner D (2009). Moving the QALY forward: rationale for change. *Value Health*, 12(Suppl 1), pp. S1–S4.

Thokala P, *et al.* (2016). Multiple criteria decision analysis for health care decision making — an introduction: Report 1 of the ISPOR MCDA Emerging Good Practices Task Force. *Value Health*, 19(1), pp. 1–13.

Van de Wetering G, *et al.* (2012). Early Bayesian modeling of a potassium lab-on-a-chip for monitoring of heart failure patients at increased risk of hyperkalaemia. *Technol Forecasting Soc Change*, 79(7), pp. 1268–1279.

Weernink MGM, *et al.* (2016). Valuing treatments for parkinson disease incorporating process utility: performance of best-worst scaling, time trade-off, and visual analogue scales. *Value Health*, 19(2), pp. 226–232.

Wissing TB, Apeldoorn AA and IJzerman MJ (2013). The expected value of bio-artificial pancreas development in view of endocrinologists "and patients" preferences. *Value Health*, 16(3), p. A169.

Chapter 10
Membranes for Regenerative Medicine in Clinical Applications

G. F. D'Urso Labate and G. Catapano*

Department of Environmental and Chemical Engineering, University of Calabria, Via Pietro Bucci, 87036 Rende (CS), Italy
*gerardo.catapano@unical.it

10.1 Introduction

Regenerative medicine (RM) is an interdisciplinary field of research and clinical applications that integrates several technological approaches, such as transplantation of human cells and tissues, cell and gene therapy, molecular medicines to stimulate endogenous regeneration, biomaterials and artificial devices, to "replace, or regenerate human cells, tissues and organs, to restore or establish normal function" [Mason & Dunnill, 2008; US Department of Health and Human Services, 2013]. Since its ultimate aim is to return the patient to full health, RM goes beyond repair, intended as the adaptation to loss of normal organs, and aims at fully restoring functions lost for any cause, be it aging, disease, trauma or congenital defects. Hence, RM therapies are potentially useful for treating a wide range of dermatological, dental, cardiovascular, orthopedic and central nervous system degenerative pathologies, traumas or congenital defects, to say but a few [PR Newswire, 2016].

The global market of RM has been boosted by recent technological advancements in such fields as stem cell therapy, tissue engineering and 3D bioprinting, and by an increasing incidence of age-related degenerative diseases, and it is expected to grow from $2.6 billion in 2012 to $6.5 billion by 2019 [Transparency Market Research, 2012]. Human cells play a central role in RM, whether they are directly recruited from the patients' body or are isolated, manipulated (e.g. gene modified, reprogrammed or expanded) and implanted. Cell scaffolding with functional (nano)biomaterials has also proven effective in fields such as skin, bladder and cornea, wound care, drug delivery and immunomodulation. However, the stringent regulations to clear RM products for clinical use and the high costs of treatments currently hinder the faster growth of this market [Transparency Market Research, 2012].

Within this framework, tissue engineering (TE) is often considered a branch of RM with more limited aims. TE is a multi-disciplinary field that aims at preparing *in vitro* biological substitutes of tissues that restore, maintain, improve or enhance tissue function after implantation [Langer & Vacanti, 1993]. Tissue substitution occurs through (i) isolation of patient's own cells from a biopsy, (ii) cell expansion *in vitro* to reach clinical mass, (iii) cell seeding in three-dimensional (3D) resorbable artificial supports (scaffolds) simulating the macroscopic shape of the missing (or failing) tissue and the microstructure of its extracellular matrix (ECM), (iv) culture in bioreactors of the cell-seeded construct with biochemical and mechanical cues guiding formation of an *in vivo*-like tissue, (v) implantation of the construct and its integration with the natural tissue surrounding the implant site, as the scaffold is resorbed.

The transport, separation and physical–chemical properties of the most recent clinical membranes make them appealing for RM and TE. Information on the possible use of membranes was gathered by searching scientific databases for papers published in the last 25 years on artificial or resorbable membranes in TE or RM. Figure 10.1 shows that the interest in the use of membranes for RM applications is growing fast. In fact, starting in 2005, the number of papers on this topic published in the years 2010–2015 has increased fivefold with respect to the years 2005–2009 [Pubmed Central, 2015]. A similar trend was found for papers published on artificial or resorbable membranes in TE,

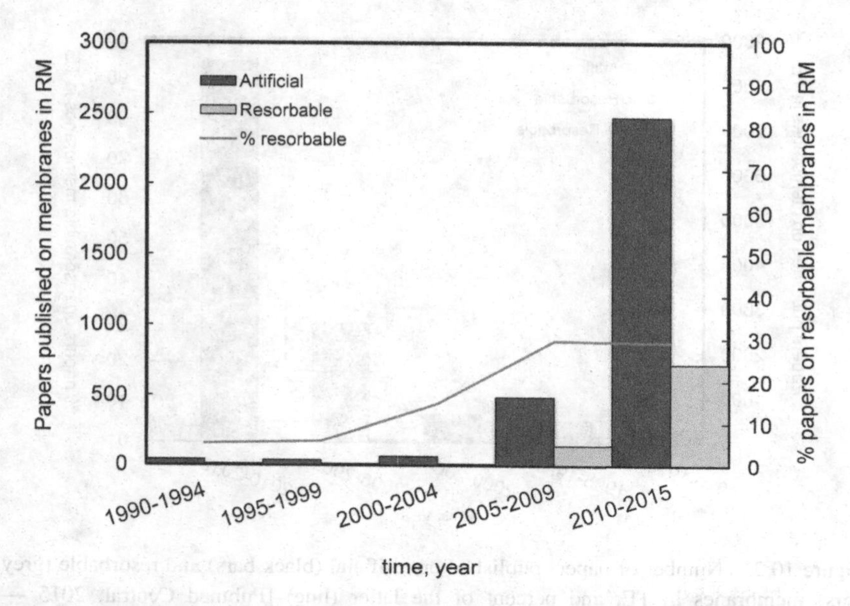

Figure 10.1. Number of papers published on artificial (black bars) and resorbable (grey bars) membranes in RM, and percent of the latter (line) [Pubmed Central, 2015 — Keywords: Artificial — (Regenerative AND Medicine) AND Membranes AND (Artificial OR Synthetic); Resorbable — (Regenerative AND Medicine) AND Membranes AND (Artificial OR Synthetic) AND (Resorbable OR Biodegradable) — Years: 1990–today].

with a threefold increase in the number of papers published in the years 2010–2015 with respect to the years 2005–2009 (Fig. 10.2) [Pubmed Central, 2015].

Some membranes are commercially available for clinical applications. Synthetic aliphatic polyester membranes (e.g. polycaprolactone, polyglycolic acid, polylactic acid, polylactic-co-glycolic acid) are used in cartilage repair. The MACI graft BioSeed-C (Biotissue Technologies, Freiburg, Germany) is a composite polylactic-co-glycolic and polydioxane membrane infiltrated with fibrin. The Cartilage Autograft Implantation System (CAIS, DePuy Mitek, Raynham, MA) uses a copolymer membrane (35% polycaprolactone–65% polyglycolic acid) structurally reinforced with a polydioxane mesh [Dewan *et al.*, 2014]. Microporous AMCA (ammonium methacrylate copolymer type A) membranes have been effectively used in the regeneration of load-bearing bone [Grin *et al.*, 2009; Mosheiff *et al.*, 2003].

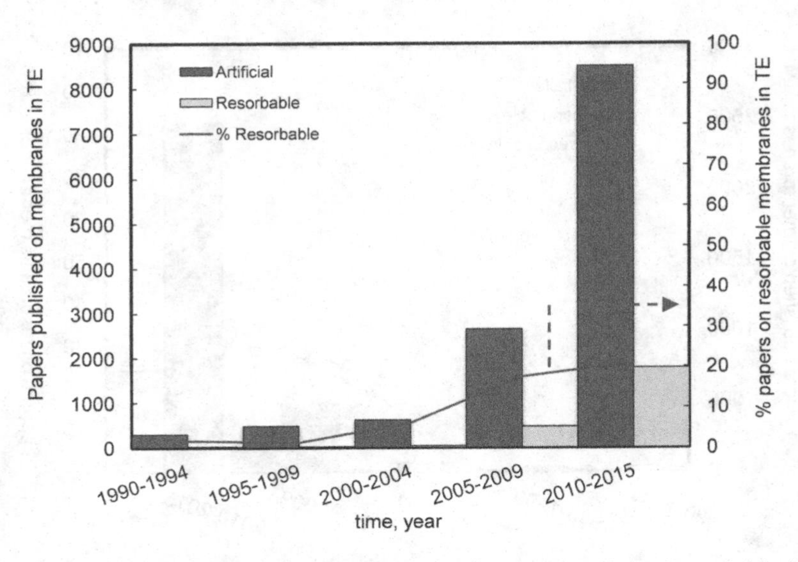

Figure 10.2. Number of papers published on artificial (black bars) and resorbable (grey bars) membranes in TE, and percent of the latter (line) [Pubmed Central, 2015 — Keywords: Artificial — (Tissue AND Engineering) AND Membranes AND (Artificial OR Synthetic); Resorbable — (Tissue AND Engineering) AND Membranes AND (Artificial OR Synthetic) AND (Resorbable OR Biodegradable) — Years: 1990–today].

Polymeric membranes have also been proposed for liver, kidney, pancreas, vascular, nerve, bone and cartilage TE [Diban & Stamatialis, 2014], as: 3D mechanical support (scaffolding) to multiple anchorage-dependent tissue-specific cell types [Unger *et al.*, 2005]; size-selective barriers to guide cell migration to tissue-specific spatial positions and enable tissue in-growth [Gentile *et al.*, 1995]; receptor-selective barriers to guide cell spatial positioning (i.e. adhesion) as in natural tissue; semi-permeable barriers to enable physiological supply of oxygen, nutrients and biochemical cues to cells and to avoid cell overgrowth [Quirk *et al.*, 2001].

A successful TE application requires that the membranes be resorbed and replaced by the cell-secreted ECM, as tissue matures. For this reason, many researchers have investigated the use of resorbable polymers for the preparation of membranes, generally in flat sheet configuration, of both natural (e.g. alginate, cellulose, collagen, chitosan) and synthetic origin (e.g. polylactic acid, polylactic-co-glycolic acid, poly-ε-caprolactone, poly(lacticacid-co-ε-caprolactone), polyethyleneglycol, poly(hydroxybutyrate-co-hydroxyvalerate), biodegradable polyurethanes, polytrimethylene carbonate). These membranes still exhibit fair-to-poor mechanical resistance and limited permeability and release degradation products that may cause local pH changes as the membrane degrades. However, it has been shown that membranes varying with regard to wall geometry and structure and transport properties may be produced [Dhandayuthapani *et al*., 2011].

Hollow fiber (HF) membranes have been proposed for replacing the nutrient supply function of the vascular network in the preparation of large TE internal organs, or when the tissue to replace has a tubular shape (e.g. intestine, urethra, blood vessels and nerves) [Diban & Stamatialis, 2014]. So far, only a couple of resorbable HF membranes have been proposed, which also suffer from the same drawbacks of those prepared as flat sheets [Diban & Stamatialis, 2014; Ellis & Chaudhuri, 2007; Meneghello *et al*., 2009]. As shown in Fig. 10.2, in most cases, technical, highly inert and chemically/mechanically resistant polymers (e.g. polyethersulfone, polypropylene, polyurethane, polyetheretherketone, polyacrylonitrile, polysulfone, polyethylene coated with ethylenevinylalcohol) have been proposed which impede graft–host integration and may cause mechanical constriction and tissue compression, long-term foreign body reactions, pain and discomfort and may limit the regenerative processes for their low permeability [Diban & Stamatialis, 2014]. As a result, membranes for TE are still at the developmental stage and have, as yet, no significant impact on the RM market.

Among the applications of membranes to RM, dental implantation and wound dressing are very interesting from a clinical point of view and have a high commercial impact. In 2012, the global dental membrane market was over $200 million with a 5–10% annual growth, and it is expected to reach $300 million by 2017 [PR Newswire, 2013]. The global wound dressing market was worth $9.9 billion in 2015 and it is expected to grow at a 6.9% rate in 2016–2022 [PR Newswire, 2017].

For this reason, in this chapter, attention is mainly focused on commercial membranes used for dental implantation and wound dressings. In the following, their requirements, structural features and use are briefly described, although not exhaustively, to provide membrane scientists with useful information for the development of the next-generation membranes for clinical applications of RM.

10.2 Membranes in RM: General Requirements

Membranes are often classified according to their properties, the most frequently used being [Catapano *et al.*, 2009]:

- the chemical nature of the material of which they are made (e.g. inorganic vs organic; synthetic vs natural);
- the morphology of the wall (e.g. symmetric vs asymmetric, dense vs porous);
- the force driving mass transport across the membrane (e.g. concentration vs pressure vs temperature transmembrane difference);
- the material's physical–chemical properties (e.g. charged vs neutral, hydrophobic vs hydrophilic);
- the separation mechanism (e.g. size vs charge).

To qualify a membrane for RM, additional properties would have to be considered that depend on the application. Tissue regeneration involves different specific cell types acting in different phases, going from inflammation, to tissue formation and remodeling. It may be deduced that the good outcome of a regenerative process strongly depends on cell behavior, migration and proliferation. Engulfment and isolation of bacteria also play a key role in the avoidance of infections during the healing process [Evans *et al.*, 2013]. Additionally, oxygen, nutrients and growth factors should easily reach the regeneration site and should support and guide cell metabolism, differentiation and functions. Within this framework, membranes can be effectively used in RM for favoring the regeneration of the treated site, by aiding and enhancing all steps of the natural healing process. In RM, membranes may be used to perform a few key functions such as:

- act as temporary perm-selective barriers to foster regeneration of, and protect, the wound or defect site. Membranes should protect the site against bacterial attack and the entrance of body fluids, while offering a large surface area for the physiological exchange of gases and nutrients;

- act as temporary guide and template for tissue regeneration. Membranes should sort cells migrating into the treated site by attracting those cells relevant for tissue regeneration (thus stimulating tissue regeneration) and by preventing the access of unnecessary or detrimental, but faster growing, cells. The membrane should also avoid cell overgrowth and maintain the shape of the tissue at the wound site.

Additionally, membranes might be used to deliver soluble biochemical cues or drugs to help avoid infections, drive cell migration and promote tissue regeneration [Thomas, 1997].

To fulfill these expectations and be successful in the clinical setting, in addition to exhibiting particular properties among those often used for their classification, membranes for RM would have to exhibit additional properties often determined by practical considerations, such as:

- cell sorting capacity;
- good interface with tissue and cells;
- easy to shape to the wound or defect contour;
- good mechanical resistance;
- easily recoverable or resorbable.

To meet all the above requirements, membranes should often exhibit contradictory properties. For example, membranes should be hydrophilic to offer a good interface to tissues or cells but should be hydrophobic to be permeable to oxygen and prevent body fluids from entering the wound site. They should be resorbable to reduce the number of surgical interventions and patient's discomfort, but resorbable materials generally exhibit poor mechanical properties and are difficult to handle during surgery. In the following, it will be briefly described how such hurdles have been solved to make membranes successful in clinical applications of RM in the field of dental implantation and wound care.

10.3 Membranes in Dental Implantation

Periodontium is a group of specialized tissues surrounding and supporting the teeth, which make it possible to keep them in the maxillary and mandibular bones. The periodontium consists of four principal components: (i) gingiva, (ii) periodontal ligament (PDL), (iii) cementum and (iv) alveolar bone, each with its own distinct functions [Kumar, 2011].

Periodontitis is a very aggressive pathology that can lead to the destruction of the periodontium. This may eventually result in tooth loss unless it is treated [Haffajee & Socransky, 2000]. Till mid-1980s, it was believed that the cells capable of regenerating the periodontium were localized in the alveolar bone only [Melcher *et al.*, 1987]. In the 1990s, it was shown that progenitor cells in the periodontium are localized in the PDL [Buser *et al.*, 1990], and implantation of physical barriers to separate the PDL from the alveolar bone to favor the healing process was started [Gottlow *et al.*, 1984]. Guided tissue regeneration (GTR) and guided bone regeneration (GBR) started this way.

In particular, in the treatment of periodontitis by GTR, an occlusive membrane is implanted between the gingival connective tissue and the PDL/alveolar bone tissue. The membrane maintains the space for blood clot stabilization and promotes periodontal tissue regeneration by preventing post-surgical epithelial cell migration into the treated site. At the same time, the membrane allows progenitor cells located in the PDL to preferentially colonize the root area and differentiate into new alveolar bone, PDL and cementum (Fig. 10.3(a)) [Wang *et al.*, 2005].

GBR aims to heal a localized lack of bone volume caused by congenital, post-traumatic, post-surgical defects or a disease. GBR is used when the augmentation and restoration of deficient alveolar ridges is needed because such deficiency compromises the function or the esthetics of the dental implant. In GBR, a filler (either a bone autograft harvested from a different site or an artificial osteogenic filler) is often used to partially replace the missing alveolar bone (Fig. 10.3(b)). GBR can be carried out prior to, or in some cases along with, the placement of dental implant [Buser *et al.*, 1993].

A successful GTR or GBR treatment depends not only on membrane properties but also relies on correctly performing a number of procedural steps, such as [Sheikh *et al.*, 2014]:

- *Good site preparation.* The gingival flaps must be properly separated and the bone cavity must be correctly filled.

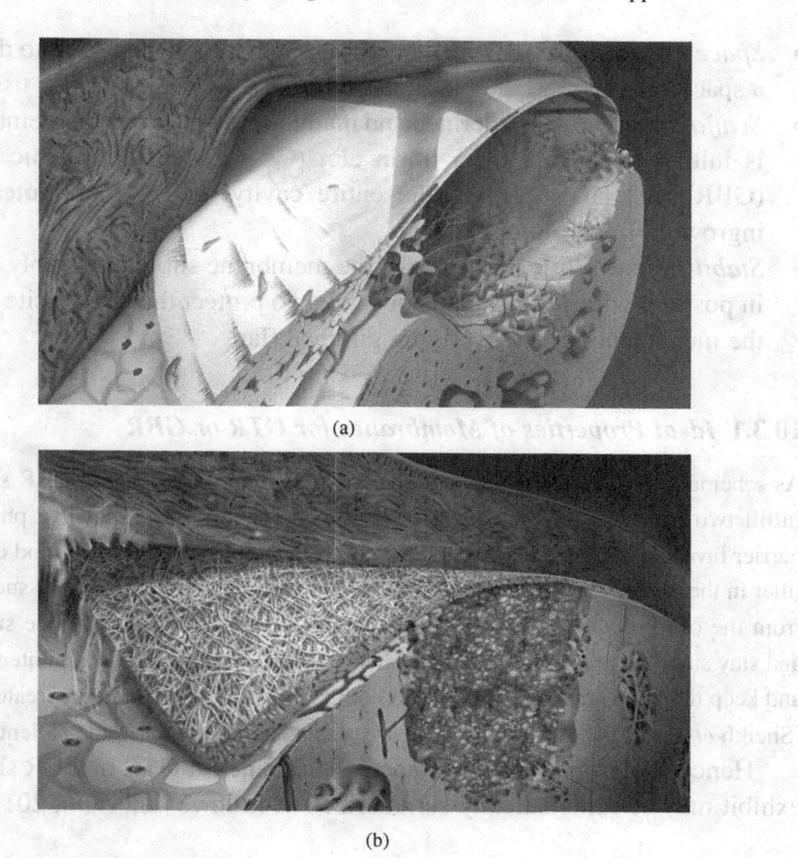

(a)

(b)

Figure 10.3. (a) Membrane positioning in GTR procedure. The membrane maintains the space for blood clot stabilization and promotes periodontal tissue regeneration by preventing migration of post-surgical epithelial cells into the treated site. At the same time, the membrane allows progenitor cells located in the PDL to preferentially colonize the root area and differentiate to new alveolar bone, PDL and cementum. Courtesy of Dental White Maker (Cancún, México). (b) Membrane positioning in a GBR procedure. A filler (either bone autograft harvested from a different site or artificial osteogenic filler) is used to partially replace the missing alveolar bone [White Maker, 2017].

- *Cell sorting and exclusion*. The barrier membrane should adhere to surrounding tissues so as to prevent gingival fibroblasts and epithelial cells from accessing the treated site and from forming fibrous connective tissue.

- *Space maintenance*. The membrane should be implanted so as to define a space isolating the alveolar bone side from the overlying soft tissue.
- *Scaffolding*. The space defined and maintained by the barrier membrane is initially occupied by a fibrin clot (GTR) or an osteogenic filler (GBR) that has to fill in the entire cavity and that promotes the ingrowth of progenitor cells.
- *Stabilization*. While tissue heals, the membrane should be stably fixed in position with sutures, nails or screws to protect the treated site from the movements of the overlying gingival flap.

10.3.1 *Ideal Properties of Membranes for GTR or GBR*

As schematically summarized above, barrier membranes for GTR or GBR should fulfill two tasks: (i) they should act as a biocompatible perm-selective physical barrier favoring migration of angiogenic and osteogenic cells into the blood clot or filler in the treated site while preventing the ingrowth of competing soft tissue cells from the overlying mucosa; (ii) the membranes should adapt to the bone surface and stay stably in place to seal the periphery of the treated site (space maintenance) and keep the bone graft materials (GBR) or the blood clot (GTR) in the treated site [Sheikh *et al.*, 2014]. Additionally, the treatment should not harm the patient.

Hence, the properties that an ideal membrane for GTR or GBR should exhibit may be schematically summarized as follows [Tal *et al.*, 2012]:

- *Biocompatibility*. The material of which the membrane is made should be safe and not cytotoxic, should not elicit immune reactions and should not cause cell lysis, or metaplastic or neoplastic changes. In the case of resorbable membranes, the degradation products should elicit minimal or no tissue reaction, and they should not negatively affect the healing process nor pose hazard to the patient.
- *Capacity to reject undesired cells and integrate well with the host tissue*. To meet both requirements, the membrane surface should exhibit different properties on either side. One membrane surface should be biomimetic and bioactive to facilitate PDL cell growth [Kim *et al.*, 2014]. The other membrane surface should be osteoconductive to positively affect bone formation toward the membrane surface [Anitua *et al.*, 2012]. This latter membrane surface should also properly adhere to bone tissue to seal the

treated site but should not allow for cell attachment to make membrane removal and recovery painless and easier.

- *Good oxygen and nutrients transfer capacity*. The membrane should not hinder oxygen and nutrients transport to tissue to prevent necrosis.
- *Good mechanical properties and stability*. The membrane mechanical properties should make it easy to apply and handle the membrane safely in the operating theater. Hence, the membrane should be resistant to tear to minimize the chance of ruptures during surgical handling and placement [Donos *et al.*, 2002], and it should be stiff enough to stably separate the gingival flap from the fibrin clot, maintain space for the new alveolar bone and PDL, and bear the pressures exerted by external forces (e.g. mastication) until the clot underneath the membrane has matured enough to provide support [Shin *et al.*, 2009]. Yet, it should be compliant enough to adapt to the contour of the treated site. In the case of resorbable membranes, their resorption rate should match the physiological rate of tissue formation, the duration of their barrier function should be predictable and they should degrade entirely after healing without leaving behind hazardous residues [Bilir *et al.*, 2007].
- *Easy recovery or resorption*. If membrane material does not degrade and resorb in the time in which it is implanted, the membrane should be easily recovered to minimize harm and suffering of the patient. Alternatively, membrane material should degrade and resorb, and should be timely replaced by the host tissue.

10.3.2 *Commercial Membranes for GTR or GBR*

The commercial attractiveness of GTR and GBR procedures has promoted the development of several membranes for this purpose. Different strategies have been adopted to try and satisfy the ideal requirements that a membrane is expected to meet. In Table 10.1, the main features of some exemplary, albeit relevant, commercial membranes for GTR and GBR are reported.

A quick analysis of such features shows that polymers (e.g. polytetrafluoroethylene, polylactic and polyglycolic acids, collagen) or metals (e.g. titanium) already certified by regulatory bodies for implantation are generally preferred to avoid new, time-intensive and costly certification procedures [ASTM International, 2016].

Table 10.1: Commercial membranes for GTR/GBR Materials.

Material	Trade name	Manufacturer	Size (max)	Thickness	Pore size	References
d-PTFE[a]	ACE	Surgical Supply	25 × 30 mm	200 μm	<0.2 μm	Kasaj *et al.* [2008]
	Cytoplast™ GBR200	Osteogenics Biomedical	25 × 30 mm	200 μm	<0.3 μm	Kasaj *et al.* [2008]
	HD Gore-Tex	W.L. Gore & Associates			0.2 μm	Barber *et al.* [2007]
	TefGen FD	Lifecore Biomedical			0.2–0.3 μm	Marouf *et al.* [2000]
e-PTFE[b]	BioBarrier	Imtec™	25 × 34 mm	125 μm	5 μm	Al Ruhaimi *et al.* [2001]
	GoreTex	W.L. Gore & Associates			5 μm	Zwahlen *et al.* [2009]
Titanium	Ti-Micromesh ACE	Surgical Supply		100 μm	1.7 mm	Rakhmatia *et al.* [2013]
	Tocksystem Mesh	Tocksystem		100 μm	0.1–6.5 mm	Rakhmatia *et al.* [2013]
	Frios® BoneShields	Dentsply Friadent	33 × 25 mm	100 μm	30 μm	Rakhmatia *et al.* [2013]

Note: [a]d-PTFE — high-density polytetrafluoroethylene. [b]e-PTFE — expanded polytetrafluoroethylene.

Multi-layer composite membranes (i.e. consisting of two or more stacked layers varying for structure, physical–chemical and mechanical properties) are often used to expose surfaces with suitable physical–chemical properties to cells or tissues on the two sides of the defect and to overcome the poor mechanical resistance of the thin barrier layers used to permit a physiological gas exchange [Gentile *et al.*, 2011]. Suitable cell–membrane interactions are also pursued by texturization or embossing of either surface to yield higher surface areas for cell attachment without altering membrane porosity [Carlson-Mann *et al.*, 1996; Proussaefs & Lozada, 2006]. Cell sorting and controlled transport of nutrients and biochemical cues across the membrane is achieved by modulating membrane preparation or post-treatment procedures to yield pores the size of which ranges from a fraction of a micron to a few millimeters [Kasaj *et al.*, 2008; Proussaefs & Lozada, 2006]. More detailed information on the membranes commercially available for GTR or GBR is reported below for a few exemplary membranes sorted by the material. In fact, commercial membranes for GTR or GBR are often, albeit roughly, classified based on the nature of the material of which they are made as non-resorbable, synthetic resorbable or natural resorbable.

Non-resorbable membranes have the advantage of being resistant to tear and easy to handle and they stably maintain their build and shape once implanted. However, they require a second surgical procedure for removal and recovery, which increases patient discomfort, as well as the costs and the duration of treatment [Aurer & Jorgic-Srdjak, 2005]. Non-resorbable membranes are available that are made of expanded polytetrafluoroethylene (e-PTFE, Gore-Tex®) [Al Ruhaimi & Dent, 2001; Zwahlen *et al.*, 2009], high-density polytetrafluoroethylene (d-PTFE) [Barber *et al.*, 2007; Kasaj *et al.*, 2008; Marouf & El-Guindi, 2000], titanium-reinforced expanded polytetrafluoroethylene (Ti-e-PTFE) and titanium meshes (Ti).

Membranes of expanded polytetrafluoroethylene feature a microstructure made of solid nodes interconnected by fine, highly oriented fibrils providing a unique porous structures. They exhibit: (i) an open microstructure collar (90% porous), which promotes connective tissue ingrowth, and, positioned coronally, is able to inhibit or retard the apical migration of epithelium during the early phase of wound healing; and (ii) an occlusive membrane (30% porous), serving as a space provider for regeneration and as a barrier against the gingival flap [Simion *et al.*, 1999]. Drawbacks of these membranes are: (i) the need for a second surgical procedure, possibly causing undesirable bone resorption, physical trauma and risk of latent or post-surgical bacterial contamination; and (ii) their stiffness, which may induce, in a high percentage of cases, dehiscence of the soft tissues with exposure of the membrane to bacterial contamination [Tempro & Nalbandian, 1993].

Membranes of high-density polytetrafluoroethylene (e.g. Cytoplast™ Regentex GBR-200 and TXT-200; TefGen-FD®) typically feature submicron (0.2–0.3 μm) pores. These membranes may be detached easily, and their high density and small pore size hinder bacterial infiltration into the treated site [Bartee & Carr, 1995]. Their use has been associated with a slow regenerative process yielding small amounts of bone [Marouf & El-Guindi, 2000].

In titanium-embossed e-PTFE membranes (Cytoplast™ TI-250; TR9W Gore-Tex®), titanium struts are embossed in e-PTFE membranes to provide better support to the overlying soft tissue and avoid its collapse into the treated site. This is reported to increase the volume of the regenerated bone. Additionally, the struts allow for precise membrane positioning under the flaps and permit minimally invasive implantation techniques [Lindfors *et al.*, 2010].

Membranes made of titanium meshes have been used for the reconstruction of large maxillary discontinuity defects [Boyne *et al.*, 1985] for their strength, rigidity, low density and corresponding low weight, and their capacity to withstand high temperatures and resist corrosion [Wang & Fenton, 1996]. In fact, titanium is generally passivated to form a protective oxide layer which confers high resistance to corrosion [ADA Council on Scientific Affairs, 2003]. Commercial titanium mesh membranes feature through-holes of size ranging from a few hundred micrometers to some millimeters [Proussaefs & Lozada, 2006; Rakhmatia *et al.*, 2013].

In recent years, the market of non-resorbable membranes for GTR or GBR is decreasing as an effect of the commercial introduction of better performing resorbable membranes [Dori *et al.*, 2007].

The use of resorbable membranes for GTR or GBR is appealing because it permits a single-step treatment, reduces patients' pain and discomfort, lowers the cost of treatment and eliminates potential surgical complications [Bottino *et al.*, 2011]. However, the release of biodegradation products may trigger tissue immune reactions which may influence the healing of the treated site and may compromise regeneration [Simion *et al.*, 1997]. Resorbable membranes are made of materials that generally exhibit fair-to-poor intrinsic mechanical properties which worsen as they biodegrade. This makes it difficult for them to remain stiff long enough to maintain the required space for bone regeneration [Zellin *et al.*, 1995]. This drawback is often overcome by filling the defect entirely with autogenous or synthetic bone graft substitutes so as to support the membrane [Avera *et al.*, 1997; Parodi *et al.*, 1996]. Alternatively, holding the membrane in place with more screws or pins than for pure fixation has been investigated with reasonable success [Selvig *et al.*, 1990]. Anyway, screws or pins have to be removed as the defect heals.

Both synthetic and natural polymers have been used for the preparation of resorbable barrier membranes for GTR or GBR. In Tables 10.2 and 10.3, some exemplary commercial resorbable synthetic and natural membranes are reported together with their resorption time, respectively.

Synthetic resorbable polymers such as polyester [von Arx *et al.*, 2005], resorbable polylactic acid (PLA) [Cutbirth, 2013], polyglycolic acid (PGA) [Milella *et al.*, 2001], poly(ε-caprolactone) [Hoogeveen *et al.*, 2009] and their copolymers [Donos *et al.*, 2002] have mainly been used for the preparation of these membranes. The Resolut® membrane consists of an occlusive membrane of a copolymer of glycolic and lactic acid laid on top of a porous web of PGA fibers [Hou *et al.*, 2004].

The occlusive membrane is intended to prevent cell ingrowth, and the porous part promotes tissue integration [Donos *et al.*, 2002]. The Epi-Guide® is a membrane designed for use as an adjunct to periodontal restorative surgeries and to assist in the regeneration of bone and periodontal tissue [Bilir *et al.*, 2007]. It is a porous 3D matrix made of D, D-L, L polylactic acid [Curasan Inc., 2015]. The barrier consists of three-stacked layers designed to maintain its architecture and structural integrity for 20 weeks after implantation with complete resorption between 6 and 12 months [Takata *et al.*, 2001].

Natural resorbable membranes are mostly produced using collagen of animal origin [Abbassi *et al.*, 2008; Duskova *et al.*, 2006; Lee *et al.*, 2015; Papaioannou *et al.*, 2011; Rothamel *et al.*, 2005], which is isolated,

Table 10.2: Commercial membranes for GTR or GBR made of synthetic resorbable materials.

Material	Trade name	Manufacturer	Size (max)	Thickness	Resorption	References
PDLA[a]	Atrisorb®	Tolmar Supply			24–48 weeks	Hou *et al.* [2004]
	Epi-Guide®	Kensey Nash Co.		3× layered	6–12 weeks	Bilir *et al.* [2007]
PLA[b]	BioCellect™ Osseo	Imtec	20 × 30 mm	200 μm	12–16 weeks	Cutbirth [2013]
PGA[c]	Biofix®	Bioscience			24–48 weeks	Milella *et al.* [2001]
Polyester	OsseoQuest™	W.L. Gore & Associates			16–24 weeks	von Arx *et al.* [2005]
PLGA[d]	Resolut®	W.L. Gore & Associates				Donos *et al.* [2002]
Polyglactin[e]	Vicryl®-Netz	Ethicon			4–12 weeks	Manuf.
PLCL[f]	Vivosorb®	Polyganics			8 weeks	Hoogeveen *et al.* [2009]

Note: [a]PDLA — poly-DL-lactic acid; [b]PLA — polylactic acid; [c]PGA — polyglycolic acid; [d]PLGA — polylactic-co-glycolic acid; [e]polygalactin-polyglycolic/polylactic acid 9:1; [f]PLCL — poly(DL-lactic acid-ε-caprolactone).

Table 10.3: Commercial membranes for GTR or GBR made of natural resorbable materials.

Material	Trade name	Manufacturer	Size (max)	Thickness	Resorption	References
Type I + Type III porcine collagen	Bio-Gide®	Geistlich Biomaterials	13 × 25 mm	200 μm	2–4 weeks	Lee *et al*. [2015]
	Ossix®	OraPharma			16–24 weeks	Lee *et al*. [2015]
	Osgide®	Curasan Inc.	30 × 40 mm		12 weeks	Manuf.
Type I bovine collagen	BioMend®	Zimmer			8 weeks	Rothamel *et al*. [2005]
	BioSorb™	3MESPE			26–38 weeks	Al Ruhaimi *et al*. [2001]
	Neomem®	Citagenix			26–38 weeks	Duskova *et al*. [2006]
	OsseoGuard®	Biomet 3i			24–32 weeks	Papaioannou *et al*. [2011]
Type I horse collagen + GAG[a]	Paroguide®	Vebas	30 × 30 mm	500 μm		Abbassi *et al*. [2008]

Note: [a]GAG — glycosaminoglycans.

purified enzymatically or by chemical extraction, and finally processed [Sheikh *et al.*, 2014]. Collagen meets many of the requirements for GTR or GBR membranes. It is poorly immunogenic, attracts and activates PDL and gingival fibroblast cells, and sorts and interacts with various cell types during the healing process [Buser & Dula, 2000]. When crosslinked, collagen membranes have been shown to last 6–8 weeks before being resorbed, thus maintaining their mechanical integrity long enough for treatment [Blumenthal, 1988].

Drawbacks of collagen-based membranes are that they quickly lose their space-maintaining ability in humid environment and, when collagen is isolated from animal tissues, they pose a potential risk of disease transmission from animals to humans [Dori *et al.*, 2007].

The Bio-Gide® membrane is an example of collagen-based commercial resorbable membrane. It is made of porcine type I and type III collagen fibers, without any organic components and/or chemicals and has a bilayer structure composed of a compact and a porous layer laid on top of one another. The compact layer has a smooth and homogeneous surface that protects against connective tissue infiltration, whereas the porous layer has an open pore surface and permits osteogenic cell migration [Kim *et al.*, 2009].

10.4 Membranes in Wound Care

A wound may be defined as a defect, or a break, in the skin caused by physical damage or by an underlying medical or physiological condition [Boateng *et al.*, 2008]. Wounds are generally classified based on the number of skin layers and the area of the skin affected [Bolton & van Rijswijk, 1991; Krasner *et al.*, 2006].

Superficial wounds are injuries that affect the epidermal skin surface only, or both the epidermis and the deeper dermal layers, including blood vessels, sweat glands and hair. The main causes of superficial wounds are cuts, abrasions, burns and blisters. They usually heal fast as a result of cells moving across the wound and replacing the skin's outermost layer, the epidermis. In superficial wounds, the injury initiates inflammation, an early stage of the healing process. Mediators involved in the inflammation process (e.g. histamine) increase the permeability of capillaries so that white blood cells can escape and blood vessels leak fluid that enters the wound where it forms the basis of the exudate. In healing wounds, the exudate promotes healing (e.g. by stimulating cell proliferation). Matrix metalloproteinases (MMPs) which break down the cell-supporting ECM are mainly inactive. Superficial wounds generally produce small amounts of exudate, whereas the amount of exudate formed may be a problem in burns. The conventional treatment of superficial or burn wounds aims to protect the wound and prevent infections. For this purpose, a cotton gauze is fixed above the wound (as such or impregnated with paraffin) with adhesive tape and is changed daily. The gauze (i.e. the dressing) promotes healing by keeping the wound clean, by absorbing the exudate, by reducing the risk of bacterial infections and by allowing for the entry of gaseous oxygen and the escape of water vapor. Dressings are also used to hide or cover a wound for cosmetic reasons. Drawbacks of conventional dressings for superficial wounds are their poor barrier properties against water and bacteria, periwound skin reaction to the adhesive, pain and discomfort, and infections [Thomas, 1997].

Deep wounds are three-dimensional deep injuries that affect also the underlying subcutaneous fat or deeper tissues (e.g. the muscles) in addition to the epidermis and dermal layers. The main causes of deep wounds are pressure (*decubitus*) ulcers, diabetic foot ulcers and post-surgery ulcers. They usually have long healing times. In deep wounds, cells start to fill in the wound cavity from the bottom, which makes the wound smaller as tissue heals. In chronic deep wounds, large amounts of exudate may form that hinder healing. In fact, this exudate contains high concentrations of inflammatory mediators and activated MMPs which break down the cell-supporting ECM and hinder the healing process. The conventional treatment of deep wounds aims at minimizing the detrimental effects and maximizing the positive effects of the exudate. For this purpose, a long cotton gauze is generally inserted in the wound cavity to absorb excess exudate and bacteria, and this is changed twice daily. The dressing promotes healing by removing excess exudate and bacteria, by preventing bacterial infections and by providing a moist wound bed to facilitate the production of granulation tissue and epithelialization. In fact, if exposed to a dry environment, wounds may rapidly lose moisture and become dehydrated. As this happens, the wound shrinks progressively, which is often associated with the onset of pain. Maintaining a moist wound bed may alleviate pain and facilitate autolytic debridement of the wound necrotic tissue. Dressings for deep wounds are often used also to minimize unpleasant odors. Dressings for superficial wounds are generally used to hide or cover treated deep wounds for cosmetic reasons. Drawbacks of conventional dressings used for deep wounds are mainly related to the fact that newly formed tissue cells often adhere to the dressing and are removed with it when it is changed. This retards healing and causes pain and discomfort. Infections and scar formation are other drawbacks [Thomas, 1997].

10.4.1 *Ideal Properties of Membranes for Wound Care*

As noted above, wound healing is a dynamic process, and the properties required of a dressing change with the features of the wound. For as much as they are effective and cheap, dressings used in conventional wound treatments are not optimal and may cause pain and discomfort, and may even retard healing.

Membranes have been developed for the treatment of both superficial and deep wound care that minimize the problems of cotton gauzes and provide additional functions to enhance healing and minimize pain and discomfort (Fig. 10.4).

Ideal membranes for the care of superficial or burn wounds should:

- act as two-dimensional (2D) perm-selective physical–chemical barriers, which allow for the permeation of oxygen, and protect the wound from dirt, bacteria and excess water to prevent infections and bad odor;
- provide a moist wound bed, to reduce pain and discomfort by ensuring adequate permeation of water vapor;
- adhere well to the wound edges, but not to wound tissue;
- act as a vehicle to locally deliver drugs or antibiotics.

Ideal membranes for the care of deep wounds should:

- remove excess exudate;
- sequester bacteria, to prevent infections, and enzymes, to prevent ECM disruption;

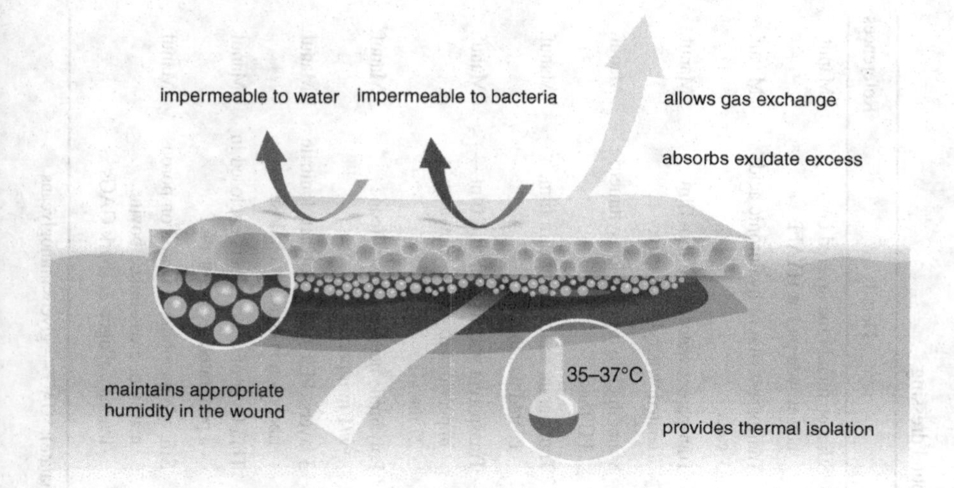

Figure 10.4. Features of an ideal dressing for wound healing. [Matopat, 2017].

- provide a moist wound bed and ensure adequate evaporation and oxygenation;
- conform to wound contour but not adhere to wound tissue;
- reduce pain and discomfort;
- act as a vehicle to locally deliver drugs or antibiotics.

10.4.2 *Commercial Membranes for Wound Care*

The analysis of the features of the membrane-based dressings reported in Tables 10.4 and 10.5 suggests that there is no membrane that is suitable for the care of all types of wounds. Few membrane-based dressings are ideally suited for the treatment of a wound during all stages of the healing process.

Successful wound management depends upon a time-varying approach to the selection and use of dressings based on the knowledge of the characteristics of a given wound and the progression of its healing combined with the knowledge of the properties of the various dressings commercially available.

Table 10.4: Membranes for superficial or burn wound dressing.

Material	Trade name	Manufacturer	Specific application	Details	References
HYAFF[a]	Hyalomatrix®	Anika Ther	Slow-healing, chronic and burn wounds	Silicone membrane layered on non-woven pad of HYAFF	Manuf.
	Jaloskin®	Fidia Adv.	Moderately exuding wounds	Transparent film of hyaluronic acid ester	Manuf.
PU[b]	Bioclusive™	Systagenix	Moderately exuding wounds	Transparent water-proof thin film coated w/acrylic adhesive	Manuf.
	Lyofoam®	Mölnlycke Healthcare	Wounds	8-mm thick hydrophobic asymmetric PU foam	Manuf.
	Opsite™	Smith & Nephew	Low exuding wounds	Transparent water-proof thin film, coated w/adhesive	Manuf.
	Tegaderm™	3M Healthcare	Catheter ports, abrasions	Transparent water-proof thin film — impervious to viruses down to 27 nm size	Manuf.
PA + Silicone	Mepitel	Mölnlycke Healthcare	Burns, blistering	Polyamide net coated w/silicone w/1 mm pores	Manuf.
PET[c]	Melolin™	Smith & Nephew	Moderately exuding wounds	3 layers (PET film + polyacrylonitrile fibers + non-woven cellulose	Manuf.
	Telfa™	Kendall	Exuding wounds	Thin layer of cotton fibers enclosed in a perforated sleeve of PET	Manuf.
Collagen & GAGs[d]	Integra®	Integra LifeSciences	Partial and full thickness wounds, trauma and draining wounds	Silicone membrane layered on porous matrix of cross-linked bovine tendon collagen & shark GAGs	Manuf.

Note: [a] HYAFF — esterified hyaluronic acid; [b] PU — polyurethane; [c] PET — poly(ethylene terephthalate); [d] GAG — glycosaminoglycans.

Table 10.5: Membrane-using commercial dressings for deep wounds.

Material	Trade name	Manufacturer	Specific application	Details	References
PU[a]	Allevyn™ Cavity	Smith & Nephew	Cavity wounds	Hydrophilic PU foam encapsulated in honeycomb PU film	Berry *et al.* [2006]
	Comfeel®	Cotoplast	Full thickness wounds	PU film containing sodium CMC* and calcium alginate	Suvarna *et al.* [2013]
	Mepilex®	Mölnlycke Healthcare	Exuding shallow wounds	Foam	Suvarna *et al.* [2013]
	PermaFoam™ Cavity	Hartmann	Cavity wounds	Open-cell phenolic foam	Cuervo *et al.* [2009]
PET	Telfa™	Kendall	Exuding wounds	Layer of cotton fiber enclosed in a perforated sleeve of PET	Manuf.
Woven acetate	Cuticerin™	Smith & Nephew	Shallow and deep wounds	Smooth gauze impregnated with ointment	Suvarna *et al.* [2013]
Non-woven alginate & CMC[b]	Maxorb®	Medline	Moderately to heavily draining wounds	Fiber monolayer	Suvarna *et al.* [2013]
Calcium alginate	Algisite™ M	Smith & Nephew	Full thickness wounds heavy exudate	Fiber monolayer	Suvarna *et al.* [2013]
Hydrogel-loaded cotton fiber	Skintegrity™	Medline	Cavity wounds	Hydrogel impregnated gauze	Suvarna *et al.* [2013]

Note: [a]PU — polyurethane; [b]CMC — carboxymethyl cellulose.

In the care of superficial wounds, the conflicting requirements of absorbing excess exudate and preventing dehydration of the wound bed have been generally balanced off by developing membranes with a bilayer (seldom three layers) structure. The upper layer in contact with air is generally a membrane made of a hydrophobic material permeable to gaseous oxygen and water vapor (e.g. silicone, polyurethane, polyethylene terephthalate) and is laminated, or glued, to a bottom layer contacting the wound tissue and made of a hydrophilic material in the form of foam or fabric (e.g. cotton fibers, esterified hyaluronic acid or resorbable materials like collagen and glycosaminoglycans) and capable of absorbing large amounts of fluids.

This is the case of the Hyalomatrix®, Mepitel™ and Integra® dressings, all of which share a thin upper membrane layer made of silicon, but differ with regard to the structure and material of the bottom foamy layer. The bottom layer is made of an ester of the hyaluronic acid (HYAFF), which is known for its angiogenic properties, as is the case of the Hyalomatrix®, or of natural proteins, such as collagen and GAGs, as is the case of the Integra®, which adds a good bioactivity to the dressing properties.

It is worth noting that the hydrophobic layer is sometimes glued to the bottom layer with low-strength adhesives so that it may be peeled off from the bottom layer when this has been fully vascularized and colonized by newly formed dermis (e.g. to permit skin grafting). Among those considered, only in the Lyofoam® dressing is the barrier layer the dense layer (or skin) of an 8 mm thick asymmetric polyurethane (PU) foam. Not recurring to a hydrogel, such as the HYAFF, the Lyofoam® absorbs limited amounts of fluid and is indicated for poorly exuding wounds, or for minor injuries and wounds in the final stages of healing.

When the exudate is not a problem, membranes may be used as such in the form of a perforated plastic film (e.g. in the Melolin™ or Telfa™ dressings) or of a vapor-permeable dense film (e.g. in the Opsite™, Tegaderm™ or Bioclusive™) to ensure wound hydration.

For the care of deep wounds with large cavities (e.g. pressure (*decubitus*) ulcers), larger wound cavities (e.g. those remaining following the excision of a pilonidal) and poorly healing or heavily exuding wounds, three-dimensional dressings are required in which membranes also play a key role [Cuervo *et al*., 2009; Suvarna & Munira, 2013]. Some of these dressings are briefly described in Table 10.5.

The development of such dressings in time is well illustrated by referring to the Allevyn™ Cavity dressing [Berry *et al*., 1996]. In fact, the original dressing consisted of highly absorbent hydrophilic polyurethane foam chips enclosed in a soft, flexible, semi-permeable and non-adherent honeycomb polyurethane film which had a surface that presented small perforations to allow for the entry of exudate and to provide highly effective wound contact. The PU chips in the Allevyn™ Cavity absorbed fourfold more than a hydrocolloid the same size, also under compression, and helped prevent bacterial contamination. The PU film enveloping the chips had perforations large enough to make it permeable to oxygen and fluids, thus helping maintain a moist wound bed. Its honeycomb surface structure made it come in close contact with the wound tissue, yet its hydrophobic character prevented adhesion to it. Thus, the dressing could be easily removed without trauma and pain to the patient. Its compliance made it conform well to awkward wound areas to dress. Moreover, the dressing was produced in a range of shapes (e.g. pillow-like or cylindrical) and sizes to better fit a given wound [Thomas, 1997]. Today, the pillow-like appearance of the Allevyn™ Cavity has given the way to a PU dressing that looks more like a patch, it has similar absorbance to the original dressing, and so it has a high compliance that makes it easy to dress wound areas awkward to reach.

Membrane-based dressings for wound care are usually more expensive than traditional cellulose-based conventional dressings (e.g. cotton gauzes), and there is general reluctance to use them in the clinics on economic grounds.

However, wounds treated with membrane-based dressings respond to treatment more rapidly, causing less pain than conventional dressings.

It is therefore important that any comparisons be made accounting for costs of the entire treatment and that the patients' right to the best possible care and quality of life be given proper consideration.

10.5 Conclusions

The increasing interest in the development and use of membranes for RM is witnessed by the number of publications on this topic, which is increasing at a faster pace than ever. This has generated a progressive increase in the global market of membranes for RM, which is gaining a significant market share of healthcare products.

Membranes are mainly used in RM for their physical–chemical, transport and separation properties. However, meeting the complex requirements specific for given treatments has forced the combination of membranes with other biomaterials and adhesives, or the introduction of post-processing techniques, to overcome the intrinsic limitations of available membranes.

It is noteworthy that many non-resorbable and resorbable membranes are already commercially available for guiding tissue regeneration in dental implantation and in wound care. The introduction in the clinical setting of resorbable membranes is slowly gaining momentum because their use strongly reduces pain and morbidity, their mechanical and barrier properties are becoming more reliable, and new materials and fabrication methods are making them less prone to tear and perforation.

However, it should be taken into consideration that success of membrane-based tissue regeneration approaches strongly depends also on the surgeons' skills (e.g. for good wound site preparation) and the proper identification of the type of wound that needs to be treated, and its specific requirements.

Acknowledgments

The study was co-funded by the Italian Ministry of Instruction and University (MIUR) (Project PRIN 2010, MIND).

References

Abbassi F, Semyari H and Haghgoo R (2008). Histological evaluation of periodontal regeneration due to using collagen membrane (Paroguide) in surgical defects of sheep teeth. *Res J Biol Sci*, 3(11), pp. 1317–1319.

ADA Council on Scientific Affairs (2003). Titanium applications in dentistry. *J Am Dent Assoc*, 134, pp. 347–349.

Al Ruhaimi KA and Dent M (2001). Augmentation of osseous-implant dehiscence with membrane alone or with a combination of bone graft and membrane. *Saudi Dent J*, 13(2), pp. 56–65.

Anitua E, Prado R, Sanchez M and Orive G (2012). Platelet-rich plasma: preparation and formulation. *Oper Techniq Orthop*, 22, pp. 25–32.

ASTM International (2016). Medical device standards and implant standards. [Online] Available at: http://www.astm.org/Standards/medical-device-and-implant-standards.html [Accessed 2015].

Aurer A and Jorgic-Srdjak K (2005). Membranes for periodontal regeneration. *Acta Stomat Croat*, 39, pp. 107–112.

Avera IS, Stampley AW and McAllister BS (1997). Histologic and clinical observation of resorbable and nonresorbable barrier membranes used in maxillary sinus graft containment. *Int J Oral Maxillofac Implants*, 12, pp. 88–94.

Barber HD, Lignelli J, Smith BM and Bartee BK (2007). Using a dense PTFE membrane without primary closure to achieve bone and tissue regeneration. *J Oral Maxillofac Surg*, 65(4), pp. 748–752.

Bartee BK and Carr JA (1995). Evaluation of high-density polytetrafluoroethylene membrane as a barrier material to facilitate guided bone regeneration in the rat mandible. *J Oral Implantol*, 21, pp. 88–95.

Berry DP, Bale S and Harding KG (1996). Dressings for treating cavity wounds. *J Wound Care*, 5(1), pp. 10–17.

Bilir A, *et al.* (2007). Biocompatibility of different barrier membranes in cultures of human CRL 11372 osteoblast-like cells: an immunohistochemical study. *Clin Oral Implants Res*, 18(1), pp. 46–52.

Blumenthal NM (1988). The use of collagen membranes to guide regeneration of new connective tissue attachment in dogs. *J Periodontol*, 59, pp. 830–836.

Boateng JS, Matthews KH, Stevens HN and Eccleston GM (2008). Wound healing dressing and drug delivery systems: a review. *J Pharm Sci*, 97(8), pp. 2892–2923.

Bolton L and van Rijswijk L (1991). Wound dressing: meeting clinical and biological needs. *Dermatol Nurs*, 3, pp. 146–161.

Bottino MC, Thomas V and Janowski GM (2011). A novel spatially designed and functionally graded electrospun membrane for periodontal regeneration. *Acta Biomater*, 7, pp. 216–224.

Boyne PJ, Cole MD, Stringer D and Shafqat JP (1985). A technique for osseous restoration of deficient edentulous maxillary ridges. *J Oral Maxillofac Surg*, 43, pp. 87–91.

Buser D and Dula AK (2000). Localized ridge augmentation with autografts and barrier membranes. *Periodontology*, 19, pp. 151–163.

Buser D, Warrer K and Karring T (1990). Formation of a periodontal ligament around titanium implants. *J Periodontol*, 61(9), pp. 597–601.

Buser D, *et al.* (1993). Localized ridge augmentation using guided bone regeneration. Surgical procedure in the maxilla. *Int J Periodont Restorative Dent*, 13, pp. 29–37.

Carlson-Mann LD, Ibbott CG and Grieman RB (1996). Ridge augmentation with guided bone regeneration and GTAM case illustrations. *Eur PMC*, 30(6), pp. 232–233.

Catapano G, *et al.* (2009). Bioreactor design and scale-up. In Eibl R, Eibl D, Pörtner R, Catapano G, Czermak P, Eds., *Cell and Tissue Reaction Engineering*, pp. 173–262.

Cuervo FM, Soriano JV, Lopez JR and Gomez TS (2009). Care for ulcers having diverse etiology prospective study on PermaFoam. *Rev Enferm*, 32(9), pp. 21–26.

Curasan Inc. (2015). *Epi-Guide bioresorbable barrier matrix — brochure*.

Cutbirth ST (2013). Full-mouth restoration of a severely decayed dentition. *Dent Today*, 32(12), pp. 68–70.

Dewan A, Gibson MA, Elisseeff JH and Trice ME (2014). Evolution of autologous chondrocyte repair and comparison to other cartilage repair techniques. *BioMed Res Int*, 2014, pp. 1–11.

Dhandayuthapani B, Yoshida Y, Maekawa T and Kumar S (2011). Polymeric scaffolds in tissue engineering application: a review. *Int J Polym Sci*, 2011(2011), pp. 1–19.

Diban N and Stamatialis D (2014). Polymeric hollow fiber membranes for bioartificial organs and tissue engineering applications. *J Chem Technol Biotechnol*, 89, pp. 633–643.

Donos N, Kostopoulos L and Karring T (2002). Alveolar ridge augmentation using a resorbable copolymer membrane and autogenous bone grafts. *Clin Oral Implants Res*, 13(2), pp. 202–213.

Dori F, *et al.* (2007). Effect of platelet-rich plasma on the healing of intra-bony defects treated with a natural bone mineral and a collagen membrane. *J Clin Periodontol*, 34(3), pp. 254–261.

Duskova M, Leamerova E, Sosna B and Gojis O (2006). Guided tissue regeneration, barrier membranes and reconstruction of the cleft maxillary alveolus. *J Craniofac Surg*, 17(6), pp. 1153–1160.

Ellis MJ and Chaudhuri JB (2007). Poly(lactic-co-glycolid acid) hollow fibre membranes for use as tissue engineering scaffold. *Biotechnol Bioeng*, 96(1), pp. 177–187.

Evans ND, *et al.* (2013). Epithelial mechanobiology, skin wound healing and the stem cell niche. *J Mech Behav Biomed Mater*, 28, pp. 397–409.

Gentile FT, *et al.* (1995). Polymer science for macroencapsulation of cells for central nervous system transplantation. *Reactive Polym*, 25, pp. 207–227.

Gentile P, *et al.* (2011). Polymeric membranes for guided bone regeneration. *Biotechnology*, 6, pp. 1187–1197.

Gottlow J, Nyman S, Karring T and Lindhe J (1984). New attachment formation as the result of controlled tissue regeneration. *J Clin Periodontol*, 11(8), pp. 494–503.

Grin A, *et al.* (2009). *In vitro* study of a novel polymeric mesenchymal stem-cell coated membrane. *J Drug Del Sci Technol*, 19(4), pp. 241–246.

Haffajee AD and Socransky SS (2000). Microbial etiological agents of destructive periodontal diseases. *Periodontol 2000*, 5, pp. 78–111.

Hoogeveen EJ, *et al.* (2009). Vivosorb as a barrier membrane in rat mandibular defects. An evaluation with transversal microradiography. *Int J Oral Maxillofac Surg*, 38(8), pp. 870–875.

Hou LT, *et al.* (2004). Polymer-assisted regeneration therapy with Atrisorb barriers in human periodontal intrabony defects. *J Clin Periodontol*, 31(1), pp. 68–74.

Kasaj A, *et al.* (2008). *In vitro* evaluation of various bioadsorbable and non-resorbable barrier membranes for guided tissue regeneration. *Head Face Med*, 4(22), pp. 1–8.

Kim SH, *et al.* (2009). The efficacy of a double-layer collagen membrane technique for overlaying block grafts in rabbit calvarium model. *Clin Oral Implants Res*, 20(10), pp. 1124–1132.

Kim JH, *et al.* (2014). Advanced biomatrix designs for regenerative therapy of periodontal tissues. *J Dent Res*, 93(12), pp. 1203–1211.

Krasner D, Kennedy KL, Rolstad BS and Roma AW (2006). The ABCs of wound care dressings. *Wound Manage*, 66, pp. 68–69.

Kumar GS (2011). *Orban's oral histology and embryology*, (Elsevier, India).

Langer R and Vacanti JP (1993). Tissue engineering. *Science*, 260(5110), pp. 920–926.

Lee SH, *et al.* (2015). The effect of bacterial cellulose membrane compared with collagen membrane on guided bone regeneration. *J Adv Periodontol*, 7(6), pp. 484–495.

Lindfors LT, Tervonen EA and Sandor GK (2010). Guided bone regeneration using a titanium-reinforced ePTFE membrane and particulate autogenous bone: the effect of smoking and membrane exposure. *Oral Surg Oral Med Oral Pathol Oral Radiol Endod*, 109, p. 825.

Marouf HA and El-Guindi HM (2000). Efficacy of high-density versus semi-permeable PTFE membranes in an elderly experimental model. *Oral Surg Oral Med Oral Pathol Oral Radiol Endod*, 89, pp. 164–170.

Mason C and Dunnill P (2008). A brief definition of regenerative medicine. *Regen Med*, 3(1), pp. 1–5.

Matopat (2017). Wound treatment [Online]. Available at: http://en.matopat-global.com/our-solutions-view/wound-treatment/ [Accessed 2017].

Melcher AH, *et al.* (1987). Cells from bone synthesize cementum-like and bone-like tissue *in vitro* and may migrate into periodontal ligament *in vivo*. *J Periodontol Res*, 22(3), pp. 246–247.

Meneghello G, *et al.* (2009). Fabrication and characterization of poly(lactic-co-glycolid acid)/polyvinyl alcohol blended hollow fibre membranes for tissue engineering applications. *J Memb Sci*, 344(1–2), pp. 55–61.

Milella E, *et al.* (2001). Physicochemical, mechanical, and biological properties of commercial membranes for GTR. *J Biomed Mater Res*, 58(4), pp. 427–435.

Mosheiff R, Friedman A, Friedman M and Liebergall M (2003). Quantification of guided regeneration of weight-bearing bones. *Orthopedics*, 26(8), pp. 789–794.

Papaioannou KA, *et al.* (2011). Attachment and proliferation of human osteoblast-like cells on guided bone regeneration (GBR) membranes in the absence or presence of nicotine: an *in vitro* study. *Int J Oral Maxillofac Implants*, 26(3), pp. 509–519.

Parodi R, Santarelli G and Carusi G (1996). Application of slow-resorbing collagen membrane to periodontal and peri-implant guided tissue regeneration. *Int J Periodont Restorative Dent*, 16, pp. 174–185.

PR Newswire (2013). RegeneCure starts clinical study using polymeric bone stimulating membrane for dental implants. [Online] Available at: http://www.prnewswire.com/news-releases/regenecure-starts-clinical-study-using-polymeric-bone-stimulating-membrane-for-dental-implants-211961891.html [Accessed 2016].

PR Newswire (2016). Regenerative medicine market is expected to reach $67.6 billion, global by 2020. [Online] Available at: http://www.prnewswire.com/news-releases/regenerative-medicine-market-is-expected-to-reach-676-billion-global-by-2020-265200801.html [Accessed 2016].

PR Newswire (2017). Global $9.98 Billion Wound Dressing Market 2016–2022-Research and Markets. [Online] Available at: http://www.prnewswire.com/news-releases/global-998-billion-wound-dressing-market-2016–2022---research-and-markets-300421984.html [Accessed 2017].

Proussaefs P and Lozada J (2006). Use of titanium mesh for staged localized alveolar ridge augmentation: clinical and histologic–histomorphometric evaluation. *J Oral Implant*, 32, pp. 237–247.

Pubmed Central (2015). Pubmed Central. [Online] Available at: http://www.ncbi.nlm.nih.gov/pmc/?term=(((regenerative+medicine)+AND+membranes)+AND+artificial)+OR+synthetic.

Quirk RA, *et al.* (2001). Poly(L-lysine)-GRGDS as a biomimetic surface modifier for poly(lactic acid). *Biomaterials*, 22, pp. 865–872.

Rakhmatia YD, Ayukawa Y, Furuhashi A and Koyano K (2013). Current barrier membranes: titanium mesh and other membranes for guided bone regeneration in dental applications. *J Prosthod Res*, 57, pp. 3–14.

Rothamel D, *et al.* (2005). Biodegradation of differently cross-linked collagen membranes: an experimental study in the rat. *Clin Oral Implants Res*, 16(3), pp. 369–378.

Selvig AK, Nilveus ER, Fitzmorris L and Khorsandi SS (1990). Scanning electron microscopic observation of cell population and bacterial contamination of membranes used for guided periodontal tissue regeneration in humans. *J Periodontol*, 61, pp. 515–520.

Sheikh Z, *et al.* (2014). Barrier membranes for periodontal guided tissue regeneration application. In Matinlinna JP, (Ed.), *Handbook of oral biomaterials* (Pan Stanford Publishing Pte. Ltd., Singapore, Singapore), pp. 605–636.

Shin RH, *et al.* (2009). Treatment of a segmental nerve defect in the rat with use of bioabsorbable synthetic nerve conduits: a comparison of commercially available conduits. *J Bone Joint Surg Am*, 91(9), pp. 2194–2204.

Simion M, Dahlin C and Blair K (1999). Effect of different microstructures of e-PTFE membranes on bone regeneration and soft tissue response: a histologic study in canine mandible. *Clin Oral Implant Res*, 10(73), pp. 73–84.

Simion M, Misitano U, Gionso L and Salvato A (1997). Treatment of dehiscences and fenestrations around dental implants using resorbable and nonresorbable membranes associated with bone autografts: a comparative clinical study. *Int J Oral Maxillofac Implants*, 12, pp. 159–167.

Suvarna K and Munira M (2013). Wound healing process and wound care dressing: a detailed review. *J Pharma Res*, 2(11), pp. 6–12.

Takata T, Wang HL and Miyauchi M (2001). Migration of osteoblastic cells on various guided bone regeneration membranes. *Clin Oral Impl Res*, 12, pp. 332–338.

Tal H, Moses O, Kozlovsky A, Nemcovsky C (2012). Bioresorbable Collagen Membranes for Guided Bone Regeneration, Bone Regeneration, In Tal H (Ed.), *InTech* [Online] Available at: https://www.intechopen.com/books/

bone-regeneration/bioresorbable-collagen-membranes-for-guided-bone-regeneration [Accessed 2017].

Tempro PJ and Nalbandian J (1993). Colonization of retrieved polytetrafluoroethylene membranes: morphological and microbiological observations. *J Periodontol*, 64(3), pp. 162–168.

Thomas S (1997). A structured approach to the selection of dressing. [Online] Available at: www.worldwidewounds.com/1997july/Thomas-Guide/Dress-Select.html [Accessed 2015].

Transparency Market Research (2012). Global regenerative medicine market set to register 12.8% CAGR due to rising tissue engineering and stem cell therapy. [Online] Available at: http://www.transparencymarketresearch.com/pressrelease/regenerative-medicines-market.htm [Accessed 2016].

Unger RE, *et al.* (2005). Growth of human cells on polyethersulfone (PES) hollow fiber membranes. *Biomaterials*, 26, pp. 1877–1884.

US Department of Health and Human Services (2013). Yesterday, today and tomorrow: NIH research timelines. [Online] Available at: https://report.nih.gov/nihfactsheets/viewfactsheet.aspx?csid=62 [Accessed 2015].

von Arx T, *et al.* (2005). Membrane durability and tissue response of different bioresorbable barrier membranes: a histologic study in the rabbit calvarium. *Int J Oral Maxillofac Implants*, 20(6), pp. 843–853.

Wang RR and Fenton A (1996). Titanium prosthodontic applications: a review of the literature. *Quintessence Int*, 27, pp. 401–408.

Wang HL, *et al.* (2005). Periodontal regeneration. *J Periodontol*, 76(9), pp. 1601–1622.

White Maker Dental S.p.A. (2017) Treatment and Tissue Oral Regeneration [Online]. Available at: http://en.dentalwhitemaker.com/service/colocacion-inmediata-del-implante-en-el-lugar-de-la-extraccion/ [Accessed 2017].

Zellin G, Gritli-Linde A and Linde A (1995). Healing of mandibular defects with different biodegradable and non-biodegradable membranes: an experimental study in rats. *Biomaterials*, 16, pp. 601–609.

Zwahlen RA, *et al.* (2009). Comparison of two resorbable membrane systems in bone regeneration after removal of wisdom teeth: a randomized-controlled clinical pilot study. *Clin Oral Implants Res*, 20(10), pp. 1084–1091.

Chapter 11
Membranes for Organs-On-Chips

M. P. Tibbe*, A. D. van der Meer†,
A. van den Berg*, D. Stamatialis‡
and L. I. Segerink*,§

* *BIOS Lab on a Chip Group, MIRA & MESA + Institutes, University of Twente, The Netherlands*

† *Applied Stem Cell Technology MIRA Institute, University of Twente, The Netherlands*

‡ *Biomaterials Science and Technology, MIRA Institute, University of Twente, The Netherlands*

§ *l.i.segerink@utwente.nl*

"Organs-on-chips are microfluidic devices for culturing living cells in continuously perfused, μm sized chambers in order to model physiological functions of tissues and organs."

Bhatia and Ingber, 2014

11.1 Introduction

This chapter describes the role of membranes in the rapidly emerging field of organs-on-chips (OOC), the reasons why specific membranes are used and where there are opportunities for improvement.

11.2 Organs-On-Chips

Understanding the human physiology is of great importance for drug development and toxicology studies. Physiological responses to drugs or toxic substances can be studied by using human bodies or similar organisms. *In vivo* studies using human bodies give relevant information about tissue response. However, these studies are considered ethically questionable and dangerous. A more common, but still ethically questioned, method to study tissue response is the use of animals. However, pharmacologists believe that animal studies can be useful tools, but results cannot always be directly translated to the clinic as 80% of candidate drugs, successfully tested in animals, fail in clinical trials [Martić-Kehl *et al.*, 2012]. One other disadvantage of *in vivo* studies is the time-consuming character. Studies can take months or even years, which makes them very costly. Furthermore, researchers are applying the 3R principle which stands for "replacement, reduction and refinement". The use of animal models should be replaced by a different method such as *in vitro* research. If this is not possible, the amount of research done *in vivo* should be reduced to a minimum and the research should be refined as much as possible to prevent unnecessary suffering of the animal.

To overcome these issues, tissue engineering (TE) recreates physiological environments of tissues or organs, to be able to study tissue responses as a result of external and internal processes [Hutmacher *et al.*, 2008]. These so-called *in vitro* models give much faster results and are less costly compared to *in vivo* studies. The first *in vitro* created tissues were conventional two-dimensional (2D) cell cultures in which cells were cultured on a flat surface, for example, on a tissue culture plate. Although this method is, because of its simplicity, widely used to analyze cells *in vitro*, it does not replicate the cellular microenvironment that is necessary for cells to function as they do *in vivo* since these cultures are not able to maintain their differentiated functions in 2D [Gallagher & Appenzeller, 1999; Manson, 2001]. A slightly more advanced 2D culture method is the Transwell® system, which consists of two compartments separated by a porous membrane. Cells can be cultured in one compartment, while a different cell type can be cultured on top of the porous membrane on the other compartment, which is placed inside the big compartment. Using this, a static co-culture system is established where the cell types are separated by an artificial barrier.

Three-dimensional (3D) cell culture models are able to partially recreate a physiologically relevant cellular microenvironment [Pampaloni *et al.*, 2007]. Huh *et al.* [2011] define 3D cell culture as the culture of living cells within engineered devices having 3D structures that mimic tissue- and organ-specific microarchitecture. Researchers were able to recreate realistic cell differentiation and reorganization *in vitro*. Stiff, pre-engineered, scaffolds were often used to culture rigid structures such as bone and cartilage prior to implantation *in vivo*. Due to mechanical cues induced by cell–material interactions, osteogenic and chondrogenic cells cultured on these scaffolds were able to keep their differentiated state [Burdick & Vunjak-Novakovic, 2008; Engler *et al.*, 2006; Ingber, 2008; Lutolf *et al.*, 2009; Paszek *et al.*, 2005; Whiteside, 2008]. Another way to retain tissues in their differentiated state is to recreate the physiological microenvironment by culturing these cells inside a synthetic or biological extracellular matrix (ECM)-like structure. This can be either a synthetic hydrogel or a naturally derived ECM-based gel.

However, recreating the microarchitecture is not sufficient to reconstitute the function of a living organ. Comparing these 2D and 3D culture systems with a normal functioning organ, it becomes clear that critical organ functions such as physiological mechanical stimuli, vascularization including the transport of immune cells and the ability to have a co-culture with a functioning microbiome for a long time period are not yet present in these *in vitro* systems. Realizing that a top–down TE approach does not provide the ability to fully recreate an organ function *in vitro*, reverse engineering provides a better opportunity to engineer a functioning organ. "Reverse engineering seeks to identify the minimal set of design principles that are necessary to reconstitute relevant functions of the whole" (quote from Ingber [2016]). Approaching these organ functions from the bottom–up gives much more possibilities to include the above-mentioned critical organ system into the *in vitro* model.

The rapid developments in microfluidic technology give us the tools to develop *in vitro* models using the well-controlled, bottom–up approach. Microfluidic devices, or "chips" are systems that consist of microchannels with the size of tens to hundreds of micrometers in which small amounts of fluids (10^{-9}–10^{-19} μL) can be processed and handled [Whitesides, 2006]. When culturing human cells in microfluidic chips, bottom–up engineering of tissue and organ physiology can be performed. The resulting devices are called "organs-on-chips". Microfluidic OOC systems provide a dynamic and mechanically relevant microenvironment for *in vitro* tissue culture.

It is necessary to understand an organ function starting with defining the basic structure of it. In the human body, practically every organ consists of a parenchymal tissue, such as epithelium or connective tissue, which forms an interface with a vascular tissue like a blood vessel. Vascularization of the parenchymal tissue is crucial for nutrient supply, immune cell delivery and to provide transport of chemical, hormonal and neural signals to the organ. Apart from this characteristic interface, all organs experience mechanical forces created either by contractions or by shear forces caused by fluid flow. In OOC research, the parenchymal–vascular interface and organ-specific mechanical stimulations are indispensable and are the starting point of every new research. The possibility to incorporate these parameters on a chip created a whole new toolbox of opportunities for *in vitro* organ research.

Due to the fast development of microengineering in the last decades, it is now possible to create microfluidic chips in a rapid and reproducible way. Using photolithography and etching, a negative mold can be created out of a solid material such as silicon. These molds can then be used for soft lithography to produce a positive replica of the mold (Fig. 11.1(a)).

Nowadays, the liquid polymer poly-dimethyl siloxane (PDMS) is often used in this process [Whitesides, 2006]. PDMS is poured onto the mold, after which the polymer/curing-agent mixture is temperature-cured. These positive replicates of the mold can be fixed onto a glass slide by hydrophilization of the glass and PDMS surfaces. The cavities in between the glass and PDMS form the microfluidic channels. Another way of creating negative molds is by applying a pattern of photoresist using photolithography (Fig. 11.1(b)). The amount of detail that can be applied onto the mold and thus onto the negative replica makes this technique very interesting for tissue culture purposes, as cells are influenced by surface texture. Using this knowledge and the possibility to apply surface texture

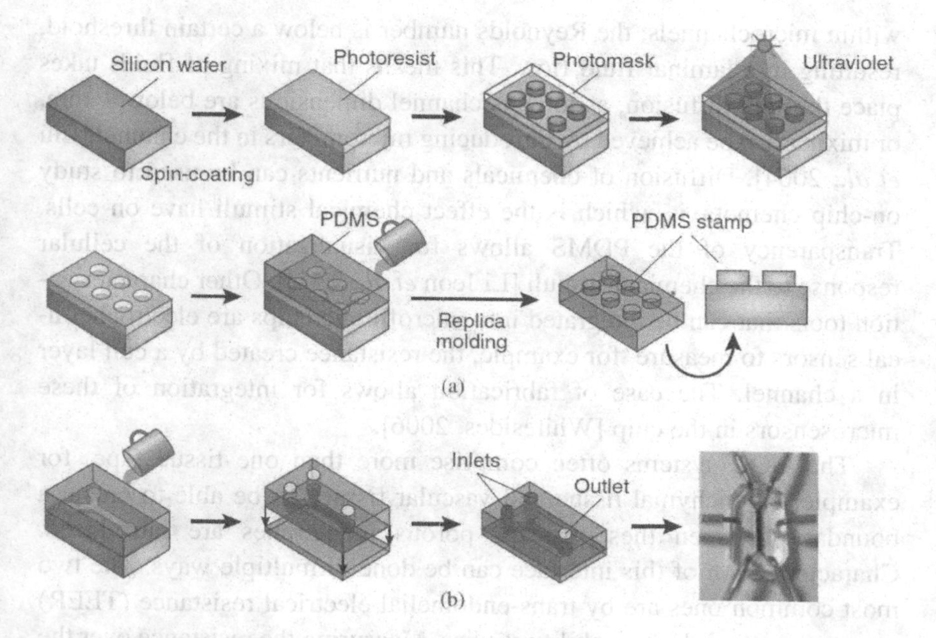

Figure 11.1. Engineering of microfluidic chips by photolithography and soft lithography. (a) Replica molding. First, a layer of photoresist is patterned onto a silicon wafer using a photomask and UV light. PDMS is then cast onto the negative photoresist mold to create a PDMS stamp. (b) PDMS is cast onto a SU-8 patterned silicon wafer after which holes are punctured in the PDMS. Prior to use, the PDMS chip is bonded with its channel side down onto a glass slide by using O_2-plasma. Reprinted with permission from Macmillan Publishers Ltd: *Nature Biotechnology* [Bhatia & Ingber, 2014], copyright 2014.

using photolithography, microfluidic channels that provide cell guidance can be engineered [Dai *et al.*, 2005]. In this way, boundaries can be created between different cell types.

The microfluidic channels also allow cells and tissues to be cultured in a 3D setting by using a hydrogel, which serves as a microenvironment that resembles the natural ECM. Gels which have a short curing time can be used in a microfluidic chip without the addition of a supportive membrane [Caliari & Burdick, 2016; Lee & Cho, 2016].

Fluid flow controllability is crucial for OOC research. As mentioned above, mechanical cues induced by fluidic shear stress are of great importance for cells to maintain their function. The Reynolds number determines the way fluid flows within a channel. Due to the small dimensions within microchannels, the Reynolds number is below a certain threshold, resulting in a laminar fluid flow. This means that mixing of fluids takes place through diffusion, as long as channel dimensions are below 1 mm, or mixing can be achieved by introducing micromixers in the channel [Liu *et al.*, 2004]. Diffusion of chemicals and nutrients can be used to study on-chip chemotaxis, which is the effect chemical stimuli have on cells. Transparency of the PDMS allows for visualization of the cellular response to the chemical stimuli [Li Jeon *et al.*, 2002]. Other characterization tools that can be integrated into microfluidic chips are electrochemical sensors to measure, for example, the resistance created by a cell layer in a channel. The ease of fabrication allows for integration of these microsensors in the chip [Whitesides, 2006].

The OOC systems often comprise more than one tissue type, for example, parenchymal tissue and vascular tissue. To be able to create a boundary between these tissues, porous membranes are introduced. Characterization of this interface can be done in multiple ways. The two most common ones are by trans-endothelial electrical resistance (TEER) measurements and permeability studies. Measuring the resistance over the boundary gives the researcher information about the state of the interface. For certain tissue types, such as the blood–brain barrier, a dense monolayer of endothelial cells is required. The integrity of this layer can be measured by TEER [Sakolish *et al.*, 2016]. Besides, the permeability can be studied by injecting a measurable substance in one channel and measuring the amount of substance going through the interface over time. The permeability and resistance of the interface can be influenced by factors such as mechanical stress and cell–cell interactions.

11.3 Current OOC Models

The first OOC models were only comprised of one tissue type cultured in a microfluidic channel. By introducing a porous membrane that separates two parallelly placed microchannels, it is possible to culture multiple tissue types in one compartmentalized chip. Current OOC models are actually compartmentalized systems containing microfluidic channels, often separated by a (porous) membrane, with on either side a cell layer of different cell types. Sensors are included in these chips for *in situ* measurements. The compartments can be individually controlled to regulate fluid flow resulting in physiologically relevant shear stresses to which the tissues are exposed. In the following sections, the function of the membrane in a number of OOC systems is described in more detail, highlighting the benefits and crucial role that membranes have in this technology [Esch *et al.*, 2015].

11.3.1 *Lung-On-Chip*

The lung consists of millions of alveoli surrounded by capillaries. Transporting oxygen from inhaled air to the blood stream is, together with the removal of carbon dioxide, one of the main functions of the lung carried out by these alveoli–capillary interfaces. When engineering the capillary oxygen uptake from air-on-chip, recreating this interface is crucial. Huh *et al.* developed a compartmentalized system comprised of two parallel PDMS channels separated by a porous, 10-μm thick PDMS membrane (pore size 0.4 μm) in which both human pulmonary microvascular endothelial and human alveolar epithelial cell lines can be cultured simultaneously to mimic the interface. Microdevices were made by soft lithography. Prior to cell culture, the PDMS microchannels were coated with an ECM coating to induce cell attachment.

Besides mimicking the cell–cell interface, a lung-on-chip system needs to mimic very well the mechanical forces present in the organ. When a lung inhales, alveoli expand, increasing the surface area over which oxygen can pass the interface. During this mechanical stretching and relaxing, epithelial and endothelial cells undergo mechanical stress which induces changes to the paracellular transport, resulting in a change in permeability of the endothelial cell layer. In the system of Huh *et al.*, this movement is mimicked by adding, parallel to the microfluidic channels and separated by a thin PDMS layer, two air-filled chambers (Fig. 11.2). By applying a vacuum in these chambers, both adherent cell layers are stretched as they do during normal inspiration. By introducing mechanical stress, together with controlled fluid flow, Huh *et al.* were also able to study the whole-organ response of a lung. In the lung-on-chip system by Huh *et al.*, the porous PDMS membrane not only functions as a barrier between two tissue types, but it also functions as a flexible substrate through which mechanical strain is transferred to the attached tissue. Stretching of the membrane induces mechanotransduction in the attached cells, leading to cytoskeletal reorganization which influences the behavior of the cells. By looking at the pulmonary inflammation reaction caused by immune cells, which can be introduced into the vascular channel, they concluded that the cells function as they would do *in vivo*. Studying such immune response *in vitro* is not possible in multi-tissue setups, such as the Transwell® systems, since those are static. When using a porous membrane, there is a possibility to study the permeability of the cell layers; however, this is limited by the pore size of the membrane. Results show that the inflammatory response, induced by nanoparticles, is more active when strain is applied to the cells.

11.3.2 *Gut-On-Chip*

Chronic intestinal disorders such as ulcerative colitis and Crohn's disease are lacking proper medicinal treatment. To test new drugs, a physiologically relevant intestinal system has to be created. The difficulty of recreating such a system lies with culturing living microbes on the luminal side of the epithelium. These so-called microbial symbionts have a major contribution in the barrier function of the intestinal epithelium layer [Arthur & Jobin, 2011; Sokol & Seksik, 2010]. To study these microbial symbionts and the influence of drugs on the intestinal system, *in vitro* systems are being developed. Simple 2D and 3D studies, such as Transwell® and polymeric scaffold systems, cannot mimic the physiologically relevant shear stress and stretch that the cells experience in the gut as a result of fluid flow and peristalsis. In these systems, it is also challenging to keep the microbes alive for longer periods of time. By using OOC technology, researchers have tried to recreate the intestinal microenvironment on a microfluidic chip. Such a system provides a platform for tissue culture as well as for the introduction of the proper mechanical cues to the tissue.

Kim *et al.* developed a gut-on-chip system by culturing gut epithelium cells under physiologically relevant conditions (Fig. 11.3). Similar to the chip designed by Huh *et al.* (Fig. 11.2), this PDMS chip consists of two microfluidic channels separated by a porous, 10-μm thin, PDMS membrane (pore size 10 μm). On both sides of the channels, vacuum chambers

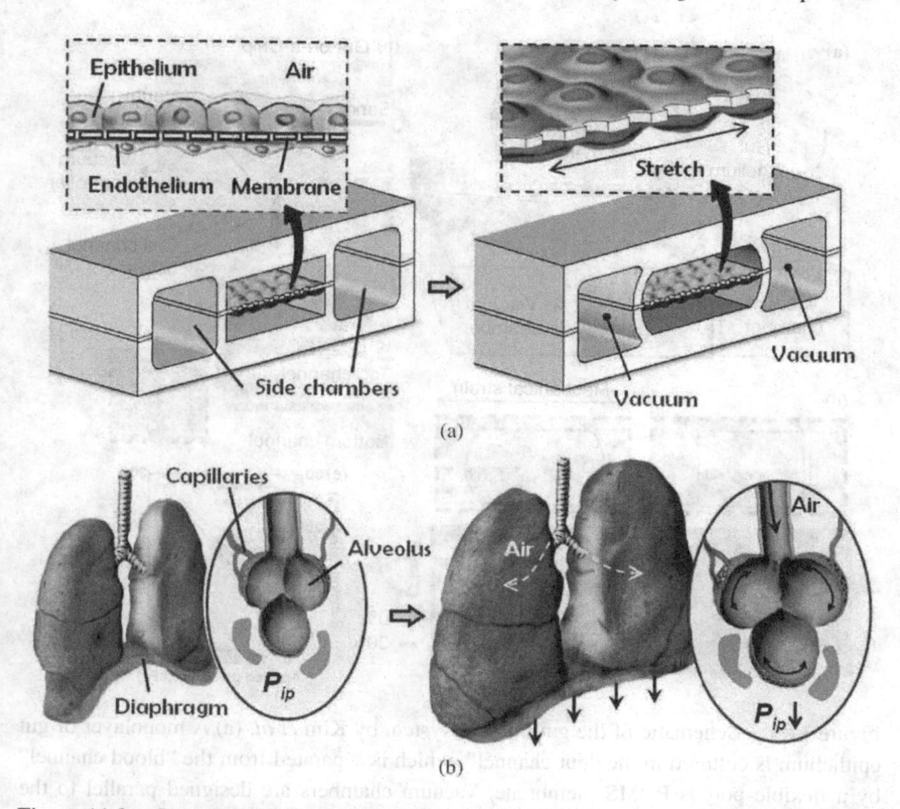

Figure 11.2. Lung-on-chip model by Huh *et al.* (a) Chip design in which two cell types, namely endothelial cells and epithelium cells, are co-cultured onto a porous PDMS membrane. By applying a vacuum in the side chambers, the membrane is stretched, causing a stretching movement in the attaching cells. (b) Inhalation in a normal lung by expansion of the alveoli. From Huh *et al.* [2010]. Reprinted with permission from AAAS.

were used to create peristaltic movement of the membrane. When cells were attached to the membrane, a 10% width increase was achieved mimicking the mechanical microenvironment in a more realistic matter. For this gut-on-chip system, cells of the human colorectal carcinoma line (Caco-2) were used to recreate the epithelial cell layer present in the intestinal tract [Kim *et al.*, 2012]. As can be seen in Fig. 11.3(d), the cells become larger in size when a mechanical strain, which increases the membrane width by 30%, is applied. The cells produce a similar amount of strain compared to the membrane as a function of the pressure applied in the vacuum chambers (Fig. 11.3(e)).

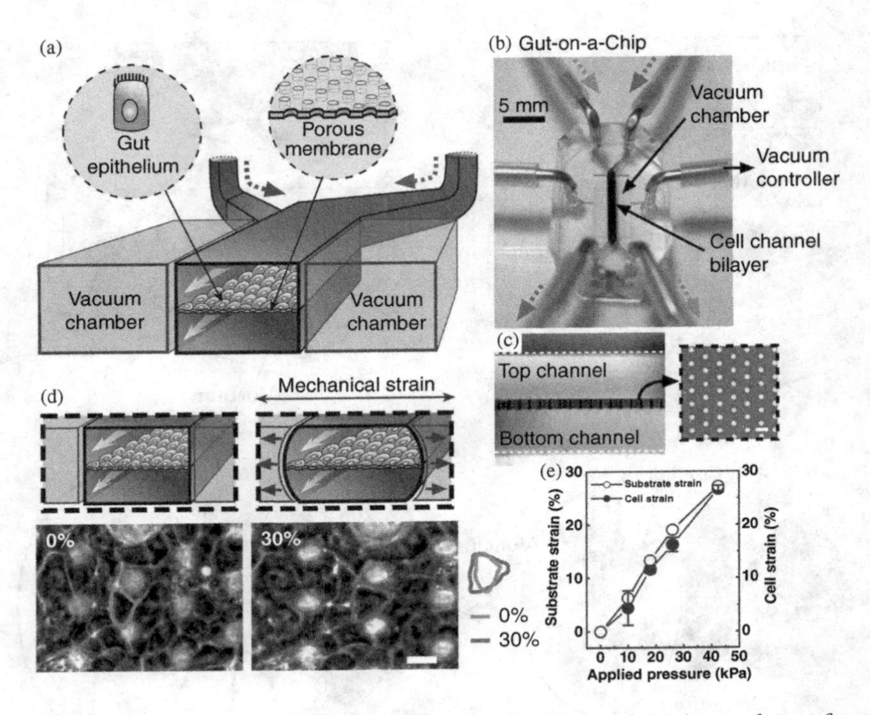

Figure 11.3. Schematic of the gut-on-chip system by Kim *et al.* (a) A monolayer of gut epithelium is cultured in the "gut channel", which is separated from the "blood channel" by a flexible porous PDMS membrane. Vacuum chambers are designed parallel to the channels to be able to apply mechanical strain to the cell layer. (b) Photographic image of the actual chip. Tubing is connected to a syringe pump with which the fluids were perfused through the chip. (c) Cross-section of the microfluidic channels (150-μm high), showing the membrane with its homogeneous pore distribution in the square inset. (d) In the top two images, a schematic is given of what happens to the membrane and cell layer when a mechanical strain is applied. In the bottom two images, the monolayer of Caco-2 cells can be seen. When a width increase of 30% is achieved (right image), the cells show a change in morphology (for both situations, one cell is framed) (scale bar is 20 μm). (e) Quantitative comparison between the strain produced in the PDMS membrane and the strain produced in the attached Caco-2 cell layer as a function of applied pressure. Reproduced from Kim *et al.* [2012] with permission of The Royal Society of Chemistry.

Although Kim *et al.* used a two-channel microfluidic device to recreate a gut-on-chip, Gumuscu *et al.* [2015] developed a microfluidic chip in which hydrogel arrays were patterned in closed microchips. By using these so-called hydrogel pockets as scaffolds for culturing intestinal epithelium, a multiplexed platform was created in which each pocket resembles a part of the intestinal lumen. This technique is currently being developed further in OOC technology.

11.3.3 *Blood–Brain Barrier-On-Chip*

In the mammalian body, there is a barrier between the central nervous system (CNS) and the circulation. This barrier present in the brain, which is called the blood–brain barrier (BBB), was first discovered by Paul Ehrlich in 1885. There are a few barrier functions which the BBB is responsible for, such as the protection of the brain from the extracellular environment and the blockage and diffusion of specific nutrients. Besides, it also maintains the homeostasis of the CNS. The BBB is formed by the interaction of multiple cell types and membranes in the context of the neurovascular unit (NVU). One NVU consists of a monolayer of brain microvascular endothelial cells (BMVECs) which are surrounded by a basement membrane and glial cells. The inner endothelial cell layer is surrounded by a basement membrane which anchors the endothelial cells and pericytes and forms a connection between these cells and the other glial cells. Structural and specialized proteins such as collagen, elastin, fibronectin and laminin form, together with proteoglycans, the basement membrane. These ECM proteins are generated and maintained by BMVECs, astrocytes and pericytes within the NVU. When the anchoring ability of the basement membrane can no longer be maintained, the tight junctions between the endothelial cells are disrupted, leading to instability of the barrier, causing BBB permeability.

Multiple research institutes have attempted to recreate this complex organ *in vitro*. Standard co-cultures using BMVECs and glial cells were carried out in Transwell® systems. These systems were also used to study passive drug transportation through the endothelial layer. Since flow is necessary to increase the physiological behavior of the endothelial cell layer [White & Frangos, 2007], OOC technology is used to recreate the BBB-on-chip. Most of these systems are comprised again of two parallel microchannels separated by a porous membrane on which different cell types can be cultured. By measuring TEER, the tightness of the BMVEC layer can be quantified. Since the resistance can be influenced by the membrane porosity, it is important to have a control study on the barrier.

This can be done by staining the tight junction complexes formed between endothelial cells. During such a staining, the tight junction protein ZO-1 is stained [Gottardi *et al.*, 1996].

One of the first BBB models was produced by Booth and Kim [2012]. Their model consists of two pieces of PDMS containing microfluidic channels separated by a polycarbonate membrane (10-μm thick, 0.4-μm pores). They were able to seed a layer of endothelial cells in the top channel, while simultaneously a murine astrocyte cell line was cultured in the other channel. A resistance of 180–280 Ωcm^2 was measured, for the endothelial cell layer on the membrane, which indicates that the barrier functions as it should. However, note that there is still no actual resistance value that defines a successful barrier. Resistance inside a microfluidic chip depends on multiple factors such as material properties and the consistency of the used liquids. In 2014, the same research group improved their first model and tested it again for TEER and permeability. This time they found a TEER value of 150 Ωcm^2 and a permeability coefficient which could be correlated to physiological brain/plasma permeability coefficients [Booth & Kim, 2014].

In 2016, van der Helm *et al.* [2016] developed a similar system in which two channels, microfabricated in PDMS, are placed perpendicularly on top of each other and the channels are separated by a polycarbonate (PC) membrane similar to that of Booth and Kim. Due to the smart chip design (Fig. 11.4), it is possible to perform a 4-point TEER measurement, which is much more accurate compared to the traditional 2-point measurement.

Both van der Helm *et al.* and Booth *et al.* use the same PC membrane which is placed horizontally in the chip [Booth & Kim, 2014; van der Helm *et al.*, 2016]. These membranes are opaque, which makes visual inspection of both channels at the same time very difficult, if not impossible, when using a bright-field microscope. The TEER and permeability measurements show that the membrane does not have a significant influence on the resistance of the BBB chip.

11.4 Membrane Properties

The type of material used for the membrane determines its properties such as elasticity, transparency, biocompatibility and cytocompatibility.

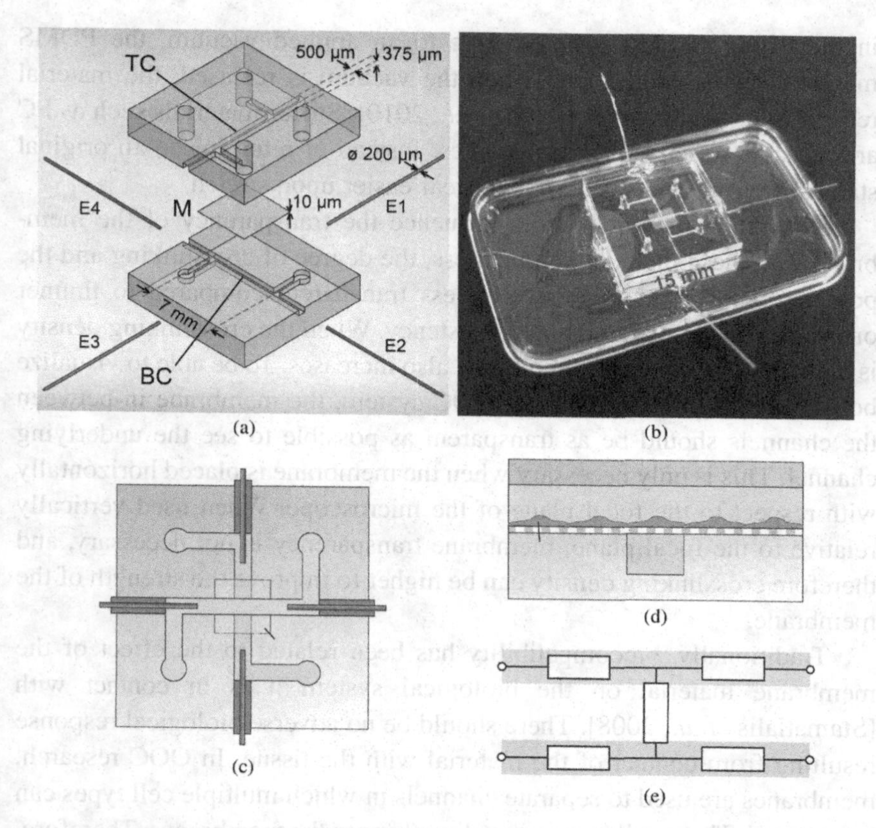

(a) (b)

(c) (d)

(e)

Figure 11.4. Schematic of the chip design by van der Helm *et al.* (a) Exploded view of the chip showing all the components, with the porous polycarbonate membrane (M) in the middle. The total culture area of the membrane suspended between the two channels is 0.25 mm². (b) Photographic image of the actual chip. (c) Schematic top view of the chip. (d) Schematic cross-section view of the chip showing endothelial cells (EC) in the top channel (TC). No cells are present in the bottom channel (BC). (e) Electrode circuit of the chip, with electrodes E1 and E3 in the TC and E2 and E4 in the BC, top channel represented by resistors R1 and R3, and the bottom channel represented by resistors R2 and R4. Resistor Rm represents the membrane and possible EC barrier. Reprinted from van der Helm *et al.* [2016] with permission from Elsevier.

Elasticity is the ability of a material body, deformed by an outer force, to return to its original shape and size when the forces causing the deformation are removed. A body with this ability is said to behave (or respond) elastically [Britannica, 2016]. Huh *et al.* used an elastic PDMS membrane in their lung-on-chip systems. Due to an applied vacuum, the PDMS membrane is stretched, and when the vacuum is released, the material returns to its original state [Huh *et al.*, 2010]. Stiffer materials such as PC are not able to withstand such forces. Instead of returning to an original state, stiffer materials can break or tear easier upon stretch.

Different structural factors influence the transparency of the membrane, and these include the thickness, the degree of crosslinking and the porosity. Thicker membranes are less transparent compared to thinner ones of the same material and consistency. When the crosslinking density is high, the opacity of the membrane also increases. To be able to visualize both channels in a two-channel OOC system, the membrane in-between the channels should be as transparent as possible to see the underlying channel. This is only necessary when the membrane is placed horizontally with respect to the focal plane of the microscope. When used vertically relative to the focal plane, membrane transparency is not necessary, and therefore crosslinking density can be higher to improve the strength of the membrane.

Traditionally, biocompatibility has been related to the effect of the membrane material on the biological system it is in contact with [Stamatialis *et al.*, 2008]. There should be no adverse biological response resulting from contact of the material with the tissue. In OOC research, membranes are used to separate channels in which multiple cell types can be cultured. These cells are grown directly onto the membranes. Therefore, it is necessary that these membranes are made of biocompatible materials. It is also possible to apply a surface treatment to the membranes so that they become biocompatible.

Apart from the biocompatibility of a material, anchorage-dependent cells and tissues need a mechanical interaction with the material surface. Integrins on the cell surface can bind to proteins located at the surface of the membrane. This integrin binding triggers an internal process in the cell, called mechanotransduction. Cells attach to the surface, pulling on it with a certain force, deforming the internal cytoskeletal structure. Deformation leads to phenotypic change, influencing the state of the cells. Stiffer materials are more suitable to culture cells from stiff tissues compared to more elastic or softer materials [White & Frangos, 2007]. To keep a cell in its differentiated state, the material stiffness should not induce a change in phenotype with regard to the cells original phenotype. Therefore, it is necessary to identify the ideal material stiffness for a specific cell type prior to the experiment. In a co-culture system such as an OOC where multiple tissues are involved, it is important to find a balance between the material properties that are suitable for both tissue types. When anchorage-dependent cells are used, it is often crucial to apply the proper surface treatment to the membrane material. To culture endothelial cells on a hydrophilic surface, attachment can be induced by applying an ECM-protein coating prior to cell seeding. This coating can, for example, be fibronectin, collagen, laminin or Matrigel™ [Chaw *et al.*, 2007; Cooke *et al.*, 2008]. Besides, by applying an O_2 plasma treatment to the used chip, the channels and the membrane become hydrophilic, which improves fluid inflow into the channels. Such treatment is especially useful when a viscous hydrogel has to be injected into a chip. Due to hydrophobic recovery, the material should be subjected to plasma treatment within a short period prior to fluid inflow. Cells, however, do not attach well to hydrophilic surfaces. So, when an O_2 plasma treatment is used prior to cell seeding, the channels and the membrane should be coated with the appropriate coating to promote cell attachment.

Surface porosity is a measure of the total pore area of a membrane; thus, it is given by the total amount of pores per surface area multiplied by the size of a single pore [Mulder, 1996]. When increasing membrane porosity, the amount of light that can pass the membrane increases too. In OOC systems, having a membrane with a high porosity and thus a good transparency allows for inspection of both channels at the same time without having to turn the chip over. Increasing the porosity will also have an influence on the membrane's electrical resistance. Besides, depending on the pore size, cells might be able to penetrate the membrane pores, blocking electrical signal propagation. However, when the porosity is high, but the pore size small, cell penetration can be avoided and electrical signals can pass easily. In OOC systems, flow of nutrients and cell-signaling molecules through the membrane is also crucial. Nutrients and small molecules are able to pass membranes with very small pores down to a few nanometers. For some tissue types, communication between tissues separated by a membrane, or even cell–cell contact, is crucial to function properly. For example, in the BBB, direct cell–cell contact between brain endothelial cells and surrounding cells (pericytes, microglia and neurons) is thought to be essential for maintenance of the barrier [Abbott *et al.*, 2010]. To achieve this cell–cell contact, the pores of the used membrane should be large enough for cells to contact the opposite site directly.

A summary of the membrane properties that play an important role in OOC systems is given in Table 11.1.

11.5 Reflection and Outlook

Although the OOC systems developed so far function properly, the rapidly emerging field of OOC still holds a lot of room for improvement. Making

Table 11.1. Overview of the most commonly used materials in OOC technology with their properties and applicability.

	Materials	PC	PDMS	Polyethylene terephthalate (PET)
	OOC systems	— BBB[1, 2, 3]	— Lung[4] — Gut[5]	— BBB[6] — Kidney[7, 8]
Properties and Applicability	Elasticity	–	++	+
	Transparency	+/–	++	++
	Biocompatibility	+	+	+
	Cell–material interaction	+/–	+/–	+
	Visualization	+/–	+	+
	TEER	+	+	+
	Porosity and pore size	Variable 0.2–8 μm	Adjustable	Variable 0.4–8 μm

Note: (–) Not applicable, (+/–) can be applicable with some adjustments, (+) good applicability, (++) perfect applicability.

[1] van der Helm *et al.* [2016].
[2] Booth and Kim [2014].
[3] Brown *et al.* [2015].
[4] Huh *et al.* [2010].
[5] Kim *et al.* [2012].
[6] Walter *et al.* [2016].
[7] Jang and Suh [2010].
[8] Nieskens and Wilmer [2016].

these systems more physiologically relevant will improve the output for which these systems are used. To achieve more realistic systems, structural and mechanical adjustments have to be made to the chips and especially to the membranes.

11.5.1 *Membrane Morphology: 2D vs 3D*

All organs have specific morphologies, from the macroscale to the microscale, all the way down to the nanoscale. When recreating the tissue microenvironment in an OOC, the organ morphology plays a crucial role in the function of the system. All systems described here consist of a planar membrane on which tissues and cells are cultured. Such a planar interface is almost nowhere to be found in the human body. Lungs consist of alveoli, which are spherical-shaped balloon-like structures that regulate, among others, the uptake of oxygen by bloodstream. In their model, Huh *et al.* did not recreate the curvature to which lung endothelial cells are exposed to in actual alveoli. This curvature can influence the compactness and the permeability of the lung epithelial cell layer and thus the uptake of factors, such as CO_2, O_2 or medication, from the blood side.

The influence of cellular compactness is also very relevant for the endothelial cells used to recreate the BBB-on-chip as it is known that the BBB contains a higher degree of tight junctions compared to other cell barriers. When recreating a brain capillary on-chip, the curvature of the membrane on which endothelial cells are cultured should be mimicking the curvature of a brain capillary. As is the case for the BBB and the lung-on-chip, the gut-on-chip as it exists now also contains a planar membrane. However, the intestine is not planar. The small intestine contains a surface structure which is based upon villi, small lobe-like structures that increase the total surface area of the small intestine enormously. The total surface area of the gastro-intestinal mucosa in an adult human is between 30 and 40 m^2. To make a realistic model for the gut-on-chip, the total surface area of the cells used for secretion and absorption should be proportional to the physiological situation. The challenge lies in creating villi-like structures in a membrane, making it non-planar. Creation of 3D membranes can be done using various methods including hot embossing, thermoforming and/or phase separation micromolding [Papenburg *et al.*, 2007;

Truckenmüller *et al.*, 2008, 2011]. Using hot embossing, it is challenging to obtain membranes that are thin enough (<10 μm) to allow for cell–cell contact. There, the polymer is heated up to its glass transition temperature, which allows for the material to be molded into the desired shape. Depending on the original pore size and porosity of the membrane, it is possible for the pores become larger or smaller during the embossing process. Depending on the microfabrication method, the choice of materials may be limited as a limited amount of materials are suitable to be molded into the desired shape. Technologies such as etching and lithography mostly use silicon-like materials, whereas polymers are being used in soft-lithography processes [Vogelaar *et al.*, 2005].

11.5.2 *Membrane Topography*

Apart from the microstructure of the membrane, surface texture can also be adjusted. This texture can vary from a nanometer-size roughness up to patterned microstructures. By patterning of the membrane surface with micrometer-sized features, cells can reorganize their cytoskeleton upon cell attachment. It has been shown that this rearrangement by cell attachment to nano- and microtopographical patterned surfaces influences stem cell differentiation and cell fate. Cell lines can be kept in their differentiated state more easily when the surface directs the cells to adapt a certain phenotype [Griffin *et al.*, 2015; Hulshof, 2016]. Cell patterning has been used to create aligned and higher-order tissues in, for example, heart-on-chip devices. In the heart-on-chip model of Zhang *et al.*, a PDMS mold is made by lithography after which a gel is imprinted, transferring micrometer-sized features onto the surface [Zhang *et al.*, 2015b].

Just like membrane morphology, thermoforming or hot embossing can be used to pattern a surface. The "topochip", developed by Unadkat *et al.*, is made by hot embossing a polylactic acid (PLA) film. A mathematical algorithm was developed to create random surface topographies on a polymer sheet to study the cellular interaction with these topographies [Unadkat *et al.*, 2011]. Another interesting method to create a surface topography in a controlled way is phase separation micromolding [Vogelaar *et al.*, 2005]. A dissolved polymer film is cast onto a mold, after this phase separation takes place, solidifying the polymer (Fig. 11.5). This

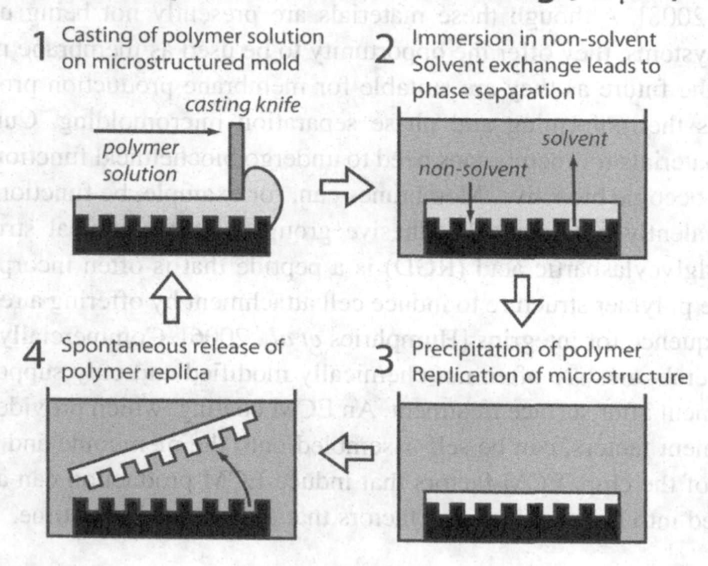

Figure 11.5. Schematic of liquid-induced phase separation micromolding process. First, a dissolved polymer is cast onto a structured mold (1). By placing the polymer into a non-solvent solution, phase inversion takes place (2). The polymer precipitates, replicating the mold's structure (3). Due to shrinkage of the created polymer film, it is released from the mold (4). Reproduced from de Jong *et al.* [2005] with permission of The Royal Society of Chemistry.

can either be liquid- or thermally induced phase separation. Phase separation micromolding allows for molding of a variety of polymers including block copolymers and biodegradable polymers. When the features of the mold are high enough to perforate the polymer film, it is possible to create an open structure which is interesting to be used as the membrane in OOC systems [de Jong *et al.*, 2005; Gironès *et al.*, 2006].

Differences in cell morphology and mechanics are a result of surface stiffness in combination with the area, and thus the topography, to which a cell is constrained [Tee *et al.*, 2011].

11.5.3 *Biochemical Functionalization of the Membrane*

There are multiple cell adhesive polymers, such as PLA, polytrimethyl carbonate (PTMC) and polycaprolactone (PCL) that are used for biomedical applications [Ulery *et al.*, 2011; van Dijkhuizen-Radersma *et al.*, 2008]. Although these materials are presently not being used in OOC systems, they offer the opportunity to be used as membrane materials in the future as they are suitable for membrane production processes such as thermoforming and phase separation micromolding. Currently used materials for membranes need to undergo biochemical functionalization to become bioactive. Membranes can, for example, be functionalized by covalently bonding cell adhesive groups to the chemical structure. Arginylglycylaspartic acid (RGD) is a peptide that is often incorporated into the polymer structure to induce cell attachment by offering a recognition sequence for integrins [Humphries *et al.*, 2006]. Commercially available membranes are often not chemically modified and only support cell attachment after surface treatment. An ECM coating, which provides cell-attachment factors, can be self-assembled onto the membrane and on the inside of the chip. ECM factors that induce ECM production can also be included into the membrane as factors that are secreted over time.

11.5.4 *Temporary Membranes*

To be able to create a system without any additional factors that can have an influence on the possible outcome of the process, temporary membranes should be used. There is a wide range of polymers that hydrolytically degrade over time. A commonly used material in TE, PLA, has a degradation time of weeks to months under cell culture conditions [Xu *et al.*, 2011; Zhang *et al.*, 2006], which is too long for OOC research. PC is another frequently used membrane material which does not degrade at all. Up till now, it is challenging to keep tissue cultures alive for longer periods in a microfluidic system, and therefore OOC systems are used for short-term experiments and drug testing. The process of creating a membrane-free system by degradation of the polymer membrane can be time-consuming, and therefore fully or partially removable membranes are preferred. Some polymers possess the ability to be degraded enzymatically. By flowing an enzyme solution over the membrane, it can be degraded faster [Banerjee *et al.*, 2014]. This way, a co-culture of different cells can be made by first seeding the first cell type against the membrane and secondly removing the membrane. If the cells produce enough ECM, they are able to form their own basal membrane on the interface between two channels after which other cell types can be added into the other channel. Another option would be the on-chip fabrication of a temporary membrane instead of placing the membrane in the chip during chip fabrication. A possible way to do this is by deprotonation of a polysaccharide which causes the polysaccharide to precipitate at the interface where it is deprotonated [Luo *et al.*, 2010]. Upon protonation of such a material, the material will become soluble again. These so-called reversible membranes can be used as temporal phase guides.

It is thought that in the ideal case, cells should be able to form their own ECM and thus their own basal membrane. This basal membrane provides the basic mechanical stability that organ tissues need. As mentioned above, the membrane surface can be used to induce ECM formation in cells. However, to be able to get the best results from an OOC system, the system should be as realistic as possible. Therefore, membrane-free systems are being studied recently. Without a membrane, cells are in direct contact with each other like they would be in the physiological situation.

Hydrogels have already been mentioned in this chapter and can be considered membrane-free systems. Cells are able to migrate through the gel interface and reach the other cell layer. Using a hydrogel, both a horizontal and a vertical interface between two channels can be created. Horizontally, the hydrogel can be injected into the channels, if this is done to create a vertical membrane, there is a possibility that the gel does not have enough time to set at the interface and it will fill both channels. To solve this problem, the company MIMETAS, developed OrganoPlates® which contain phase guides that guide two liquids exactly along the middle axis of the chip [Jang *et al.*, 2015]. Using hydrogels is already a big step in the direction of realistic membrane-free OOC devices, but still they introduce an unnatural element into the system.

11.5.5 *Improving Membranes for OOC Research*

OOC research is an exciting field of *in vitro* research in which there is still a lot of room for improvement. Considering membrane-containing systems, more research is needed to improve the structural, mechanical and chemical structure of the membranes to make the system more physiological. The latest idea to create membrane-free OOC systems can be of great importance for the development of new lab-on-chip applications. Therefore, other techniques, such as interfacial polymerization or deprotonation of polysaccharides, should be studied more [Luo *et al.*, 2010; Zhang *et al.*, 2015a]. These techniques and their applications in a microfluidic chip are currently being studied thoroughly.

List of Abbreviations

2D	two dimensional
3D	three dimensional
BBB	blood–brain barrier
BMVEC	Brain microvascular endothelial cells
Caco-2	colorectal adenocarcinoma cells
CNS	central nervous system
ECM	extracellular matrix
NVU	neurovascular unit
OOC	organ-on-chip
PC	polycarbonate
PCL	polycaprolactone
PDMS	poly-dimethyl siloxane
PET	polyethylene terephthalate
PLA	polylactic acid
PTMC	polytrimethyl carbonate
RGD	arginylglycylaspartic acid
TE	tissue engineering
TEER	trans-endothelial electrical resistance

References

Abbott NJ, Patabendige AAK, Dolman DEM, Yusof SR and Begley DJ (2010). Structure and function of the blood–brain barrier. *Neurobiol Disease*, 37(1), pp. 13–25.

Arthur JC and Jobin C (2011). The struggle within: microbial influences on colorectal cancer. *Inflamm Bowel Diseases*, 17(1), pp. 396–409.

Banerjee A, Chatterjee K and Madras G (2014). Enzymatic degradation of polymers: a brief review. *Mater Sci Technol*, 30(5), pp. 567–573.

Bhatia SN and Ingber DE (2014). Microfluidic organs-on-chips. *Nat Biotechnol*, 32(8), pp. 760–772.

Booth R and Kim H (2012). Characterization of a microfluidic *in vitro* model of the blood–brain barrier ([small mu]BBB). *Lab on a Chip*, 12(10), pp. 1784–1792.

Booth R and Kim H (2014). Permeability analysis of neuroactive drugs through a dynamic microfluidic *in vitro* blood–brain barrier model. *Ann Biomed Eng*, 42(12), pp. 2379–2391.

Britannica, E. (2016, 21 June). Elasticity. from http://www.britannica.com/science/elasticity-physics.

Brown JA, Pensabene V, Markov DA, Allwardt V, Neely MD, Shi M, Britt CM, Hoilett OS, Yang Q, Brewer BM, Samson PC, McCawley LJ, May JM, Webb DJ, Li D, Bowman AB, Reiserer RS and Wikswo JP (2015). Recreating blood–brain barrier physiology and structure on chip: a novel neurovascular microfluidic bioreactor. *Biomicrofluidics*, 9(5), p. 054124.

Burdick JA and Vunjak-Novakovic G (2008). Engineered microenvironments for controlled stem cell differentiation. *Tissue Eng Part A*, 15(2), pp. 205–219.

Caliari SR and Burdick JA (2016). A practical guide to hydrogels for cell culture. *Nat Meth*, 13(5), pp. 405–414.

Chaw KC, Manimaran M, Tay FEH and Swaminathan S (2007). Matrigel coated polydimethylsiloxane based microfluidic devices for studying metastatic and non-metastatic cancer cell invasion and migration. *Biomed Microdev*, 9(4), pp. 597–602.

Cooke MJ, Phillips SR, Shah DS, Athey D, Lakey JH and Przyborski SA (2008). Enhanced cell attachment using a novel cell culture surface presenting functional domains from extracellular matrix proteins. *Cytotechnology*, 56(2), pp. 71–79.

Dai J, Guan Y-X, Wang S-L, Wu Z-Y and Fang Z-L (2005). Feature characterization of microfabricated microfluidic chips by PDMS replication and CCD imaging. *Anal Bioanal Chem*, 381(4), pp. 839–843.

de Jong J, Ankone B, Lammertink RGH and Wessling M (2005). New replication technique for the fabrication of thin polymeric microfluidic devices with tunable porosity. *Lab on a Chip*, 5(11), pp. 1240–1247.

Engler AJ, Sen S, Sweeney HL and Discher DE (2006). Matrix elasticity directs stem cell lineage specification. *Cell*, 126(4), pp. 677–689.

Esch EW, Bahinski A and Huh D (2015). Organs-on-chips at the frontiers of drug discovery. *Nat Rev Drug Discov*, 14(4), pp. 248–260.

Gallagher R and Appenzeller T (1999). Beyond reductionism. *Science*, 284(5411), pp. 79–79.

Gironès M, Akbarsyah IJ, Nijdam W, van Rijn CJM, Jansen HV, Lammertink RGH and Wessling M (2006). Polymeric microsieves produced by phase separation micromolding. *J Membrane Sci*, 283(1–2), pp. 411–424.

Gottardi CJ, Arpin M, Fanning AS and Louvard D (1996). The junction-associated protein, zonula occludens-1, localizes to the nucleus before the maturation and during the remodeling of cell–cell contacts. *Proc Natl Acad Sci USA*, 93(20), pp. 10779–10784.

Griffin MF, Butler PE, Seifalian AM and Kalaskar DM (2015). Control of stem cell fate by engineering their micro and nanoenvironment. *World J Stem Cells*, 7(1), pp. 37–50.

Gumuscu B, Bomer JG, van den Berg A and Eijkel JCT (2015). Photopatterning of hydrogel microarrays in closed microchips. *Biomacromolecules*, 16(12), pp. 3802–3810.

Huh D, Hamilton GA and Ingber DE (2011). From three-dimensional cell culture to organs-on-chips. *Trends Cell Biol*, 21(12), pp. 745–754.

Huh D, Matthews BD, Mammoto A, Montoya-Zavala M, Hsin HY and Ingber DE (2010). Reconstituting organ-level lung functions on a chip. *Science*, 328(5986), pp. 1662–1668.

Hulshof GFB (2016). Topochip: technology for instructing cell fate and morphology via designed surface topography. University of Twente, Enschede, DOI 10.3990/1.9789036541220.

Humphries JD, Byron A and Humphries MJ (2006). Integrin ligands at a glance. *J Cell Sci*, 119(19), pp. 3901–3903.

Hutmacher D, Woodfield T, Dalton P and Lewis J (2008). Scaffold design and fabrication. In Clemens van Blitterswijk PT, Anders Lindahl, Jeffrey Hubbell, David F. Williams, Ranieri Cancedda, Joost D. de Bruijn and Jérôme Sohier, (Eds.), *Tissue engineering,* Chapter 14 (Academic Press, Burlington), pp. 403–454.

Ingber DE (2008). Can cancer be reversed by engineering the tumor microenvironment? *Sem Cancer Biol*, 18(5), pp. 356–364.

Ingber DE (2016). Reverse engineering human pathophysiology with organs-on-chips. *Cell*, 164(6), pp. 1105–1109.

Jang M, Neuzil P, Volk T, Manz A and Kleber A (2015). On-chip three-dimensional cell culture in phaseguides improves hepatocyte functions *in vitro*. *Biomicrofluidics*, 9(3), p. 034113.

Jang K-J and Suh K-Y (2010). A multi-layer microfluidic device for efficient culture and analysis of renal tubular cells. *Lab on a Chip*, 10(1), pp. 36–42.

Kim HJ, Huh D, Hamilton G and Ingber DE (2012). Human gut-on-a-chip inhabited by microbial flora that experiences intestinal peristalsis-like motions and flow. *Lab on a Chip*, 12(12), pp. 2165–2174.

Lee H and Cho D-W (2016). One-step fabrication of an organ-on-a-chip with spatial heterogeneity using a 3D bioprinting technology. *Lab on a Chip*, 16(14), pp. 2618–2625.

Li Jeon N, Baskaran H, Dertinger SKW, Whitesides GM, Van De Water L and Toner M (2002). Neutrophil chemotaxis in linear and complex gradients of interleukin-8 formed in a microfabricated device. *Nat Biotechnol*, 20(8), pp. 826–830.

Liu YZ, Kim BJ and Sung HJ (2004). Two-fluid mixing in a microchannel. *Int J Heat Fluid Flow*, 25(6), pp. 986–995.

Luo X, Berlin DL, Betz J, Payne GF, Bentley WE and Rubloff GW (2010). *In situ* generation of pH gradients in microfluidic devices for biofabrication of freestanding, semi-permeable chitosan membranes. *Lab on a Chip*, 10(1), pp. 59–65.

Lutolf MP, Gilbert PM and Blau HM (2009). Designing materials to direct stem-cell fate. *Nature*, 462(7272), pp. 433–441.

Manson SM (2001). Simplifying complexity: a review of complexity theory. *Geoforum*, 32(3), pp. 405–414.

Martić-Kehl MI, Schibli R and Schubiger PA (2012). Can animal data predict human outcome? Problems and pitfalls of translational animal research. *Eur J Nucl Med Mol Imaging*, 39(9), pp. 1492–1496.

Mulder M (1996). Transport in membranes. In *Baisc Principles of Membrane Technology* (Kluwer Academic Publishers: Dordrecht, The Netherlands), pp. 210–230.

Nieskens TTG and Wilmer MJ (2016). Kidney-on-a-chip technology for renal proximal tubule tissue reconstruction. *Eur J Pharmacol*, 790, pp. 46–56.

Pampaloni F, Reynaud EG and Stelzer EHK (2007). The third dimension bridges the gap between cell culture and live tissue. *Nat Rev Mol Cell Biol*, 8(10), pp. 839–845.

Papenburg BJ, Vogelaar L, Bolhuis-Versteeg LAM, Lammertink RGH, Stamatialis D and Wessling M (2007). One-step fabrication of porous micropatterned scaffolds to control cell behavior. *Biomaterials*, 28(11), pp. 1998–2009.

Paszek MJ, Zahir N, Johnson KR, Lakins JN, Rozenberg GI, Gefen A, Reinhart-King CA, Margulies SS, Dembo M, Boettiger D, Hammer DA and Weaver VM (2005). Tensional homeostasis and the malignant phenotype. *Cancer Cell*, 8(3), pp. 241–254.

Sakolish CM, Esch MB, Hickman JJ, Shuler ML and Mahler GJ (2016). Modeling barrier tissues *in vitro*: methods, achievements, and challenges. *EBio Med*, 5, pp. 30–39.

Sokol H and Seksik P (2010). The intestinal microbiota in inflammatory bowel diseases: time to connect with the host. *Curr Opin Gastroenterol*, 26(4), pp. 327–331.

Stamatialis DF, Papenburg BJ, Gironés M, Saiful S, Bettahalli SNM, Schmitmeier S and Wessling M (2008). Medical applications of membranes: drug delivery, artificial organs and tissue engineering. *J Membrane Sci*, 308(1–2), pp. 1–34.

Tee S-Y, Fu J, Chen CS and Janmey PA (2011). Cell shape and substrate rigidity both regulate cell stiffness. *Biophys J*, 100(5), pp. L25–L27.

Truckenmüller R, Giselbrecht S, Rivron N, Gottwald E, Saile V, van den Berg A, Wessling M and van Blitterswijk C (2011). Thermoforming of film-based biomedical microdevices. *Adv Mater*, 23(11), pp. 1311–1329.

Truckenmüller R, Giselbrecht S, van Blitterswijk C, Dambrowsky N, Gottwald E, Mappes T, Rolletschek A, Saile V, Trautmann C, Weibezahn KF and Welle A (2008). Flexible fluidic microchips based on thermoformed and locally modified thin polymer films. *Lab on a Chip*, 8(9), pp. 1570–1579.

Ulery BD, Nair LS and Laurencin CT (2011). Biomedical applications of biodegradable polymers. *J Polym Sci Part B*, 49(12), pp. 832–864.

Unadkat HV, Hulsman M, Cornelissen K, Papenburg BJ, Truckenmüller RK, Carpenter AE, Wessling M, Post GF, Uetz M, Reinders MJT, Stamatialis D, van Blitterswijk CA and de Boer J (2011). An algorithm-based topographical biomaterials library to instruct cell fate. *Proc Natl Acad Sci*, 108(40), pp. 16565–16570.

van der Helm MW, Odijk M, Frimat J-P, van der Meer AD, Eijkel JCT, van den Berg A and Segerink LI (2016). Direct quantification of transendothelial electrical resistance in organs-on-chips. *Biosensors Bioelectron*, 85, pp. 924–929.

van Dijkhuizen-Radersma R, Moroni L, Apeldoorn AV, Zhang Z and Grijpma D (2008). Degradable polymers for tissue engineering. In Clemens van Blitterswijk PT, Anders Lindahl, Jeffrey Hubbell, David F. Williams, Ranieri Cancedda, Joost D. de Bruijn and Jérôme Sohier (Ed.), *Tissue engineering*, Chapter 7 (Academic Press, Burlington), pp. 193–221.

Vogelaar L, Lammertink RGH, Barsema JN, Nijdam W, Bolhuis-Versteeg LAM, van Rijn CJM and Wessling M (2005). Phase separation micromolding: a new generic approach for microstructuring various materials. *Small*, 1(6), pp. 645–655.

Walter FR, Valkai S, Kincses A, Petneházi A, Czeller T, Veszelka S, Ormos P, Deli MA and Dér A (2016). A versatile lab-on-a-chip tool for modeling biological barriers. *Sensors Actuators B*, 222, pp. 1209–1219.

White CR and Frangos JA (2007). The shear stress of it all: the cell membrane and mechanochemical transduction. *Philos Trans Roy Soc B*, 362(1484), pp. 1459–1467.

Whiteside TL (2008). The tumor microenvironment and its role in promoting tumor growth. *Oncogene*, 27(45), pp. 5904–5912.

Whitesides GM (2006). The origins and the future of microfluidics. *Nature*, 442(7101), pp. 368–373.

Xu L, Crawford K and Gorman CB (2011). Effects of temperature and pH on the degradation of poly(lactic acid) brushes. *Macromolecules*, 44(12), pp. 4777–4782.

Zhang YS, Aleman J, Arneri A, Bersini S, Piraino F, Shin SR, Dokmeci MR and Khademhosseini A (2015b). From cardiac tissue engineering to heart-on-a-chip: beating challenges. *Biomed Mater (Bristol, Engl)*, 10(3), p. 034006.

Zhang Y, Benes NE and Lammertink RGH (2015a). Visualization and characterization of interfacial polymerization layer formation. *Lab on a Chip*, 15(2), pp. 575–580.

Zhang Z, Kuijer R, Bulstra SK, Grijpma DW and Feijen J (2006). The *in vivo* and *in vitro* degradation behavior of poly(trimethylene carbonate). *Biomaterials*, 27(9), pp. 1741–1748.

Index

B

C

Printed in the United States
By Bookmasters

Printed in the United States
By Bookmasters